Pediatric Nutrition in Clinical Practice

Pediatric Nutrition in Clinical Practice

William C. MacLean, Jr., M.D.

and

George Graham, M.D.

School of Medicine
Department of Pediatrics
Gastroenterology and Nutrition Unit and
School of Hygiene and Public Health
Division of Human Nutrition
Johns Hopkins University
Baltimore, Maryland

ADDISON-WESLEY PUBLISHING COMPANY
Medical/Nursing Division • Menlo Park, California
Reading, Massachusetts • London • Amsterdam
Don Mills, Ontario • Sydney

Sponsoring Editor: Richard W. Mixter
Production Coordinator: Nancy Sjoberg
Copy Editor: Linnea Dayton
Cover and Book Design: Michael A. Rogondino

Library of Congress Cataloging in Publication Data

MacLean, William C.
    Pediatric nutrition in clinical practice.

    (Clinical practice series)
    Bibliography: p.
    Includes index.
    1. Children—Nutrition. 2. Malnutrition in children.
3. Nutrition disorders in children. I. Graham, George,
1923- . II. Title. III. Series. [DNLM: 1. Child
nutrition. 2. Infant nutrition. 3. Nutrition disorders
—In infancy and childhood. WS 115 M1635p]
RJ206.M253   613'.0432   82-4067

ISBN 0-201-15900-7   AACR2

ABCDEFGHIJ-MA-898765432

The authors and publishers have exerted every effort to ensure that drug selection and dosage formulations and composition of formulas set forth in this text are in accord with current recommendations and practice at the time of publication. However, in view of ongoing research, changes in government regulations, the reformulation of nutritional products, and the constant flow of information relating to drug therapy and drug reactions, the reader is urged to check product information on composition or the package insert for each drug for any change in indications of dosage and for added warnings and precautions. This is particularly important where the recommended agent is a new and/or infrequently employed drug.

The paper in this book meets the guidelines for permanence and durability of the Committee on Production Guidelines for Book Longevity of the Council on Library Resources.

Addison-Wesley Publishing Company
Medical/Nursing Division
2725 Sand Hill Road
Menlo Park, California 94025

To Betsy, Rachel,
Paige, and Simone

Publisher's Foreword

The **Clinical Practice Series** provides current clinical information in a practical and accessible format. Each title in the series addresses an important topic in modern primary care medicine. Essential pathophysiology is presented in the context of clinical material; the emphasis is always on sound diagnosis and management. Recommendations on when to refer are often included.

Clinical Practice Series authors are authoritative clinicians from a variety of distinguished medical centers. Each manuscript receives extensive critical review and commentary from our consulting physicians, many of whom have worked with us to develop the editorial goals and design of the series.

The format of this volume provides direct access to information on two levels—quick reference and in-depth study. Open the book to the beginning of any chapter. **Brief chapter contents** guide you to the topics of immediate interest. The **chapter overview** summarizes the chapter's content and purpose. **Marginal notes** distill facts and opinions from the text and offer critical commentary when appropriate. **Tables** and **figures** summarize data and provide quick visual references. No other series offers such accessibility to practical information and comprehensive coverage of clinically important topics.

Look for these published and immediately forthcoming volumes in the Clinical Practice Series:

PUBLISHED

Behavioral Medicine in General Medical Practice
Clinical Psychiatry in Primary Care
Diabetes Mellitus: Problems in Management
Diagnosis and Management of Cancer
Diagnosis and Management of Obstetric Emergencies
Diagnosis and Management of Pulmonary Disease
Diagnosis and Management of Stroke and TIAs
Infectious Diseases in General Medical Practice
Pediatric Nutrition in Clinical Practice
Perinatal Medicine: Practical Diagnosis and Management
Practical Rheumatology
The Practice of Preventive Health Care
Psychosocial Aspects of Medical Practice: Children and Adolescents
Skin Diseases: Diagnosis and Management in Clinical Practice
To Make the Patient Ready for Anesthesia

FORTHCOMING

Death and Dying
Diagnosis and Management of Pelvic Infections
A Family Approach to Health Care of the Elderly
Nutritional Management in Clinical Practice
A Physician's Guide to Coronary Heart Disease Prevention
Practical Rehabilitation Medicine
Psychological Aspects of Medical Practice: Adults and the Elderly

Contents

Foreword   *Harold E. Harrison, M.D.*   viii

Preface   x

Chapter 1   Goals of Good Nutrition and Assessment of
Nutritional Status   1
Goals of Good Nutrition   2
Assessment of Nutritional Status   4
Assessment of Food Intake   16
Recommended Dietary Allowances   19

Chapter 2   Principles of Nutrition   22
Energy   23
Protein   24
Fats   30
Carbohydrates   32
Vitamins   34
Minerals   43
Osmolality of the Diet   48
Renal Solute Load   49

Chapter 3   Breast-Feeding the Normal Infant   54
Trends in Breast-Feeding   55
Reasons to Breast-Feed   56
Contraindications to Breast-Feeding   64

	Physiology of Lactation	65
	Clinical Management of Breast-Feeding	67
	Maternal Medication and Breast-Feeding	74
Chapter 4	Formula-Feeding the Normal Infant	79
	Uses of Infant Formulas	80
	Cow-Milk Formulas	80
	Skim Milk	85
	Goat Milk	86
	Soy-Based Formulas	87
	Choice of Formula	90
	Management of Bottle-Feeding	91
Chapter 5	Solid Foods	99
	When to Introduce Solids	100
	Sequence of the Addition of Solid Foods	104
	Additives in Commercial Baby Foods	109
	Homemade Baby Food	111
	Foods Generally Not Fed to Young Infants	112
	Additional Issues Concerning the Feeding of Solid Foods	114
Chapter 6	Feeding of the Preschool Child, Older Child, and Adolescent	117
	Feeding the Preschool Child	118
	Children's Attitudes Toward Food	121
	Nutritional Status of Preschool Children	123
	Preadolescent Children	124
	Nutritional Requirements of Adolescents	124
	"Junk Food"	129
Chapter 7	Vegetarianism in Children	132
	Factors Affecting Vegetarianism	133
	Types of Vegetarianism	134
	Nutritional Problems in Vegetarianism	135
	Zen Macrobiotics	143
	Management of the Vegetarian Child	145
	Natural Foods, Organic Foods, and Megavitamins	147
Chapter 8	Iron Deficiency and Other Nutritional Anemias	151
	Iron Balance	152
	Dietary Requirements for Iron	156
	Iron Deficiency	162
	Other Nutritional Anemias	169

Chapter 9	Lactose Intolerance and Milk Intolerance	176
	Lactose Intolerance	177
	Milk-Protein Intolerance and Milk Allergy	188
Chapter 10	Protein-Energy Malnutrition (PEM)	197
	Marasmus	198
	Kwashiorkor	201
	Classification and Diagnosis of PEM	205
	Changes in Gastrointestinal Function in PEM	209
	Effect of PEM on Ultimate Stature	209
	Effect of PEM on Subsequent Mental Development	210
	Anorexia Nervosa	213
Chapter 11	Nutritional Management of Malabsorption and Malnutrition	218
	Normal Mechanisms of Digestion and Absorption	219
	Malabsorption and Malnutrition in Infancy	223
	Malabsorption and Malnutrition in the Older Child	238
Chapter 12	Feeding the Premature Infant	241
	Gastrointestinal Function of the Premature Infant	242
	Nutrient Requirements of the Premature Infant	244
	Feeding the Premature Infant	247
Chapter 13	Obesity	254
	Definition of Obesity	255
	Energy Balance	257
	Origins of Obesity	259
	Morbidity Associated with Obesity	261
	The Relationship of Childhood Obesity to Adult Obesity	262
	Management of Obesity	263
Appendix A	Restricted Diets	266
Appendix B	Nutrition History for Infants	275
Appendix C	Nutritional Status Assessment	278
Appendix D	Calorie Count–Food Record	280
Index		281

Foreword

As in all branches of science there have been peaks and valleys in the science of nutrition, especially in its applications to medicine. During the first half of this century nutritional science made dramatic contributions to the health of our population. The concept of essential amino acids, the discovery of vitamins (those organic compounds required in minute quantities for the normal functioning of cellular systems) and the discovery of trace minerals (the minerals also needed in minute amounts for cell functions) gave physicians the tools to combat specific nutritional deficiencies. Rickets and scurvy, the most common vitamin deficiencies of infants and children in this country, were eradicated. Pellagra, a major vitamin-deficiency disease in the southeastern section of the United States was conquered. And in Asia the common deficiency disease beri-beri was markedly reduced in incidence.

The practice of infant and child feeding was strikingly altered by the advances in nutritional science. Fortification of cow's milk with vitamin D and of white flour, breadstuffs, and cereals with vitamins and minerals guaranteed that children eating these foods would obtain needed nutrients not available in unfortified foods. Commercially prepared infant-feeding preparations became available, providing satisfactory nutrition for infants not being breast-fed, that is, most of the infants in the United States.

Malnutrition was still a major problem in many parts of the world, but in this country those specific nutritional disorders with immediate dramatic manifestation became rarities. As a result, the teaching of nutritional science in our medical schools was no longer emphasized, and physicians lost interest in nutritional science. The science itself, however, was not dormant. Research took a new turn—the examination of the long-term consequences of current dietary habits, as, for example, the high intakes of sodium chloride, saturated fatty acids, and calories and the reduced ingestion of indigestible carbohydrates, or fiber. The possibility of prevention of atherosclerosis, cancer of the bowel, and hypertension by changes in nutritional practice was considered. Because medical practitioners were relatively indifferent to or uneducated in nutritional science, nonmedical sources rushed in to fill the vacuum. Books on diets became best sellers; proponents of megavitamin treatment, or of other unusual diets, developed a large following; and newspaper columns provided a major source of nutritional advice for many people.

It is apparent that physicians must again become interested in nutritional science in order to be able to supply the balanced advice concerning diets and nutritional needs sought by patients and their families. This book by William MacLean and George Graham, who are both pediatricians and nutritional scientists, combines the necessary theoretical information for understanding the chemistry and physiology of nutrients and the application of this information to the nutritional needs of individuals throughout the growing period. The practical advice is sound and well balanced, and it recognizes differing points of view in areas of incomplete knowledge. But withal it is concrete and unequivocating. The sections on the feeding of infants, whether infants are breast-fed or given prepared feedings, are sufficiently detailed to help the practitioner handle the day-to-day problems of infant feeding. Other chapters also offer information necessary to provide sound advice to families who are concerned about the food habits of older children and adolescents. This book provides all health practitioners concerned about nutritional requirements during growth with a valuable source of the knowledge needed to counsel and instruct families concerning proper dietary practices.

Harold E. Harrison, M.D.
Professor Emeritus of Pediatrics
Johns Hopkins University
School of Medicine
and
Former Pediatrician-in-Chief
Baltimore City Hospitals
Baltimore, Maryland

Preface

One of the first concerns of a new mother is how best to feed her baby. She is likely to seek advice on nutrition from the primary care practitioner. Most physicians feel comfortable advising mothers regarding feeding during the first year of life, although the advice given is frequently based more on tradition than on sound nutritional principles. Beyond the first year, mothers are left pretty much on their own. Few physicians have had much formal nutrition education during their training. As a result it may be difficult to provide sound guidance and to answer questions on nutrition from parents who are exposed to a confusing and often contradictory lay literature on the subject.

This book was written to provide a nutritionally sound and practical approach to normal nutrition and common nutritional problems for practitioners dealing with patients from diverse ethnic and social backgrounds. It is not a comprehensive reference book. Unlike most nutrition textbooks, it does not approach the subject through a review of individual nutrients. Rather it is patient oriented. We hope it will prove valuable to primary care physicians, pediatricians, nurse practitioners, and house officers.

The first two chapters deal with "the basics"—essential nutrition knowledge that is presupposed in the rest of the book. The rest of the first half of the book addresses the feeding of normal infants and children. The book provides a variety of ways of feeding children adequately and advice on nutrition that is not rigid but adheres to basic principles. Vegetarianism is treated as an approach to diet that is compatible with nutrition but that presents problems that both practitioners and parents need to be aware of.

The second half of the book deals with nutritional problems commonly encountered in pediatric practice. Iron deficiency anemia is the most frequently encountered nutrient deficiency in otherwise healthy children; a separate chapter is devoted to this subject. Lactose and milk intolerance, often suggested as potential diagnoses, are in fact rare according to strict diagnostic criteria. The relative merits of approaches used to confirm these conditions are discussed.

Many chronic illnesses result in protein-energy malnutrition (marasmus and kwashiorkor), although these conditions are frequently unrecognized; Chapter 10 details these syndromes. Chapter 11 gives a physiologic approach to the dietary management of undernutrition and the other common pediatric diseases that produce malabsorption and, subsequently, poor nutritional status.

Although most small premature infants are cared for in specialized centers, the nutrition of the premature infant over 1500 g is appropriately the responsibility of the primary care practitioner. Chapter 12 examines the nutrient needs of these infants and how they differ from those of the term infant. It also addresses the adequacy of breast milk and specialized infant formulas for meeting these needs.

Obesity continues to increase in importance as the most common form of malnutrition in the United States. The relationship of obesity in infancy to obesity in later life is reappraised in Chapter 13, and the complex cultural and nutritional factors that contribute to obesity are addressed.

In producing this book there has been a third unnamed collaborator, Mrs. Marguerite Taylor, without whose constant willingness to dig out references and to type and retype manuscript our efforts would not have taken final form. We would also like to thank the editorial staff of Addison-Wesley for leading us through the complexities of creating a book.

William C. MacLean
George Graham

1 Goals of Good Nutrition and Assessment of Nutritional Status

Contents

Goals of Good Nutrition   2

Assessment of Nutritional Status   4

Height and Weight   4

Head Circumference   7

Growth Standards   7

Interpretation of Growth Data   9

Growth Velocity Curves   9

Triceps Skinfold   10

Mid-arm Circumference   12

General Examination   13

Laboratory Assessment   13

Assessment of Food Intake   16

Dietary Recall and Food Diary   16

Assessment During Hospitalization—The Calorie Count   18

Goals of Assessment   18

Recommended Dietary Allowances   19

Overview

Practitioners and parents alike are exposed to ever-increasing amounts of nutrition information and misinformation. There is a preoccupation with good nutrition and often an unrealistic expectation of what good nutrition can do. This chapter provides guidelines for assessing nutritional status using standard growth charts and a few simple additional anthropometric or laboratory measurements. The use and abuse of Recommended Dietary Allowances in assessing food intakes are explained.

GOALS OF GOOD NUTRITION

Good nutrition is not an end in itself. As physicians and parents alike have become more interested in and "sophisticated" about various aspects of nutrition, many have lost sight of what good nutrition is and what role good nutrition can reasonably be expected to play in the overall health of the child. The basic four food groups of 30 years ago have gradually been replaced by a much more complicated set of rules for "good nutrition." Mothers today no longer follow nutritional patterns passed from generation to generation. Rather, with the best interests of their children at heart, they try to adjust eating habits in accord with the confusing and often conflicting body of fragmentary nutrition knowledge to which they are exposed. Most mothers today are aware of the controversies surrounding sodium intake, consumption of cholesterol and animal fat, "empty calories," complex versus simple sugars, food additives and behavior, and dietary fiber. Rarely is a mother neutral regarding these topics. In fact, it is fair to say that in many cases what used to be a healthy interest has turned into a preoccupation with "good" nutrition.

> In many cases what used to be a healthy interest has turned into a preoccupation with "good" nutrition.

This preoccupation with nutrition has had several consequences. As already mentioned, many parents and physicians have come to expect too much of "good" nutrition. The well-nourished child is seen as somehow endowed with an extraordinary ability to ward off infections, as better able to concentrate in school, and as potentially protected to a large degree from many diseases prevalent among adults. The national nutrition goals recently set forth by the U.S. Senate Select Committee on Nutrition have reinforced this view by suggesting that changes in our dietary habits would markedly decrease the incidence of dental caries, hypertension, atherosclerosis and its sequelae, and cancer of the colon.

All of these expectations are to some extent based on factual information. *Severely* malnourished children, for example, are more susceptible to infection and are apathetic, but the severity of malnutrition in which these functional derangements have been documented is rarely encountered in children in this country except in association with chronic disease. Similarly, there are individuals with hyperlipidemia whose condition does respond to

Nutrition is just one environmental factor interacting with the child's genetic make-up.

The preoccupation with the consequences of under-nutrition is one of many factors that have elevated obesity to the number one nutritional problem among children.

Attempts to prevent obesity may lead to poor diets.

Although neither under-nutrition nor overnutrition is desirable, the range of food intake providing adequate nutrition between these extremes is not as narrow as many think it to be.

dietary modification, but they are a small minority. In this case, as in most, the genetic make-up of the individual interacts with a multiplicity of environmental factors, among them nutrition, in determining the health of the child. It is unrealistic, then, to expect changes in food habits alone to alter markedly the prevalence of most diseases.

The preoccupation with the consequences of undernutrition is one of many factors that have elevated obesity to the number one nutritional problem among children. Because most of us overeat as adults, we have inflated ideas about the amount of food that a healthy child should eat. Portions served to children are usually much larger than they need to be. Dessert is used as the ultimate inducement for the child to clean his plate. Failure to maintain a high level of consumption is seen as potentially subjecting the child to the dangers of malnutrition. Even by generous standards, most children in the United States are fed excessive amounts of calories and protein. Many parents supplement the diet with vitamins and minerals "just in case." These practices most certainly contribute to the increasing prevalence of obesity and may establish poor eating habits that are carried throughout life.

More and more parents and physicians *are* concerned with the growing trend toward obesity. Not infrequently, however, well-intentioned efforts to prevent obesity lead to equally poor nutrition—for example, feeding infants skim-milk-based diets that are hypocaloric and low in essential fatty acids. Here again, in an effort to eschew one extreme, another extreme position is embraced. Efforts to prevent obesity are often centered only on the energy *intake* side of the equation with little regard to the factors influencing energy *utilization*.

None of this discussion should be construed to mean that good nutrition is not important. It is, as long as we maintain a sense of perspective. Good nutrition can and should facilitate the growth and development of a healthy child. Although neither undernutrition nor overnutrition is desirable, the range of food intake providing adequate nutrition between these extremes is not as narrow as many think it to be. Early in life the range of acceptable foods is narrow; yet the range of intake that maintains adequate nutrition is quite wide. Later in childhood, as taste and food preferences become developed, there are numerous acceptable means of nourishing the child. The role of the physician is to guide parents and children within this range, balancing the principles of good nutrition with the food preferences, habits, and lifestyle of the family.

To advise parents appropriately, the practitioner must reach conclusions in his or her own mind in two areas. First, the physician must be able to make an objective assessment of the child's nutritional status. Second, the physician must be able to ascertain the child's food intake and how this intake relates to some standard of desirable intake. Nutritional status is much more easily evaluated than food intake, especially for those not trained in nutrition per se. More important, good nutritional status is the outcome we are primarily interested in.

Nutritional status is affected by more than food intake alone.

Nutritional status is affected by more than food intake alone. Food intake may be adequate, but malabsorption may be present. Chronic infection may prevent efficient utilization of nutrients, or chronic diseases, such as congestive heart failure, may increase the nutrient requirements of the child. In practice, then, if nutritional status is judged to be adequate, one can be relatively sure that food intake, absorption, and utilization are acceptable and that the necessity of a detailed dietary history is obviated to a large extent.

A brief nutritional history is always indicated regardless of nutritional status, since the child may be thriving despite inadvisable nutritional practices.

A brief nutritional history is always indicated regardless of nutritional status, since the child may be thriving despite inadvisable nutritional practices. If nutritional status is poor, food intake must be ascertained in detail, although one should keep in mind that intake is only one of a variety of possible causes of poor nutritional status.

ASSESSMENT OF NUTRITIONAL STATUS

In most cases nutritional status can be evaluated on the basis of anthropometric measurements in conjunction with one or two readily available laboratory determinations. Measurement of height, weight, and head circumference is routine for physicians who care for infants and children. The nutritionist adds the measurement of skinfold thickness and mid-arm circumference. All five of these measurements can be made by a nurse or an aide who has been specifically trained. As the use of these measurements becomes routine, the physician will gain more confidence and sophistication in interpreting anthropometric data as they relate to the child's nutritional state.

Height and Weight

Accurate determination of height at each well baby visit is essential.

Accurate determination of height (or recumbent length up to the age of two years) at each well baby visit is essential. A surprising number of infants are referred for evaluation of failure to thrive whose serial values for length are not available. Height or length is difficult to measure accurately, especially for the young infant. Proper equipment makes the task easier. The most sophisticated piece of equipment for measuring length in newborns is the

Figure 1-1

Infantometer (Figure 1-1).* The Infantometer allows the infant's head to be fixed while a sliding footboard with a direct reading meter is moved up to the feet. With such an instrument, reproducible length measurements with an error of approximately 2–3 mm can be obtained. The Infantometer is expensive and probably impractical for a busy office, but it is certainly useful for the physician with a large number of premature infants in his or her practice.

Figure 1-2

For most routine measurements an examining table with a steel measuring tape and a right-angle footboard (Figure 1-2) is sufficient. As with the Infantometer, the measurement is obtained with the infant's head fixed against the headboard by one observer while a second observer holds the knees in extension and brings the right angle up to the feet. The mean of several determinations should be used.

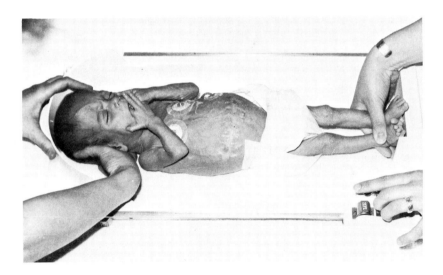

Figure 1-1   Measuring the length of an infant with an Infantometer.

*The Infantometer is available from Pfister Import-Export, Inc., 450 Barrell Ave., Carlstadt, NJ 07072. Skinfold calipers are also available from the same company.

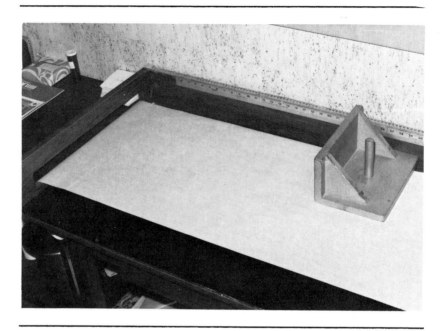

Figure 1-2 Standard examining table adapted for accurate measurement of length.

For older children the traditionally used measuring devices attached to most office scales are inadequate. Although an instrument similar to the infantometer is available for measuring height in older children and adults, a steel tape measure on the wall is still the best routine method. With the child's heels flat on the floor and both feet and buttocks against the wall, a right angle is placed on the head and the wall. Our experience has been that measurements made in this way are often several centimeters in excess of those obtained while "on the scale." In a 30-month old boy, for example, this difference is sufficient to move height from the 25th to the 50th percentile.

A steel tape measure on the wall is still the best routine method for measuring height.

Weight should also be recorded routinely at each office visit. Scales should be checked with standard weights from time to time to maintain accuracy. In a busy office with more than one scale, scales should be adjusted to give comparable weights. As long as these precautions are taken, weight is a very reproducible measurement.

Weight should be recorded routinely at each office visit.

Head Circumference

Head circumference is measured in the occipitofrontal diameter in all infants. We recommend using the same tape that is used to measure mid-arm circumference, since reading the measurement is far easier than with a standard tape, and the measurement may be done without having to overlap the tape at an angle, a maneuver that falsely increases the reading. Head circumference is of relatively less value in the assessment of nutritional status than are height and weight. In undernutrition the head circumference will generally be appropriate for the length. We have found the measurement of head circumference to be useful primarily as a clue to underlying diseases that may account for alterations in nutritional status; for example, a large head may be indicative of hydrocephalus or of a subdural hematoma in an infant whose weight and length are suboptimal.

Growth Standards

Both height and weight should be plotted on a standard growth chart.

Both height and weight should be plotted on a standard growth chart. The recently published National Center for Health Statistics (NCHS) Standards are gaining wide acceptance. There are several practical advantages to these new growth charts. One is that height after the age of two years is standardized for standing height rather than recumbent length, which is, in fact, how height is usually measured in the office in this age group. A second advantage is the weight-for-height chart. The normal weight or range of weights for any height is relatively independent of age between about one and five years. We instinctively tend to worry more about the 29-month-old whose height is at the 25th percentile and whose weight is just below the 5th percentile than we do about a 21-month-old with height and weight at the 90th and 25th percentiles, respectively. Both these children are 88 cm tall and weigh 10.5 kg. The weight-for-height chart shows that both have a weight for height well within the normal range.

Only by the recording of serial measurements can one deduce anything about the rate of linear growth or weight gain. For this reason recording height and weight at each routine visit is essential.

The NCHS charts, like most growth standards used in clinical practice, are charts of height or weight attained rather than of growth velocity. Only by the recording of *serial* measurements can one deduce anything about the rate of linear growth or weight gain. For this reason recording height and weight at each routine visit is essential. Even with serial data, one must bear in mind that these charts are statistical descriptions of the growth of a population of children. One cannot equate height or weight above or below any given percentile with good nutrition or lack thereof. We often ascribe more health significance to these charts than is warranted: a child growing below the 5th percentile is more likely to be evaluated for failure to thrive than one growing at the 25th percentile. Yet the former could be well nourished and could be fulfilling his or her genetic potential while the latter might be growing suboptimally. The physician must interpret the data if they are to be of value. Knowledge of the heights and weights of parents and siblings is essential in making a judgment about the meaning of the data.

> Height for age, weight for age, and weight for height tell us different things about the child's nutritional status.

Height for age, weight for age, and weight for height tell us different things about the child's nutritional status. Height is, in general, the best indicator of the child's long-term nutrition. Steady linear growth is the single most reassuring indicator of the adequacy of the child's diet. Linear growth is usually accompanied by an increase in lean body mass and consequently is more "nutritionally demanding" than simply gaining weight. Changes in weight may imply growth or may only reflect increased or decreased fat stores. Because weight can be lost and regained several times, variation in weight is generally a better indicator of short-term and recent changes in nutrient intake than of long-term changes. This is especially so when weight is expressed as a function of height rather than of age.

Wasting and stunting A child whose weight is low for age may be of normal height for age or may be short for age. The child who has a very low weight for height is termed "wasted." Wasting usually indicates that the child has grown adequately in length overall but has had a recent nutritional insult that has either slowed the rate of weight gain or has resulted in weight loss.

> The child who has a very low weight for height is termed "wasted."

> A child whose weight and height are both low for age but whose weight is appropriate for height is termed "stunted."

A child whose weight and height are both low for age but whose weight is appropriate for height is termed "stunted." The child who is moderately stunted is usually not at an increased risk of complications from undernutrition. He or she requires chronic rather than acute management. This child may be a so-called hypocaloric dwarf, whose growth has adapted to nearly adequate intakes of a generally well-balanced diet. The stunted child may also be genetically short, have growth hormone deficiency, or have any of a number of diseases, none of which is responsive to nutritional intervention.

Overweight At the other end of the scale is the child whose weight is excessive. If weight for height is normal—that is, the child is tall and heavy—the child may be genetically large. If weight for height

The obese child who is short is rarely so because of poor nutrition.

is excessive, the child is most likely obese. In the short child who is fat, poor nutrition is infrequently the cause of the poor linear growth. This combination more often results from underlying systemic diseases, especially of a genetic or endocrine nature.

Interpretation of Growth Data

Three notes of caution are needed at this point regarding the interpretation of height and weight data. The first is that infants frequently cross percentile lines of both height and weight during the first year, often tending to drift to the mean. Within reason this should not be cause for alarm. No hard and fast rule can be laid down as to when to become concerned. This judgment must be made using a variety of information on the child's food intake and health in general. Second, the NCHS growth standard for infants was derived from infants who were predominantly bottle-fed and for whom the early introduction of solid food was the rule rather than the exception. Breast-feeding appears to be gaining popularity again, and the breast-fed infant tends to gain weight a bit more slowly and often tends to be a bit leaner. Breast-fed infants double their birth weight later than bottle-fed infants. Consequently, as we see more infants being exclusively breast-fed for longer periods of time, we may see more infants at the lower end of the percentiles than in the past. This shift may not be indicative of an inadequacy of human milk but rather of a tendency to overfeed the bottle-fed infant.

Infants frequently cross percentile lines of both height and weight during the first year.

Finally, because the NCHS charts were derived from a racially mixed population, they do not properly reflect the normal growth spurt that occurs at the time of puberty. Different racial groups and individuals within groups experience onset of puberty at different ages. When averaged for the growth charts, these individual variations tend to cancel each other out and therefore the rapid growth seen in individuals at this time is not apparent from the charts. The stage of sexual development must be kept in mind when assessing the growth of adolescent boys and girls.

Growth Velocity Curves

Up to this point we have been discussing charts that plot height and weight attained. Although some estimate of the rate of growth can be derived from these charts, there are occasions when it is useful to have a standard against which to judge the velocity of growth. Tanner and his coworkers (1966) have published such standards for British children. Although velocity standards have not found their way into routine use in clinical practice, we have found them useful when assessing the growth of older children. Whereas the growth spurts at puberty are not reflected well in the usual charts of attained height and weight, they are quite clearly shown on standards for rates of growth. In following children with chronic illness, such as Crohn's disease or diabetes mellitus, in whom growth retardation is often present, the use of these standards has been found to be a sensitive means of assessing growth problems.

Triceps Skinfold

Skinfold or fatfold thicknesses have been measured in nutrition surveys for a number of years. The skinfold measurement is becoming a part of the in-hospital assessment of nutritional status and is

Skinfold measurement is useful in office practice, especially when obesity is a possibility.

useful in office practice, especially when obesity is a possibility. Because the amount of fat deposited differs in various parts of the body, a number of standardized sites have been used for the measurement of skinfold thickness, including the triceps, biceps, subscapular, and suprailiac skinfolds. When only a single site is to be used, the skinfold measured is that over the triceps area of the left arm, midway between the acromion and the olecranon.

Although skinfold measurements are relatively easy to make, a certain amount of practice is required before reproducibility is obtained. There are several types of sensitive (and rather delicate) instruments on the market. The most commonly used are the Holtain caliper and the Lange caliper. Either one of these instruments is acceptable for routine office use, although both are rather expensive. Recently a plastic model of reasonable accuracy has been developed. Its low cost and easy availability may make measurement of skinfolds more routine.

The actual measurement is carried out with the child sitting comfortably. An assistant holds the left arm flexed at a right angle. Once the arm is relaxed, the person making the measurement grasps a layer of skin and subcutaneous tissue approximately one centimeter above the point at which the measurement is to be taken. The skin is pulled up slightly and the caliper is applied to the

Figure 1-3

fold created (Figure 1-3). Because fat tissue is compressible, the reading is taken after several seconds. As with other anthropometric measurements, two or preferably three readings should be made and the mean of these values used.

Skinfold thickness increases with age and correlates well with the percentage of body weight as fat.

Skinfold thickness increases with age and correlates well with the percentage of body weight as fat. Data on triceps skinfold thickness obtained during the Ten State Nutrition Survey are shown in Table 1-1. Notice that after the age of about one year the median skinfold thickness is relatively constant for both sexes

Table 1-1

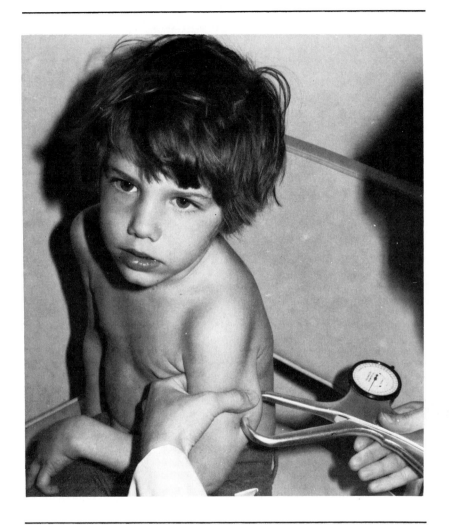

Figure 1-3 Measuring the triceps skinfold with the Holtain caliper.

until the time of puberty. It is also apparent that triceps skinfold reflects well the differences between boys and girls in body fat deposition at the time of puberty. In practice, a low value for triceps skinfold in an obviously poorly nourished child adds little critical information. As will be discussed later, the principal value of the skinfold measurement in clinical practice is in differentiating the large child with a normal percentage of body fat from the obese child. As a general rule, children with skinfold measurements above

Table 1-1 Percentiles for triceps skinfolds

Age group	Age midpoint, years	Triceps skinfold percentiles, mm									
		Males					Females				
		5th	15th	50th	85th	95th	5th	15th	50th	85th	95th
0.0–0.4	0.3	4	5	8	12	15	4	5	8	12	13
0.5–1.4	1	5	7	9	13	15	6	7	9	12	15
1.5–2.4	2	5	7	10	13	14	6	7	10	13	15
2.5–3.4	3	6	7	9	12	14	6	7	10	12	14
3.5–4.4	4	5	6	9	12	14	5	7	10	12	14
4.5–5.4	5	5	6	8	12	16	6	7	10	13	16
5.5–6.4	6	5	6	8	11	15	6	7	10	12	15
6.5–7.4	7	4	6	8	11	14	6	7	10	13	17
7.5–8.4	8	5	6	8	12	17	6	7	10	15	19
8.5–9.4	9	5	6	9	14	19	6	7	11	17	24
9.5–10.4	10	5	6	10	16	22	6	8	12	19	24
10.5–11.4	11	6	7	10	17	25	7	8	12	20	29
11.5–12.4	12	5	7	11	19	26	6	9	13	20	25
12.5–13.4	13	5	6	10	18	25	7	9	14	23	30
13.5–14.4	14	5	6	10	17	22	8	10	15	22	28
14.5–15.4	15	4	6	9	19	26	8	11	16	24	30
15.5–16.4	16	4	5	9	20	27	8	10	15	23	27
16.5–17.4	17	4	5	8	14	20	9	12	16	26	31

Source: Frisancho, A. R. 1974. Triceps skinfold and upper muscle size norms for assessment of nutritional status. *Am. J. Clin. Nutr.* 27:1052–1058. Data are from the Ten State Nutrition Survey and are for white children.

the 95th percentile should be considered obese. The problem of defining obesity is discussed in Chapter 13.

Mid-arm Circumference

The mid-arm circumference is measured at the same point that the triceps skinfold measurement is taken. Although mid-arm circumference can be measured with a standard steel tape, a special tape for this purpose simplifies the measurement considerably. Mid-arm circumference measurements are principally of value in younger children since normal values for this measurement vary little between the ages of one and four years. Mid-arm circumference can be used in conjunction with the triceps skinfold measurement to calculate the arm muscle area. Mid-arm circumference correlates quite closely with weight for age and weight for height. For this reason, we do not recommend the routine use of mid-arm circumference measurement, reserving it for situations in which nutritional status appears marginal and an additional indicator is desired.

General Examination

In addition to the anthropometric measurements done at the beginning of the physical examination or often before the physician sees the child, the general physical examination can provide many clues to nutritional deficiency. Among variables to be noted are hair color and texture (checking for signs of kwashiorkor), scleral color (vitamin A deficiency or carotenemia), mottling of the enamel (fluorosis), tachycardia (thiamin deficiency) and liver enlargement (kwashiorkor or nutritional recovery syndrome). Few physical findings, however, are pathognomonic of any nutritional syndrome. Pallor is as often associated with a normal hemoglobin concentration as not. Angular stomatitis in children in the U.S. is more often than not completely unrelated to a deficiency of B vitamins. As in making any diagnosis, one looks for a constellation of physical findings in the appropriate clinical situation that points to a nutritional disorder. As a rule, with the exception of undernutrition or mild marasmus, most of the deficiency diseases seen in the United States are associated with significant underlying chronic illness or its treatment, and it is children with these problems that require the most careful scrutiny from a nutritional point of view.

> Most of the deficiency diseases seen in the United States are associated with significant underlying chronic illness or its treatment.

Laboratory Assessment

Biochemical assessment is used primarily for undernutrition, which in the United States is most often protein-energy malnutrition (usually secondary to chronic diarrhea or diseases such as cystic fibrosis), iron deficiency, and, more recently again, rickets. A complete discussion of protein-energy malnutrition is found in Chapter 10.

The biochemical assessment of nutritional status has become extremely sophisticated and is generally more complex than the primary care physician requires. In most instances only a few simple and routinely performed laboratory determinations are required to complete the assessment of the child's nutritional status. In specific situations where there is reason to suspect a deficiency of a trace mineral or vitamin, laboratory confirmation should be sought. In these instances, however, it is wise to consult someone familiar

> In most instances only a few simple and routinely performed laboratory determinations are required to complete the assessment of the child's nutritional status.

with the specific tests and their interpretation. Although analysis of hair zinc, for example, has gained popularity, topical contamination may make the determination unreliable. Simple serum or plasma levels of the nutrient in question are not always an accurate reflection of sufficiency or deficiency. For example, a low serum copper in a child with poor protein nutriture is not always indicative of copper deficiency. Often the child has adequate stores of copper, but the plasma concentration of ceruloplasmin, the protein to which 90% of copper is bound, is low. A parallel phenomenon occurs with retinol (vitamin A) and its transport protein, retinol-binding protein.

Total protein/albumin The determination of serum total protein and albumin concentrations is important in the assessment of undernourished children because these values, in combination with anthropometrics and the physical examination, serve to differentiate marasmus from kwashiorkor. Different serum proteins have been found to have different sensitivities to dietary influences. For example, the serum globulins are maintained in normal or elevated concentrations in most malnourished children, probably because of repeated exposures to infection. Serum albumin concentrations drop when protein nutriture is inadequate or when excess salt and water are retained. Several other proteins, such as prealbumin and transferrin, are also sensitive to dietary influences. Measurement of these latter two proteins may offer some theoretical advantage in the assessment of nutritional status because of their shorter half lives, but because such measurements are not readily available in many laboratories we prefer to rely on serum total protein and albumin concentrations.

> Measurement of serum albumin concentration is the simplest means of assessing protein status.

The serum total protein should be thought of as a screening tool. Serum total protein can easily be estimated in the office setting using a hand-held refractometer. For initial screening this procedure is perfectly satisfactory. Because the globulins can have a disproportionate influence on the refractometer reading, however, this value can be misleading. If the value obtained by refractometer is low (less than 5 g/dL), a more exact determination should be requested. If findings in the history or physical examination suggest potential problems, an exact determination may be desirable regardless of the value obtained in the office.

Other biochemical indicators There are many other biochemical indicators of nutritional status that are occasionally useful. The question arises whether the determination of plasma amino acids adds anything to the assessment of nutritional status. In general, the answer is no. The total concentration of plasma amino acids and the concentration of individual amino acids have been found to correlate quite closely with serum albumin concentration in children being admitted to hospital for undernutrition. For a routine examination, plasma amino acid determination is an expensive and unnecessary test.

The 24-hour urinary creatinine excretion correlates well with lean body mass if the patient is on a creatine-free diet for several days before and during the collection. In children who are having a 24-hour urinary creatinine done for the determination of creatinine clearance, it may be of interest to determine the creatinine height index.* However, we rarely find it necessary to use the creatinine height index, relying more on anthropometric measurements.

Whether or not a child is iron deficient is the decision that must be made most frequently regarding vitamin or mineral nutrition.

Hematocrit/hemoglobin Whether or not a child is iron deficient is the decision that must be made most frequently regarding vitamin or mineral nutrition. Iron deficiency is discussed fully in Chapter 8. A variety of laboratory determinations may be used singly or in combination to assess the iron status of the child. Hematocrit and hemoglobin concentration are the most readily available tests, and, if results are above generally accepted norms, they are sufficient in themselves. In borderline cases it may be more difficult to assess iron status, and a peripheral smear, serum iron and unsaturated iron binding capacity, free erythrocyte protoporphyrin, or serum ferritin may be required. The problems surrounding the sensitivity and specificity of these tests, singly and in combination, are covered later.

No other laboratory determinations can be recommended, as a general rule. The exception is obvious: children whose specific diagnoses are known to be associated with deficiencies of one or more of the vitamins or minerals. For example, more rigorous assessment of the nutritional status of vitamins A, D, K, and E would be indicated in the infant with malabsorption of fat, such as in cystic fibrosis, biliary atresia, or celiac disease. For most children in the office, the proper interpretation of serial data on height for age, weight for age, weight for height, triceps skinfold thickness perhaps, and the hematocrit and total serum protein are all that is required to make a sound judgment regarding the child's nutritional status.

---

*Standards for the creatinine height index, relating the amount of muscle mass to the height of the child, have been published by Viteri and Alvarado (1970).

ASSESSMENT OF FOOD INTAKE

Some inquiry into the nutritional habits of the family and of the child in particular should be made at every visit. When the child's nutritional status is obviously good, nothing more than a qualitative assessment is required. Such assessment gives the practitioner a chance to pinpoint areas of potential undernutrition or overnutrition before they have a gross effect on nutritional status.

When obvious undernutrition or overnutrition is present, a quantitative assessment of food intake is required.

When obvious undernutrition or overnutrition is present, a quantitative assessment of food intake is required. In the young infant, failure to gain weight during a period of one month or suboptimal weight gain for three months is an indication that a detailed dietary history is needed. In the toddler, poor linear growth or weight gain during a three-month period may not require a thorough evaluation for failure to thrive, but a careful assessment of food intake is nevertheless indicated. All children whose weight-for-height or triceps skinfold values are above the 95th percentile should have a careful dietary history taken. As with the anthropometric measurements, much of this history can be obtained by a nurse-practitioner, nurse, or other office aide specifically trained for the purpose.

An assessment of food intake can be obtained by the following means:

24-hour dietary recall

Food diary

Calorie count

Weighed intake

Dietary Recall and Food Diary

The simplest method of determining food intake is the dietary history, sometimes referred to as the 24-hour recall method. This approach can be surprisingly accurate, as in quantitating the intake of an exclusively bottle-fed three-month-old, or it can be of almost no value whatsoever, as in the case of the exclusively breast-fed infant. For older infants and children consuming a mixed diet, the

Dietary recall depends heavily on the parent's ability as a historian.

accuracy depends heavily on the parent's ability as a historian. Parents who are precise in other aspects of their child's medical history will probably provide accurate food intake data. Nevertheless, most of us would be hard pressed to give an accurate account of the quantities of food our children consumed last night at the dinner table. In obtaining the dietary history, one seeks to quantitate with reasonable accuracy what the child actually eats.

To do this one needs information about what is eaten on specific days. Asking the mother to describe her child's "typical" day yields excellent data on what she thinks her child eats but little useful information on actual food intake.

The accuracy of the dietary history can be improved by several means. The simplest of these is the use of a food diary, in which the parents record all the foods eaten by the child and the approximate quantities of each. In cultures where the selection of foods is limited and the diet is relatively monotonous, food models are used to gauge quantity. In the United States this is often impractical and it makes more sense to ask parents to estimate portions in reference to standard measures used in the kitchen— tablespoons, cups, baby food jars, and so on. A second approach is to do dietary recalls at successive visits. Studies comparing the accuracy of the recall method with more objective measures of food intake have shown that mothers improve their accuracy once they are aware that the information will be asked for. Just as parents with second or third children become more skilled at observing the course of an acute illness and communicating it to the physician, so the parent who is asked for a diet history at each visit will become more reliable in this area.

Use of a food diary will give more accurate information than dietary recall.

The parent who is asked for a diet history at each visit will become more reliable in this area.

The recall and food diary methods have major limitations. First, parents may tell the physician what they think the physician wants to hear. This is especially true when food deprivation is a form of child abuse. Not infrequently infants who are failing to thrive and whose dietary history suggests that their food intake should be adequate gain weight rapidly when they are admitted to hospital and fed "as they had been at home."

Parents may tell the physician what they think the physician wants to hear.

Second, the diet on the day recalled may be atypical. This is not a common problem in the younger infant, whose diet is relatively constant from day to day. However, in the older child, as in the adult, food intakes vary enormously from meal to meal and day to day. Meal composition and even the number of meals change in many families on weekends, for example, and are frequently unrepresentative of food consumed during the rest of the week. Dietary recalls are often defended for use in surveys of populations, where the large number of people studied serves to cancel out some of the variation. Day-to-day variation can be a major problem, however, when assessing an individual child's food intake.

The diet on the day recalled may be atypical.

The food diary provides a more objective record of food intake over a period of days and consequently is more likely to be representative of the child's true intake. In some instances, the request to keep a food diary may alter the child's diet substantially. Because the mother is being "observed" in every sense as much as the child, there is a subconscious desire to serve a well-balanced diet and to ensure that it is eaten.

Assessment During Hospitalization— The Calorie Count

The diet of a hospitalized child is somewhat more easily assessed. Most hospitals offer a selection of foods from which the child (or parent) can choose a diet that will mimic to some extent the foods eaten at home. A good clinical dietitian can accurately estimate food intake by calculating the difference between the amount of food served and the food returned uneaten on the tray. The calorie count in hospital has the major advantage that the parents and child are usually unaware that intake is being assessed. The major drawback is that children eat differently in hospital—foods served may not closely parallel those usually served at home.

The calorie count in hospital has the major advantage that the parents and child are usually unaware that intake is being assessed.

Goals of Assessment

The goal of any assessment of food intake is an ultimate calculation of the diet in nutritional terms—that is, a conversion of food eaten (source) to nutrients consumed. In cases of failure to thrive or obesity, calorie and protein intakes are the primary concern. The determination of nutrient intakes by the breast-fed infant is nearly impossible in routine practice. Calculation of nutrient intakes is relatively simple in the formula-fed infant. Standard modified cow milk formulas provide 67 kcal and 1.5 g protein per 100 mL. Soy-based and other specialized infant formulas similarly provide 67 kcal/dL. Protein content varies. The compositions of a number of the commonly used infant formulas are found in Tables 4–2 and 4–3. Given the amounts of baby foods consumed, energy, protein, and iron intakes can be calculated using composition tables available on request from the major manufacturers of baby food. Estimation of intakes by older children is more difficult because food is not consumed from standard-sized jars. Portion sizes must be estimated. Composition is obtained from food composition tables, which are available from the United States Department of Agriculture.* Once calculated, these intake data must be analyzed as to their adequacy; that is, these nutrient intakes must be measured against some standard.

Nutrient intakes must be measured against some standard.

---

*Watt, B. K. and Merrill, A. L. 1963. *Composition of foods: agricultural handbook no. 8.* Washington, D. C.: Agricultural Research Service, United States Department of Agriculture. Available from the Superintendent of Documents, U. S. Government Printing Office, Washington, DC 20402. Stock No. 001-000-00768-8.

RECOMMENDED DIETARY ALLOWANCES

The usual standard used by nutritionists and physicians for analyzing the nutritional adequacy of a diet is the Recommended Dietary Allowances (RDAs) of the Food and Nutrition Board of the National Research Council, National Academy of Sciences.* Uses and abuses of the RDAs abound. Since few people understand what the RDAs are, how they were derived, and what their intended purpose is, it is worth taking a moment to cover these areas.

The first set of RDAs was published in 1943; periodic revisions have been made since then. With the exception of the recommendation for energy intake, the RDAs are the suggested intakes of individual nutrients that will meet the needs of nearly all healthy people. That is to say, for example, that if everyone were to consume the recommended amount of vitamin A, almost everyone would get enough. The RDA should not be confused with the individual's requirement for a nutrient. The RDAs for each age group are determined, in theory, by taking the average individual's requirement for a nutrient and, using the standard deviation around this value, increasing the amount recommended so as to be adequate for 97.5% of the population (+2.2 standard deviations). It is obvious, then, that most people will actually require less than the RDA. This fact is generally not recognized. It is common to read nutrition surveys that conclude, for example, that because 40% of school children were consuming less than the Recommended Dietary Allowance for iron, iron deficiency was rampant in this group. However, it is obvious that most healthy children could consume less iron than the recommended allowance and still meet their actual requirements. The relevant questions are: *how much* less than the RDA is being taken in, and, more important, is there any demonstrable iron deficiency in the children when assessed by more direct means?

> With the exception of the recommendation for energy intake, the RDAs are the suggested intakes of individual nutrients that will meet the needs of nearly all healthy people.

> Most people will actually require less than the RDA.

---

*To confuse matters, the Food and Drug Administration (FDA) has derived the United States Recommended *Daily* Allowances (USRDAs) for use in nutrition labeling. These RDAs are derived from those of the National Academy of Sciences, but they lump infants and children under four years together in one group and children over four years and adults in another. The USRDAs are those used for baby food jars and cereal boxes, and more and more consumers use them as a guide to buying. Our discussion concerning the need or desirability of a child's consuming enough to meet the RDAs of the NAS applies equally to the USRDAs.

The RDA for energy is unique.

As mentioned above, the RDA for energy is unique. Rather than being the energy intake that should meet the needs of nearly all healthy individuals, it is the suggested *average* requirement for the population as a whole. The latest set of RDAs (1979) includes *ranges* of recommended energy intakes, making these RDAs more useful for physicians dealing with individual children. All recent committees that have assessed the requirement for energy have implied that energy intake is well regulated by energy output, mediated through appetite. As we will discuss in the chapter on obesity in childhood, there is good evidence to the contrary.

RDAs can be useful guides. It must be acknowledged, however, that they are the result of a committee weighing available scientific data. Different scientists often interpret the same data differently, and consequently the RDAs represent a value judgment, albeit an informed one, by the committee. Through the years the RDAs for individual nutrients have gone up and down depending on available data and the make-up of the committee.

It should now be clear that when the food and nutrient intakes of most healthy children are calculated and then compared with the Recommended Dietary Allowances more often than not the diet will be found to be "insufficient" in one or a whole variety of nutrients. This is not prima facie evidence for nutritional deficiency. In fact, with the exception of the RDA for energy, the lack of RDAs that give us ranges of acceptable nutrient intakes often makes it difficult to know whether or not the child's diet is adequate. The problem is further compounded because the RDAs are based on age rather than on size, are only for healthy individuals, and may differ substantially from the requirements or desirable intakes for the child who is ill or growing poorly— the situations in which the physician most often needs an answer.

Nutrient intakes markedly below the Recommended Dietary Allowances cannot be overlooked. These substandard intakes should alert the physician to special areas that may require more detailed assessment. When the calculated intake for a nutrient is only slightly below the RDA, our approach has been to place more weight on the objective evidence of the child's nutritional status than on historical data concerning food intake.

Suggested Reading

Frisancho, A. R. 1974. Triceps skin fold and upper arm muscle size norms for assessment of nutritional status. *Am. J. Clin. Nutr.* 27: 1052–1058.

Harper, A. E. 1978. Dietary goals—a skeptical view. *Am. J. Clin. Nutr.* 31:310–321.

Parsons, H. G.; Francoeur, T. E.; Howland, P., et al. 1980. The nutritional status of hospitalized children. *Am. J. Clin. Nutr.* 33:1140–1146.

Tanner, J. M.; Whitehouse, R. H.; and Takaishi, M. 1966. Standards from birth to maturity for height, weight, height velocity and weight velocity: British children, 1965. *Arch. Dis. Child.* 41:454–471; 613–635.

Viteri, F. E., and Alvarado, J. 1970. The creatinine height index: its use in the estimation of the degree of protein depletion and repletion in protein-calorie malnourished children. *Pediatrics* 46: 696–706.

2 Principles of Nutrition

Contents

Energy 23
Protein 24
   Protein Quality and Its Measurement 25
   Protein Requirements 28
   Protein Intakes by American Children 30
Fats 30
   Types and Sources 30
   Essential Fatty Acids 32
Carbohydrates 32
   Clinical Importance of Carbohydrates 32
   Types of Carbohydrates 33
Vitamins 34
   Vitamin A 34
   Vitamin D 36
   Vitamin E 38
   Vitamin K 38
   B Vitamins 39
   Ascorbic Acid 42
Minerals 43
   Calcium and Phosphorus 43
   Sodium and Potassium 45
   Trace Minerals 46
Osmolality of the Diet 48
Renal Solute Load 49

Overview

Nutrition cannot be just an abstract science for the practitioner caring for children. For this reason this book approaches nutrition primarily from a clinical point of view, addressing the specific questions of both normal and abnormal nutrition that arise in day-to-day practice. There is nonetheless a body of basic nutrition knowledge that underlies clinical practice. This chapter covers the principles of nutrition with two objectives in mind: (1) providing a framework for understanding the specific approaches to clinical situations detailed later, and (2) because it is impossible to cover all clinical situations in any book, providing a basis for solving other clinical problems the practitioner may encounter.

ENERGY

One of the most important purposes of food intake is the provision of adequate amounts of energy to support the body's ongoing metabolic processes. With current concerns about the adequacy of intakes of specific macronutrients and micronutrients, the importance of energy intake is often forgotten. Most of the energy stored in proteins, fats, and carbohydrates is converted biochemically to heat. This energy is not entirely wasted, because it serves to maintain body temperature. Even when our metabolism is operating at maximum efficiency, only 35%-40% of the energy stored in food can be converted biochemically to a useful form. A large percentage of this biochemical energy must be used to maintain the basal metabolic rate. Voluntary activity also claims a large part. Energy that remains after these two requirements are met is available for synthesis of and storage in new tissue—that is, for growth.

> Only 35%-40% of the energy stored in food can be converted biochemically to a useful form.

In the past, when one was speaking of energy in nutritional terms, it was common to refer to "calories." In strict terms the calorie is a unit of measure of heat energy. But just as we speak of protein rather than its unit of measure, grams, it is preferable to speak of energy rather than its unit of measure, calories. However, the terms energy and calories will be used interchangeably in this book. To complicate matters further, some nutritionists are moving to drop the calorie as the measure of energy used. In the future the joule, a measure of work, will be used more and more frequently. One kilocalorie equals 4.184 kilojoules (kj). One thousand kilocalories equals 4.184 megajoules (Mj).

> Table 2-1
> Protein and fat ingested in amounts above those needed to meet requirements for nitrogen and essential fatty acids are metabolized to provide energy.

Protein, fat, and carbohydrate can all be catabolized to provide energy. The generally accepted energy conversion values are listed in Table 2-1. Minimum amounts of both protein and fat must be ingested to meet requirements for nitrogen and essential fatty acids. Amounts consumed above these requirements are metabolized to provide energy.

Table 2-1 Commonly accepted energy values

Macronutrient	kcal/g
Protein	4
Fats	
Long chain	9
Medium chain	8
Short chain	5.3
Carbohydrates	4

It is common to hear the term "empty calories" used in a pejorative sense when referring to certain foods. However, with the exceptions, perhaps, of sugar and pure vegetable oil, there are few foods that provide only calories (energy). More importantly, nearly 90% of the energy ingested in food each day is necessarily utilized to maintain temperature, activity, and growth. For the nutritionist then, assuring that energy requirements (Table 2-2) are met is just as important as assuring an adequate intake of, for example, essential amino acids or vitamin C, because without sufficient energy none of the other nutrients in the diet can be utilized efficiently.

Table 2-2

PROTEIN

Protein is a component of all living organisms. Proteins are composed of chains of amino acids. Of the 20 amino acids important in human nutrition at least ten cannot be synthesized by the human body and therefore must be provided in the diet. These essential amino acids are listed in Table 2-3. Although the body is unable to synthesize methionine or cystine, the conversion of either one to the other is possible and occurs regularly. Consequently, an increased intake of one may compensate for a decreased intake of the other. Similarly, tyrosine may be converted to phenylalanine. Histidine is probably essential for the young infant. Taurine, an amine derived from cystine, may also be essential for the infant. The question of the essentiality of taurine is important to resolve because casein, the predominant protein in most cow-milk infant formulas, is low in taurine. In contrast, the proteins in human milk and the whey of cow milk all provide large quantities of taurine, which suggests that an intake of taurine higher than that provided in most formulas may be desirable for the infant.

Table 2-3

Table 2-2 Recommended energy and protein intakes*

Category	Age (years)	Weight (kg)	(lb)	Height (cm)	(in)	Energy needs (with range) (kcal)	(Mj)	Protein (g)
Infants	0.0–0.5	6	13	60	24	kg × 115 (95–145)	kg × .48	kg × 2.2
	0.5–1.0	9	20	71	28	kg × 105 (80–135)	kg × .44	kg × 2.0
Children	1–3	13	29	90	35	1300 (900–1800)	5.5	23
	4–6	20	44	112	44	1700 (1300–2300)	7.1	30
	7–10	28	62	132	52	2400 (1650–3300)	10.1	34
Males	11–14	45	99	157	62	2700 (2000–3700)	11.3	45
	15–18	66	145	176	69	2800 (2100–3900)	11.8	56
Females	11–14	46	101	157	62	2200 (1500–3000)	9.2	46
	15–18	55	120	163	64	2100 (1200–3000)	8.8	46
Pregnancy						+300		+30
Lactation						+500		+20

Source: Recommended Dietary Allowances, 9th ed. 1980. Reproduced with the permission of the National Academy of Sciences, Washington, D.C.

*Energy allowances for children through age 18 are based on median energy intakes of children these ages followed in longitudinal growth studies. The values in parentheses are 10th and 90th percentiles of energy intake, to indicate the range of energy consumption among children of these ages.

Protein Quality and Its Measurement

Protein quality refers to the ability of protein in the diet to meet the body's requirements for essential amino acids.

Estimates of amino acid requirements for infants up to the age of six months are based on the essential amino acid pattern of human milk.

Protein quality refers to the ability of protein in the diet to meet the body's requirements for essential amino acids. The ratio of essential amino acids to total amino acids and the balance among the individual essential amino acids are both components of protein quality. The requirement for essential amino acids varies somewhat with age and is higher in the infant and small child than in the older child or adult. Estimates of amino acid requirements for infants up to the age of six months are based on the essential amino acid pattern of human milk. Estimates of the requirements for the older child are based on the results of nitrogen balance measurements and growth studies.

Several generalizations can be made about dietary proteins. Animal proteins in general contain all the essential amino acids in ratios that meet the requirements for each. The possible exception is a protein such as casein failing to meet the requirement for taurine, if it is truly essential. A lower percentage of essential

Table 2-3 Estimated essential amino acid requirements for infants and children, and the FAO/WHO reference pattern

Amino Acid	Infants (mg/g protein)	School children (mg/g protein)	Provisional scoring patterns (mg/g protein)
Histidine	14	0	0
Isoleucine	35	37	40
Leucine	80	56	70
Lysine	52	75	55
Methionine + cystine	29	34	35
Phenylalanine + tyrosine	63	34	60
Threonine	44	44	40
Tryptophan	8.5	4.6	10
Valine	47	41	50
TOTAL	372.5	325.6	360

Source: FAO/WHO. 1973. Energy and protein requirements. In: *Report of a joint FAO/WHO ad hoc expert committee,* Tech. Rep. Ser. No. 522, FAO Nutr. Meetings Rep. Ser. No. 52, WHO, Geneva.

Nearly all vegetable proteins are somewhat deficient in at least one of the essential amino acids.

amino acids is found in vegetable proteins. In addition, nearly all vegetable proteins are somewhat deficient in at least one of the essential amino acids. As a group, the cereals (wheat, rice, barley, and so on) are deficient in lysine. Threonine may also be low in some cereals, especially rice. The legumes, important vegetable sources of protein, are all relatively deficient in methionine. Interestingly, cereals are good sources of the sulfur-containing amino acids, while the legumes are good sources of lysine. When cereals and legumes are consumed together, the proteins of each balance the essential amino acid deficiencies of the other. The cereal-legume model (rice and beans, tortillas and beans) has in large part met the protein requirements of most of the world's population for thousands of years.

Differences in digestibility of animal and vegetable proteins are important in determining their nutritional value.

One additional difference between animal and vegetable proteins should be mentioned. Although not traditionally considered an element of protein quality, the differences in digestibility of animal and vegetable proteins are important in determining their nutritional value. Vegetable proteins not only contain a lower percentage of essential amino acids, but most of them, unless processed, are also substantially less digestible than animal proteins, reducing even further the bioavailability of both essential and unessential amino acids. Essential amino acid deficiencies and reduced digestibility become important when one considers the protein adequacy of vegetarian diets for children.

Protein quality can be estimated in a number of ways. It is important to note that there is not always good agreement among estimates made by the several means used to determine protein quality.

Amino acid score The simplest method of estimating protein quality is the calculation of an amino acid score. This is done by comparing the essential amino acid content of a protein to a reference pattern. The reference pattern describes the contents and balance of essential amino acids of a theoretical protein that should satisfy all amino acid requirements. The reference pattern used most frequently is the provisional scoring pattern of the Food and Agriculture Organization/World Health Organization (Table 2–3). The essential amino acid present in lowest concentration relative to the reference pattern is termed the first–limiting amino acid. The amino acid score is the content of the first–limiting amino acid expressed as a percentage of the desirable intake. There are several disadvantages to using the amino acid score to assess the dietary adequacy of proteins in clinical practice. Most diets contain proteins from a variety of sources; this allows for complementarity—the excess essential amino acids of one protein offsetting the deficiencies of another protein. In addition, the digestibility factor is completely disregarded in computing the amino acid score.

> The essential amino acid present in lowest concentration relative to the reference pattern is termed the first–limiting amino acid.

Protein efficiency ratio (PER) The protein efficiency ratio (PER) has been used for years as a standard measure of protein quality for laboratory animals. The PER is the amount of weight gained during a dietary period, generally about one month, divided by the protein intake in grams. A control group fed casein is always run and usually yields a value of about 2.5. The determination of the PER is a useful first step in determining the quality of a protein. The relative values of proteins as determined by PER often parallels their apparent values in human nutrition. Because the digestive systems and essential amino acid requirements of the rat differ considerably from those of the human, however, there is not a strict correlation between PER and actual protein quality for the human.

Nitrogen balance The value of a dietary protein to the human depends on its ability to support nitrogen balance and growth. Therefore, nitrogen balance studies in humans are sometimes used to assess protein quality. The nitrogen balance study is carried out as follows: a predetermined amount of protein is fed; all stool and urine are collected and the nitrogen content of each is determined; the apparent absorption of nitrogen is calculated by subtracting fecal nitrogen from nitrogen intake; and urinary nitrogen is subtracted from the amount of nitrogen absorbed to give the value for apparent nitrogen. The values for absorption and retention of nitrogen are termed "apparent" because obligatory losses of nitrogen in urine and stool and losses of nitrogen in sweat and integument are rarely corrected for. It is also possible to calculate the percentage of absorbed nitrogen retained. This is sometimes referred to as the biological value of the protein. Because in the nitrogen balance technique, any nitrogen not found in urine or stool is assumed to have been retained in the body, this technique always tends to overestimate the amount of nitrogen retained. Nitrogen balance studies are of value in determining the relative quality of proteins for human nutrition but are not the best way of determining whether an individual's protein requirements are being met. In the infant and child, growth is dependent upon and extremely sensitive to the intake of dietary protein. Consequently, longer term growth studies are useful in determining protein requirements. However, such studies are expensive and cumbersome to carry out and therefore are rarely done.

> The nitrogen balance technique always tends to overestimate the amount of nitrogen retained.

Protein Requirements

The minimal amount of protein needed to supply adequate quantities of individual essential amino acids and to provide adequate amounts of nitrogen is termed the protein requirement. This requirement is usually expressed in terms of high–quality animal protein. When proteins of poor digestibility or lower quality are consumed, the requirement for protein increases proportionately. Protein requirements have traditionally been expressed in grams per kilogram body weight per day. There is general agreement on the protein requirement of infants during the first six months of life, because it has been based on the amount of protein that would be consumed by an exclusively breast-fed infant. Protein requirements for children beyond this age have been estimated by expert committees. The concept of the recommended dietary allowance for protein and other nutrients was discussed in Chapter 1.

> The protein requirement is usually expressed in terms of high–quality animal protein. When proteins of poor digestibility or lower quality are consumed, the requirement for protein increases proportionately.

Because infants and children grow at different rates at different ages, when one expresses protein requirements in terms of grams per kilogram per day, the protein requirement appears to vary considerably with age. In clinical practice it is cumbersome to approach protein requirements in this fashion. There is considerable evidence that protein requirements and the utilization of protein depend

In clinical practice it is preferable to express protein requirements as a percentage of total energy intake.

heavily on energy intake. The infant who is consuming 150 kcal/kg/day will require more protein than the infant who is consuming 100 kcal/kg/day. Thus, in clinical practice it is preferable to express protein requirements as a percentage of total energy intake. For example, human milk is approximately 1% protein; that is, it provides 1 g protein per 100 mL of milk. Each gram of protein will provide 4 calories. One hundred mL of milk contains approximately 67 calories. Therefore, the percentage of energy supplied by protein in human milk is approximately 6%. In making these calculations it is important not to confuse the concept of a diet containing 6% protein with one containing 6% *of energy* as protein. The former refers to the concentration, by weight, of protein in the diet, while the latter indicates the fraction of the total dietary energy provided by protein. A sample calculation is shown in Table 2-4. In this example with human milk, a 1% protein diet contains 6% protein-energy (protein-calories).

Table 2-4

A value of 6%-8% of calories as protein is the lowest acceptable level of protein intake.

This value—6% protein-calories—probably represents the lower limit of acceptable protein intake for the healthy infant or child. Because few proteins match the protein quality of human milk, a more appropriate value for a safe level of intake is no less than 8% of total energy as high-quality protein. Most commercial infant formulas contain approximately 9% of total energy as protein. Thus, as the infant consumes more human milk or formula, the absolute amount of protein will increase while the percentage of total calories as protein will remain constant. In approaching clinical problems, it is rarely necessary to provide more than 8% of total energy as high-quality protein, regardless of the child's age. If the 8% protein-energy requirements are used in practice, it is unnecessary to refer constantly to tables of recommended protein intakes for children of different ages.

Table 2-4 Calculation of percentage of energy supplied by protein

Protein (g/dL) $\times$ 4 kcal/g = Protein (kcal/dL)

Protein (kcal/dL) $\div$ total kcal/dL = % protein kcal

Example: Human milk contains 1% protein and 67 kcal/dL. Calculate the % protein kcal:

$$1 \text{ g/dL} \times 4 = 4 \text{ kcal/dL}$$

$$4 \div 67 = 6\% \text{ protein kcal}$$

Protein Intakes by American Children

Table 2-5

Intakes of protein by children in the United States are generally well above the 8% of energy recommended above. Data from the Ten-State Nutrition Survey for protein and energy intakes are shown in Table 2-5. They suggest that at the 10th percentile protein intake by boys 1–3 years old is approximately 11% of dietary energy. At the nintieth percentile protein intake approaches 20% of total calories as protein. This range of protein intakes was virtually the same for both Black and White children of both "higher" and "lower" socioeconomic groups and appeared to result primarily from differences in milk consumption by children at the two extremes. Given the avowed purpose of the Ten-State Survey to look at food intakes and nutritional status of the less advantaged segments of the American population, it is apparent

In general, protein intakes of children in the United States are more than adequate.

that, in general, protein intakes of children in the United States are more than adequate. Although there is still no conclusive documentation indicating that excessive protein intakes by normal children are in any way harmful, it must be recognized that more than half of the protein in the diets of many American children is catabolized to energy. For many families this is an unnecessarily expensive means of meeting energy requirements.

FATS

Types and Sources

Fat is a major source of dietary energy, providing more than twice as many calories per gram as protein and carbohydrate. In addition, certain unsaturated fatty acids cannot be synthesized by the human body and must be supplied by fat in the diet.

Certain unsaturated fatty acids cannot be synthesized by the human body.

Dietary fat is mainly in the form of triglycerides, although cholesterol and phospholipids are also consumed. Approximately 48% of the energy in human milk and in most formulas is supplied by fat. Fat provides between 35% and 50% of total energy in the diet of older children and of adults in the United States. The intake of fat in mixed diets is quite closely associated with consumption of animal protein. In children this reflects milk consumption to a large extent, but meats such as beef and veal may contain 30% to 40% of their energy in the form of fat. Adequacy of energy intakes becomes a consideration in vegetarian diets, in which almost all fat is in the form of separated fats or oils.

Table 2-5 Estimated energy and protein intakes of U.S. children

Age, race, sex, and income*	Energy intake† (kcal/kg/day)	Protein intake† (g/kg/day)	Protein energy† (%)
1-3 years			
White males			
$0-500	627-2,046	29-100	11.2-20.0
$1,000+	927-2,216	34-88	12.0-20.8
Black males			
$0-500	688-1,817	22-77	11.6-20.4
$1,000+	812-2,445	31-103	12.0-20.4
12-16 years			
White males			
$0-500	1,297-3,974	39-142	9.2-19.6
$1,000+	1,568-4,674	56-194	11.2-20.0
Black males			
$0-500	891-3,541	31-127	10.0-20.0
$1,000+	1,112-4,354	39-171	11.2-20.8

Source: Modified from Ad hoc Committee to Review the Ten-state Nutrition Survey. 1975. Reflections of dietary studies with children in the Ten-state Nutrition Survey of 1968-1970. *Pediatrics* 56:320-326. Copyright American Association of Pediatrics. Data for girls did not differ substantively.

*Per capita income of family

†Presented as ranges; values shown are for the tenth and nintieth percentiles.

The triglyceride molecule is composed of three fatty acid molecules attached by an ester linkage to the three-carbon glycerol skeleton. Most dietary triglycerides are long-chain triglycerides, which contain fatty acids with 16 to 20 carbon atoms in their chains. Triglycerides in which the fatty acids are predominantly 8 to 12 carbons long are termed medium-chain triglycerides. Medium-chain triglycerides occur in high concentrations in certain types of vegetable oils—for example, coconut oil. These medium-chain triglycerides can be separated and are marketed commercially. Because of the difference in the way medium-chain triglycerides are absorbed, they are much better assimilated than long-chain triglycerides in many forms of steatorrhea.

Medium-chain triglycerides are much better assimilated than long-chain triglycerides in many forms of steatorrhea.

Essential Fatty Acids

Linoleic acid and alpha-linolenic acid, both having 18 carbons, are essential fatty acids for humans. Arachidonic acid, containing 20 carbons, is sometimes referred to as an essential fatty acid, but it can be synthesized in the human body when adequate amounts of linoleic acid are consumed. Essential fatty acids play a key role in the synthesis of prostaglandins. The fatty acids that are essential for the human body are abundant in human milk (up to 7%–8% of energy), are synthesized by many plants, and are present in large quantities in vegetable oils.

Although there is not complete agreement on the amounts of essential fatty acids required, at least 1% of total energy in the diet must be in the form of essential fatty acids if signs of deficiency are not to develop. The American Academy of Pediatrics suggests that 3% of total energy from essential fatty acids is a safer allowance, and we concur with this recommendation.

Vegetable oils tend to be high in polyunsaturated fatty acids. Because these polyunsaturated molecules are susceptible to oxidation, they increase the requirement for vitamin E (alpha–tocopherol), a natural antioxidant. In practical terms, most dietary sources of polyunsaturated fatty acids are excellent sources of vitamin E as well; consequently, an increased intake of one usually leads to a corresponding increase in intake of the other.

> Three percent of dietary energy should be supplied by essential fatty acids.

CARBOHYDRATES

Carbohydrates serve as a source of energy and provide fiber. There are no essential carbohydrates for humans, with the exception of ascorbic acid, which is thought of as a vitamin because of the small quantities required. Carbohydrates supply approximately 50% of dietary energy in the American diet. This figure is closer to 70% in many other parts of the world, where fat intakes are low.

> Carbohydrates supply approximately 50% of dietary energy in the American diet.

Clinical Importance of Carbohydrates

Carbohydrates are involved in several problems seen clinically. One such problem is reduced lactose absorption. An age–related and genetically determined diminution of intestinal lactase activity in Blacks and Orientals makes many of the older children and adults in these racial groups lactose malabsorbers. In addition, most infants and small children suffer a marked reduction in intestinal lactase activity following acute episodes of diarrhea.

(Lactose intolerance is discussed fully in Chapter 9.) Another instance of the clinical importance of carbohydrate is the relationship of dietary sucrose to certain illnesses—for example, dental caries or type IV hyperlipemia. Finally, the importance of fiber to normal gastrointestinal function is being increasingly appreciated.

Types of Carbohydrates

The simplest carbohydrates are the monosaccharides, such as glucose, fructose, and galactose. There is little dietary intake of monosaccharides per se except in fruits. Monosaccharides also exist as components of the disaccharides and of the more complex dietary carbohydrates, and their intake is primarily in these forms. There are three disaccharides of clinical importance: maltose, sucrose, and lactose. The component monosaccharides of these sugars are shown in Table 2-6. Little maltose is actually consumed in the form of the disaccharide. Most of it is derived by digestion of more complex carbohydrates. Sucrose intakes vary considerably depending on cultural dietary habits and socioeconomic status. Lactose occurs naturally only in milk.

Table 2-6

The more complex carbohydrates—starches—are all formed from polymers of glucose (Table 2-6). Amylose is one type of starch; it normally contains between 400 and 1200 glucose molecules in an unbranched chain. Amylopectin in plants and glycogen in the human

The more complex carbohydrates are all formed from polymers of glucose.

Table 2-6 Components of dietary carbohydrates

Carbohydrates	Component monosaccharides	Chain length
Starches	Glucose	
Amylose	Glucose (linear)	up to 1200
Amylopectin	Glucose (branched)	up to 5000
Dextrins	Glucose (linear)	5-10
Maltotriose	Glucose	3
Disaccharides		2
Maltose	Glucose	2
Sucrose	Glucose-fructose	2
Lactose	Glucose-galactose	2

are more complex, having chains that branch off approximately every 12–25 glucose molecules. The biochemical linkages between the glucose molecules in amylose, amylopectin, and other starches are all alpha linkages and are consequently susceptible to enzymatic hydrolysis by salivary and pancreatic amylases. Complex carbohydrates such as cellulose have beta linkages between glucose molecules and are indigestible by the human body. As a class carbohydrates with beta linkages are generally thought of as dietary fiber.

Dextrins are short-chained polymers of glucose containing five to ten glucose molecules. Dextrins are not consumed to any large extent in natural foods but rather are an intermediate product of the hydrolysis of starch by amylase. Dextrins have gained popularity in the manufacture of special infant formulas used to treat malabsorption. Dextrins provide nearly the same amount of energy per gram as the disaccharides. Because of their longer chain length, however, they are osmotically less active. Dextrins appear to be well tolerated by most infants. In addition to being a component of many specialized infant formulas, dextrins are now marketed specifically for use in altering formulas or in preparing special diets. The principles involved in using products such as these are discussed more fully in Chapter 11.

VITAMINS

Vitamins are nutrients that the body needs in small amounts. Nutritionists divide vitamins into two general groups: fat-soluble vitamins and water-soluble vitamins. The fat-soluble vitamins—vitamins A, D, E, and K—dissolve in fats, and therefore they are supplied by dietary sources containing fats. The B vitamins, folic acid and ascorbic acid are water-soluble vitamins.

Vitamin A

Biological function Vitamin A, retinol, has several specific functions in human nutrition. The best known of these is the role that retinal, the aldehyde of retinol, plays in the visual cycle. Retinal is critical to the functioning of the rods in the retina. Retinol deficiency is associated with poor visual perception in dim light, or night blindness. Vitamin A is also thought to be important in the maintenance of mucous membrane integrity. In other animals there is a clear relationship between vitamin A, protein, and growth. Recent evidence suggests that this same relationship may exist for humans.

Vitamin A in the diet may be taken in as preformed vitamin A or as the provitamin carotene.

Animal and vegetable sources   Vitamin A in the diet may be taken in as preformed vitamin A or as the provitamin carotene. All preformed vitamin A, retinol, is of animal origin. There are numerous carotenes present in plants, the most familiar being the beta-carotenes. Beta-carotene biochemically resembles two molecules of retinal joined end to end. Its hydrolysis in the enterocyte provides the basic molecule with vitamin A activity. (Carotenes absorbed intact are unable to be hydrolyzed later and have no vitamin A activity.) Because carotenes do not provide the same amount of vitamin A activity as retinol does, all forms of vitamin A are quantified as retinol equivalents. That is, 1 μg of retinol is equal to 1 retinol equivalent. The corresponding retinol equivalency of beta-carotene is 6 μg. In the past, vitamin A quantities were expressed as international units: One retinol equivalent is equal to 3.3 IU of retinol or 10 IU of beta-carotene.

Because retinol is stored in the livers of most animals, liver is an excellent dietary source of vitamin A. Milk is also a good source. The carotenes are widely distributed in vegetables with orange, red, or yellow color, although not all have provitamin A activity. Many greens, such as spinach and beet greens, are also good sources of carotene. Because vitamin A is fat soluble, its absorption parallels quite closely the absorption of dietary fat. Once in the plasma, retinol is transported on a plasma protein known as retinol-binding protein. Most retinol goes to the liver for storage until it is required at other sites.

Vitamin A deficiency is almost never seen in isolation.

Hypovitaminosis/hypervitaminosis A   Vitamin A deficiency is practically unheard of in the United States. Epidemiologically, vitamin A deficiency is almost never seen in isolation. Rather, the deficiency occurs naturally only in association with severe forms of protein-energy malnutrition. Night blindness, the most reliable clinical indicator of vitamin A deficiency, is difficult to test for in young children. The child is usually asked to pick out specific objects from a box under conditions of dim light. Bitot's spots, while not pathognonomic, are nearly so in young children, and they provide more objective evidence of vitamin A deficiency than does the test. Serum retinol levels below 10 μg/dL are considered "deficient." Although levels this low are not invariably associated with clinical disease, they require treatment.

Excess intake of carotene is associated with elevated plasma-carotene levels and a yellow-orange hue of the skin. There appears to be no physiologic impairment associated with excess carotene intake. In contrast, excessive intake of retinol on either an acute or a chronic basis can be harmful. Acute hypervitaminosis A produces a pseudotumor cerebri syndrome. More chronic overingestion initially causes a variety of nonspecific symptoms such as irritability and anorexia. Later, skin lesions (including desquamation of skin from the palms and soles), hair loss, tenderness on palpation of long bones, and radiologic evidence of hyperostosis occur.

Table 2-7

The recommended dietary allowance for vitamin A ranges between 400 and 1000 retinol equivalents per day depending on the age of the child (Table 2-7). Daily ingestion of five to ten times the RDA over a period of months is required before signs of vitamin A intoxication appear.

Vitamin D

Function and metabolism   Vitamin D may be thought of as both a vitamin and a hormone. Insofar as exogenous intake is required to assure an adequate supply, cholecalciferol (vitamin D_3) qualifies as a vitamin. The human skin, however, is capable of synthesizing vitamin D under optimal conditions. The irradiation by ultraviolet light of 7-dehydrocholesterol produces cholecalciferol, which is then reabsorbed. When produced on the skin and then transported to a distal site of action, vitamin D fulfills the definition of a hormone.

In almost all instances a dietary source of vitamin D is needed.

The proportion of vitamin D supplied to a child by endogenous production depends directly on exposure to sunlight. This in turn depends on the geographic region in which the child lives, on the child's skin color, and on his or her day-to-day habits. As a general rule, endogenous production is not sufficient to meet the child's requirements for vitamin D, except perhaps in tropical latitudes. Consequently, in almost all instances a dietary source of vitamin D is needed.

Regardless of the source, once absorbed, the vitamin D molecule is transported to the liver, where it is hydroxylated at the 25 position, and then to the kidney, where hydroxylation at the 1 position occurs. The 1, 25–dihydroxy–vitamin D then travels to various sites, where, by affecting a change in protein synthesis, it exerts specific actions on movements of calcium across membranes.

Hypovitaminosis/hypervitaminosis D   In vitamin D deficiency there is decreased absorption of calcium. In turn, a decreased serum calcium concentration stimulates parathromone secretion. The secondary hyperparathyroidism that results is responsible for many of the signs and symptoms associated with vitamin D deficiency. The signs and symptoms of rickets are well covered in most pediatric textbooks.

Chronic intakes of excessive amounts of vitamin D are toxic. Symptoms include loss of appetite, irritability, and constipation.

Table 2-7 Recommended dietary allowances of vitamins for children of different ages

| | Infants | | Children | | | Adolescents | | | |
| | | | | | | Female | | Male | |
Vitamin	0-6 mo	6-12 mo	1-3 years	4-6 years	7-10 years	11-14 years	15-18 years	11-14 years	15-18 years
Retinol (A)—RE*	420	400	400	500	700	800	800	1000	1000
Calciferol (D)—μg†	10	10	10	10	10	10	10	10	10
α-tocopherol (E)—mg	3	5	5	6	7	8	8	8	10
Vitamin K—μg	12	10-20	15-30	20-40	30-60	50-100	50-100	50-100	50-100
Thiamin (B_1)—mg	0.3	0.5	0.7	0.9	1.2	1.1	1.1	1.4	1.4
Riboflavin (B_2)—mg	0.4	0.6	0.8	1.0	1.4	1.3	1.3	1.6	1.6
Pyridoxine (B_6)—mg	0.3	0.6	0.9	1.3	1.6	1.8	2.0	1.8	2.0
Cobalamin (B_{12})—μg	0.5	1.5	2.0	2.5	3.0	3.0	3.0	3.0	3.0
Folacin—μg	30	45	100	200	300	400	400	400	400
Niacin—mg NE‡	6	8	9	11	16	15	14	18	18
Biotin—μg	35	50	65	85	120	100-200	100-200	100-200	100-200
Pantothenic acid—mg	2	3	3	3-4	4-5	4-7	4-7	4-7	4-7
Ascorbic acid (C)—mg	35	35	45	45	45	50	60	50	60

Source: Recommended Dietary Allowances, 9th ed. 1980. Reproduced with the permission of the National Academy of Sciences, Washington, D.C.

*Re = retinol equivalent. See p. 35 for definition.

†10 g cholecalciferol = 400 IU Vitamin D.

‡NE = niacin equivalent. See p. 41 for definition.

Hypercalcemia usually results. Excessive maternal intake of vitamin D during pregnancy has been associated with failure to thrive and hypercalcemia (mild syndrome) and with congenital aortic stenosis in association with an elfin facies (severe syndrome).

The recommended dietary allowance for vitamin D varies little with age and is generally set at 400 IU per day. Many American infants receive several times this amount with no apparent ill effects. Dietary sources of vitamin D include liver and liver oils. Fortified milk is a major source of vitamin D in the diet of American children. The question of the adequacy of the vitamin D content of human milk is discussed in Chapter 3.

Vitamin E

Antioxidant function There are seven naturally occurring tocopherols that have vitamin E activity. The most active of these is alpha-tocopherol, which functions primarily as a natural antioxidant in the human. Polyunsaturated fatty acids (PUFA) are easily oxidized. Vitamin E protects against their oxidation. Increased dietary intakes of PUFA increase the requirements for vitamin E in the diet. Similarly, the requirement for vitamin E can be reduced experimentally if other lipid antioxidants are fed. Selenium, for example, decreases the need for vitamin E.

Source Tocopherols may function as natural antioxidants in foods as well. The content of tocopherols in plants seems to vary directly with the content of unsaturated fatty acids, especially linoleic acid. As a general rule, foods that provide large amounts of PUFA are also good sources of vitamin E. Natural variations and losses of vitamin E through processing and cooking do occur, however.

Vitamin E deficiency in pediatrics is clinically significant primarily in the nutrition of the premature infant.

Deficiency Vitamin E deficiency in pediatrics is clinically significant primarily in the nutrition of the premature infant. A hemolytic anemia associated with skin lesions and edema has been encountered in infants consuming diets rich in PUFA, relatively low in vitamin E. The condition has been found to be aggravated by increased intakes of iron. In addition to the hemolytic anemia seen in premature infants, increased excretions of creatine, indicating muscle breakdown, and increased hemolysis have been seen in older children and adults with presumed vitamin E deficiency.

The requirement for vitamin E is best expressed in relation to the PUFA content of the diet. An intake of 0.6 mg d-alpha-tocopherol per gram of PUFA is sufficient to prevent deficiencies. Infant formulas and human milk provide adequate amounts of vitamin E for full-term newborns and older infants. The vitamin E content of formula may be inadequate for premature infants if iron-fortified formula is used. In general, animal products are low in both polyunsaturated fatty acids and in vitamin E. There is generally little concern about dietary intakes of vitamin E past the newborn period except in children with diseases producing steatorrhea.

Vitamin K

Factors II, VII, IX, and X are all vitamin K dependent.

The K vitamins are a group of structurally related compounds that are required for the normal synthesis of four of the clotting factors synthesized in the liver. Factors II, VII, IX, and X are all vitamin K dependent.

Because vitamin K is widespread in both plant and animal food, dietary vitamin K deficiency is almost never seen past the newborn period. The infant *in utero* receives relatively small amounts of vitamin K from its mother. Synthesis of vitamin K in the intestine, an important source of vitamin K in older individuals, begins only after the fecal flora is well established. For this reason, all newborn infants are treated with vitamin K shortly after birth. Vitamin K deficiency in older infants and children occurs only in association with malabsorption syndromes or chronic antibiotic administration.

Because it has been difficult to assess the relative importance of dietary intake of vitamin K and that of production of vitamin K by the intestinal microflora, recommended dietary allowance for vitamin K has not been established.

B Vitamins

Thiamin Thiamin (vitamin B_1) is a water-soluble compound integrally involved in energy metabolism—in particular, the oxidative decarboxylation of pyruvate and alpha-ketoglutarate. More than 80% of thiamin in the body is in the form of thiamin pyrophosphate, the compound involved in these decarboxylations. Because thiamin is so directly related to carbohydrate metabolism and energy production, the requirement for thiamin varies directly with energy intake and metabolic rate. For example, diseases such as thyrotoxicosis that increase the metabolic rate also increase the dietary requirement for thiamin.

The requirement for thiamin varies directly with energy intake and metabolic rate.

Thiamin deficiency results in beriberi, a disease that is extremely uncommon in the United States. Dietary deficiency of thiamin is virtually unheard of in the United States except in association with cult diets and with excessive consumption of alcohol. Thiamin is widely distributed in a variety of foods, including beef, pork, wheat and whole grains, rice, and legumes. The recommended dietary allowance for thiamin varies from 0.3 mg/day for infants to approximately 1.5 mg/day for adolescent males.

Riboflavin Riboflavin (vitamin B_2) is an important component of flavin mononucleotide (FMN) and of flavin adenine dinucleotide (FAD), both coenzymes involved in electron transport and energy production. Unlike that for thiamin, the requirement for riboflavin does not seen to be altered markedly by variations in either energy intake or metabolism. Clinically, riboflavin deficiency is a curiosity characterized by a variety of nonspecific physical findings including angular stomatitis and glossitis, both of which are more frequently associated with other conditions. Excessive corneal vascularization resulting from riboflavin deficiency has been described in both rats and humans. Dairy products and meats are excellent sources of riboflavin. Whole grains and vegetables are also important sources.

Pyridoxine Pyridoxine (vitamin B_6) in the form of pyridoxal phosphate plays an important role as a coenzyme in the metabolism of virtually all the amino acids. It is also involved to a lesser extent in carbohydrate metabolism. The requirement for pyridoxine appears to be more closely related to protein intake than to carbohydrate intake, however. Clinical pyridoxine deficiency and dependency in infants is associated with irritability and convulsions. Microcytic anemia, seborrhea–like skin lesions, cheilosis, glossitis, and peripheral neuropathies have also been seen in older individuals as a result of pyridoxine deficiency.

Signs and symptoms of pyridoxine deficiency have been reported in adults on chronic isoniazid (INH) therapy. Although pyridoxine deficiency associated with INH therapy is mentioned with regard to pediatric patients, we have not been able to find reports of problems in the pediatric age group. Oral contraceptives also affect the vitamin B_6 status of the individual. Subclinical changes in tryptophan metabolism seen in women taking oral contraceptives are corrected by supplementation with pyridoxine. Routine supplementation with B_6 for women taking oral contraceptives has not been recommended.

Vitamin B_{12} The term vitamin B_{12} refers to a variety of cobalt-containing compounds similar to cyanocobalamin. The function of vitamin B_{12} is integrally linked to folic acid metabolism. Vitamin B_{12} appears to play an important role in the recycling of folic acid derivatives back into the folic acid pool. A deficiency of vitamin B_{12} is associated with megaloblastic anemia and peripheral neuropathy as well as with gastrointestinal changes.

Vitamin B_{12} is the only vitamin for which there are no vegetable dietary sources.

Vitamin B_{12} is the only vitamin for which there are no vegetable dietary sources. As a result, dietary vitamin B_{12} inadequacy is a problem in strict vegetarian diets (see Chapter 7). Food fad diets that markedly limit the intake of animal protein may also lead to deficiency. Another point of practical clinical importance is that vitamin B_{12} is one of the few compounds obligatorily absorbed in the terminal ileum. Children who have diseases affecting the terminal ileum, such as Crohn's disease, or who have had resection of the ileum—for example, following perforation with necrotizing enterocolitis—are likely to develop vitamin B_{12} deficiency unless the vitamin is administered regularly in parenteral form.

Vitamin B_{12} is one of the few compounds obligatorily absorbed in the terminal ileum.

Virtually all foods of animal origin supply vitamin B_{12}. The concentration of vitamin B_{12} in human milk closely parallels the level in maternal plasma. Consequently, vitamin B_{12} deficiency in the nursing mother may create a deficiency in her infant. The situation in which this is most likely to occur is in vegetarian mothers nursing their infants.

Folacin Folacin is a generic term for folic acid and similar compounds with folic acid activity. Tetrahydrofolic acid, the active form of folacin, is involved in a variety of reactions in intermediary metabolism that affect the transfer of one–carbon units. It plays a role in the synthesis of purines and of pyrimidine neucleotides and also in the interconversions of several of the essential and non-essential amino acids. Folic acid deficiency produces a megaloblastic anemia indistinguishable from that produced by vitamin B_{12} deficiency. In folic acid deficiency, however, there are no associated neurologic signs or symptoms. Folic acid is found in a variety of both animal and vegetable foods, including most meats, poultry, eggs, and dark green leafy vegetables. Because folic acid is water soluble and heat labile, excessive cooking or processing of these foods may reduce the folic acid available from them. Folic acid deficiency is uncommon in the pediatric patient except in association with diseases producing severe generalized malabsorption. However, goat milk contains very little folic acid, and folic acid deficiency has been reported in children fed goat milk for suspected allergy to cow milk.

Niacin Niacin refers to both nicotinic acid and nicotinamide. Niacin, in the form of coenzyme I (NAD) and coenzyme II (NADP), plays an important role in many reactions in the Krebs cycle. Because of this integral link of niacin to energy metabolism, the requirement for niacin varies directly with energy intake.

The human body can convert the essential amino acid tryptophan to niacin.

The intake of niacin per se is not an absolute dietary requirement for humans. The human body can convert the essential amino acid tryptophan to niacin. Consequently, an adequate intake of high-quality protein reduces the dietary requirement for niacin. Because of this convertibility, the niacin content of any food is usually expressed in terms of niacin equivalents (NEs). An intake of 60 mg of tryptophan has been estimated to be the equivalent of an intake of 1 mg of niacin. The interconversion of tryptophan to niacin is also influenced by the leucine and pyridoxine contents of the diet.

Inadequate dietary intake of niacin or tryptophan results in pellagra, a disease characterized by weakness, lassitude, anorexia, and the three D's: dermatitis, diarrhea, and dementia. Pellagra was common in the southern part of the United States during the early decades of the 20th century, and it is still encountered frequently among poor alcoholics. It is otherwise a curiosity today in this country. Although all mixed diets provide adequate amounts of niacin and tryptophan, improper vegetarian diets or fad diets could provide inadequate intakes of available niacin. The dietary requirement for niacin varies between 6.6 mg (NEs)/1000 kcal and 8 mg (NEs)/1000 kcal.

Biotin Biotin is a water–soluble vitamin of the B complex that plays an important role in fatty acid synthesis. Because biotin is found in nearly all foods, dietary deficiency is not a concern in mixed diets. Raw egg albumin binds biotin in the intestine, so that consumption of large amounts of raw egg white makes biotin unavailable to the body. Synthetic diets to which biotin is not added could also conceivably product biotin deficiency.

Panthothenic acid Panthothenic acid is a critical component of coenzyme A. As such, it is important in the intermediary metabolism of proteins, fats, and carbohydrates. Because of the ubiquitous distribution of panthothenic acid in nature, dietary deficiency of this B vitamin is rarely seen.

Ascorbic Acid

The inability to convert glucose to ascorbic acid is a metabolic defect that primates share with diverse other species, such as the guinea pig, fruit-eating bat, and rainbow trout. The lengthy list of biological functions of vitamin C includes a role in collagen formation and in the formation of neurotransmitters such as norepinephrine. Vitamin C also plays an important role in hematopoiesis (increasing iron absorption) by increasing the transfer of iron from transferrin to ferritin and also by increasing conversion of folic acid to an active form. Vitamin C also appears to be an antioxidant and may slightly reduce the requirements for vitamins A and E and for certain of the B vitamins.

Inadequate intake of ascorbic acid results in scurvy. This disease was seen frequently in pediatric practice in the past. The breast-fed infant receives adequate amounts of vitamin C if the mother's diet is normal. If scurvy develops in breast–fed infants, it characteristically occurs shortly after weaning, because the body is unable to store vitamin C. Scurvy has been associated both with inadequate intakes of vitamin C and with the destruction of vitamin C in formula and juices by overzealous sterilization. The clinical description of scurvy is well covered in most pediatric textbooks.

Experts do not agree on the dietary requirement for vitamin C. Intakes of more than 10 mg of ascorbic acid per day appear to prevent scurvy. Intakes greater than 80 mg per day produce no further increase in the plasma level of ascorbic acid because ascorbic acid, with a T_m below that of glucose, is lost through the renal tubules. The recommended dietary allowance for vitamin C is shown in Table 2-7.

Virtually everyone is aware of the value of citrus fruits as sources of ascorbic acid. Ascorbic acid is also found in substantial amounts in foods such as broccoli, spinach, cauliflower, lima beans, and potatoes. Potatoes, for example, have a vitamin C concentration close to that of grapefruit. Because potatoes are consumed in large quantities by many individuals, they are an important source of vitamin C in the diet.

Because foods such as potato, broccoli, and spinach are often eaten in large quantities, they are important sources of vitamin C.

MINERALS

Many minerals are necessary for human nutrition. Some—calcium, phosphorus, sodium, and potassium—are needed in relatively large amounts. Others, although essential, are needed only in trace amounts.

Calcium and Phosphorus

Calcium　Calcium is the cation present in highest concentration in the body. Most body calcium is structurally incorporated into bone. The small amount of calcium that is soluble in body fluids plays an important role in regulating the excitability of nerves and muscles and in normal coagulation. The dietary requirement for calcium is influenced by several factors.

Although there is not complete agreement on the subject, the calcium:phosphorus ratio seems to be important in determining the dietary need for calcium, especially in the neonate with immature parathyroids. This ratio is felt to be important because of its effect on absorption of calcium from the gastrointestinal tract. The calcium and phosphorus content and the calcium:phosphorus ratio for human milk, cow milk, and infant formula are shown in Table 2-8. All three diets have a calcium:phosphorus ratio greater than 1:1. Of the three, human milk has the lowest calcium content but the highest calcium:phosphorus ratio. Because phytates, which

Table 2-8

Table 2-8 Calcium and phosphorus contents of several milks and formulas

Diet	Ca (mg/L)	P (mg/L)	Ca:P
Human milk	340	162	2.1:1
Cow milk	1240	950	1.3:1
Infant formula*	420–550	312–460	1.2–1.3:1

*Range for Enfamil, Similac and SMA.

contain large amounts of phosphorus, tend to bind calcium in the intestinal tract and decrease calcium absorption, they must be taken into account when considering the calcium intakes of vegetarians.

Finally, there is evidence from studies in adults that the level of protein in the diet markedly affects urinary excretion of calcium. Increased protein intakes are associated with urinary calcium excretions many times higher than those seen with a low-protein diet. This phenomenon has not been well studied in the pediatric age group.

For infants and most children in the United States the major dietary source of calcium is either milk or infant formula. Other good dietary sources of calcium are greens, sesame, kale, and soybean flour (see Table 7–4).

Phosphorus Because phosphorus is present in virtually all foods, the adequacy of dietary phosphorus intake is rarely questioned. However, there is some question as to whether the phosphorus content of human milk is sufficient for the rapidly growing premature infant (see Chapter 12).

Excessive phosphorus intake in early infancy can cause problems. Cow milk has been associated with tetany of the newborn infant, because the milk has a high concentration of phosphorus. In such instances, the high phosphorus intake increases the serum concentration of phosphorus and consequently lowers that of calcium, resulting in hypocalcemia. The immature parathyroid glands of some infants are unable to respond to this stress as they would in the older child.

> The adequacy of dietary phosphorus intake is rarely a question except when human milk is fed to small premature infants.

Dietary intake of phosphorus is lower than that of calcium so long as milk or formula is being consumed. With the addition of cereals or solid foods to the diet, the phosphorus intake increases markedly. In older children, for whom milk is not the major source of dietary energy intake, phosphorus intakes may be several times higher than those of calcium, with no ill effect.

Sodium and Potassium

Table 2-9

Intakes of sodium and potassium are never lower later in life than they are in the exclusively breast-fed infant.

Dietary requirements for sodium and potassium (Table 2-9) are met in virtually all natural diets. Relative to cow milk and infant formula, human milk is low in both these minerals. Intakes of sodium and potassium are never lower later in life than they are in the exclusively breast-fed infant. However, these low intakes have been considered acceptable for infants up to the age of six months. There is no evidence of a requirement for added salt in the diets of older omnivorous infants and children. The taste for sodium chloride and the use of table salt as a condiment are largely acquired habits. There are groups that do not use table salt, preferring to use potassium chloride instead.

Table 2-9 Recommended dietary allowances of minerals for children of different ages

| | Infants | | Children | | | Adolescents | | | |
| | | | | | | Females | | Males | |
Mineral	0-6 mo	6-12 mo	1-3 years	4-6 years	7-10 years	11-14 years	15-18 years	11-14 years	15-18 years
Sodium (mg)	115–350	250–750	325–975	450–1350	600–1800	900–2700	900–2700	900–2700	900–2700
Potassium (mg)	350–925	425–1275	550–1650	775–2325	1000–3000	1525–4575	1525–4575	1525–4575	1525–4575
Calcium (mg)	360	540	800	800	800	1200	1200	1200	1200
Phosphorus (mg)	240	360	800	800	800	1200	1200	1200	1200
Iron (mg)	10	15	15	10	10	18	18	18	18
Magnesium (mg)	50	70	150	200	250	300	300	350	400
Zinc (mg)	3	5	10	10	10	15	15	15	15
Copper (mg)	0.5–0.7	0.7–1.0	1.0–1.5	1.5–2.0	2.0–2.5	2.0–3.0	2.0–3.0	2.0–3.0	2.0–3.0
Iodine (μg)	40	50	70	90	120	150	150	150	150

Source: Recommended Dietary Allowances, 9th ed. 1980. Reproduced with the permission of the National Academy of Sciences, Washington, D.C.

Sodium and potassium are important nutritionally for several reasons. Because these cations are the major determinants of extracellular and intracellular osmolality, their intake and excretion are important determinants of water balance. The relationship of these intakes to renal solute load is discussed later in this chapter. Excess intake of sodium throughout life may or may not be a factor in the development of essential hypertension.

Trace Minerals

Iron Although not generally thought of as such, iron is indeed a trace mineral relative to the other major minerals of the body. However, iron is of major importance from a nutritional point of view. Iron deficiency is one of the few remaining areas of concern with regard to undernutrition in the United States. For this reason, iron nutrition is covered separately in Chapter 8.

Iron deficiency is one of the few remaining areas of concern with regard to undernutrition in the United States.

Zinc Zinc is an essential nutrient for the human. A large proportion of total body zinc is located in bone. Zinc is also found in high concentration in nucleic acids. Many pancreatic enzymes and enzymes important in intermediary metabolism are zinc metalloenzymes. What appears to be zinc deficiency has been reported in the Middle East. Children with apparent zinc deficiency manifested strikingly short stature and sexual infantilism, both of which were reversed after hospitalization and therapy with zinc. Whether there is any significant dietary zinc deficiency in this country is a subject of considerable confusion. Hambidge and his coworkers (1972) determined hair zinc levels in 250 children less than 17 years of age living in the Denver area. In ten (5.3%) of 132 children over 4 years of age the values were less than 70 ppm, which is the lower limit of normal according to these authors. Seven of the ten had a history of poor appetite. Eight had heights that fell at or below the 10th percentile; the other two were at the 25th and 75th percentiles. Diminished taste acuity (hypogeusia) was found in five of six children tested. The child whose height was at the 25th percentile showed no change of taste acuity. The tallest child was not tested. When the five children with hypogeusia were treated with zinc, they showed improved taste discrimination. The meaning of these data is unclear for several reasons. Hair zinc levels are normally quite high at birth and fall rapidly during the first year, increasing gradually thereafter. Because shorter children presumably eat less, zinc levels in their hair might be expected to increase more slowly. Finally, zinc status is difficult to assess, and the validity of using hair or plasma zinc concentrations is very much in question.

Because zinc in bone is not readily mobilized, a daily dietary source of zinc is essential.

Because zinc in bone is not readily mobilized, a daily dietary source of zinc is essential. Both human milk and commercial infant formula are good sources of zinc for the infant. For the older child dairy products, meat, and seafood are also good sources. Cereals, vegetables, and fruit are relatively poor sources. In addition, the phytate content of many of these foods reduces the bioavailability of zinc in the diet. The recommended dietary allowance for zinc is shown in Table 2–9.

Copper Copper is an essential mineral for the human body, playing a role in the normal development of bone, of the central nervous system, and of connective tissue. Ceruloplasmin, the major copper-containing protein in plasma, is thought to act as a ferroxidase, increasing iron absorption from the intestinal tract. Copper also plays a role in hemoglobin synthesis. Copper deficiency in humans has been characterized by neutropenia, resistant anemia, and bone lesions that often resemble scurvy. Because copper is avidly reabsorbed from the intestinal tract and recycled, dietary copper deficiency is extremely uncommon in the United States. There are three clinical situations in which the practitioner should consider copper deficiency: the small premature infant given an insufficient copper intake because of formula modification, the child given long-term treatment with parenteral alimentation solutions with a low copper content, and the child with severe chronic diarrhea, whose intestinal losses may not have been offset by adequate dietary intakes. Copper intakes by most children in the United States are more than adequate. As a general rule, foods that are good sources of iron are also good sources of copper. Human milk contains about 33% more copper than is found in cow milk.

There are three clinical situations in which the physician should consider copper deficiency.

Other Minerals We are just beginning to appreciate the importance of several other trace minerals in human nutrition. The relationship of iodine intake to thyroid function has been recognized for some time, but we are only beginning to uncover the roles played by many other trace minerals in intermediary metabolism. Chromium, for example, is now known to play an important part in carbohydrate metabolism, in part through its interaction with insulin. Chromium supplementation in some experimental settings improves glucose tolerance. The importance of these findings in future treatment of diabetes is uncertain.

A description of the functions of metals such as cobalt, manganese, selenium, and molybdenum is beyond the scope of this book. All of these trace elements have been found as parts of metalloenzymes or as cofactors of reactions in intermediary metabolism.

OSMOLALITY OF THE DIET

In addition to paying attention to the content of specific nutrients in the diet, the practitioner must bear in mind two other aspects of diet calculation, especially when dealing with small infants or with infants and children with compromised intestinal tracts. The two are the osmolality of the diet and the renal solute load (Table 2-10).

Table 2-10

The osmolality of a diet is a measure of the osmotic pressure that the diet will exert when it comes into contact with the semipermeable membranes of the intestinal tract. Osmolality of the diet is determined by the number of particles of solute dissolved in water, the solvent of most of the diet. A number of the constituents of the diet contribute its osmolality. These constituents include protein, carbohydrate, many of the vitamins, and the minerals. Increasing the dietary content of any of these nutrients without increasing water in the diet concommitantly increases the osmolality. Because lipid is not miscible with water, it exerts no osmotic force. Consequently, increasing the amount of fat in the diet does not affect the osmolality.

Osmolality is dependent on particle number.

Because osmolality is dependent on particle number, the molecular form of protein and carbohydrate in the diet is an important factor in determining the osmolality. For example, a formula containing whole protein will have a lower osmolality than a similar one providing the same amount of nitrogen in the form of peptides or free amino acids. Similarly, the use of starch or dextrins in a formula will result in lower osmolality than will the use of the same quantity of carbohydrate in the form of disaccharides.

Recent experimental data suggest that all the physiologic events of digestion and absorption that take place in the duodenum and beyond occur at slightly above isotonicity, about 350–450 milliosmoles/kg water, the osmolality decreasing farther down the small intestine. The traditional concern with hypertonic diets is that they will induce an increased movement of water into the small intestine as the body attempts to dilute the intestinal contents to isotonicity. This flux of water into the lumen will increase motility, causing the fluid to be moved rapidly downstream, the end result being diarrhea. Whether this concern is warranted, even with diets with osmolalities up to 700 milliosmoles, has recently been questioned. Nevertheless, some studies have related the occurrence of necrotizing enterocolitis in premature infants to the feeding of concentrated formulas.

Human milk, cow milk, and all the standard infant formulas are hypotonic or isotonic relative to plasma. Some of the

Table 2-10 Dietary alterations affecting osmolality and renal solute load

Nutrient alteration	Effect on osmolality	Effect on renal solute load
Protein		
Increase intake as whole protein	↑	↑
Decrease intake as whole protein	↓	↓
Constant intake—substitute peptides or free amino acids for whole protein	↑	0
Fat		
Increase or decrease intake	0	0
Carbohydrate		
Increase intake	↑	0
Decrease intake	↓	0
Constant intake		
Increase percentage from monosaccharides and disaccharides	↑	0
Decrease percentage from monosaccharides and disaccharides, substituting dextrins or starch	↓	0
Minerals		
Increase intake	↑	↑
Decrease intake	↓	↓

The importance of hypertonicity in causing diarrhea in infants has probably been overestimated.

therapeutic formulas, such as those with mixtures of free amino acids, are slightly hypertonic. The importance of hypertonicity in causing diarrhea in infants has probably been overestimated. As a general rule, we do not worry about diets whose osmolalities are 350–450 milliosmoles/kg water or less, except when they are to be fed by tube directly into the duodenum or jejunum. For routine oral feeding, formulas with osmolalities up to this level are nicely tolerated.

RENAL SOLUTE LOAD

Some of the attention paid to osmolality of the diet would better be given to the concept of renal solute load: the end products of intermediary metabolism that must be excreted via the kidney. The urine becomes more concentrated when more solute must be excreted relative to the amount of water available to the kidney. If the osmotic load of the diet relative to free water exceeds the ability of the kidney to concentrate, an osmotic diuresis results, leading to dehydration. Calculation of renal solute load is particularly important for the practitioner dealing with normal infants, whose ability to concentrate during the first several months can be relatively poor if they are on a low-protein diet. Consideration of renal solute load is also important with infants requiring highly concentrated diets because of restrictions on the permissible volume of intake. Two common examples of the problem with concentrated diets are the child with short gut, whose intestine tolerates only small volumes, and the child with congestive heart failure, in whom fluid overload may be a problem.

Ziegler and Fomon (1971) have suggested that, for practical purposes, the potential renal solute loads of the diet for full term and older infants can be calculated using the dietary contents of protein, sodium, chloride, and potassium (Table 2-11). The amino acids in dietary protein that are not used to synthesize new tissue will be catabolized to urea, which must be excreted through the kidneys. Approximately 4 milliosmoles of solute will be generated for every gram of protein ingested. Small amounts of all minerals ingested are retained for growth. In the net balance, however, the excretion of sodium, chloride, and potassium nearly equals their intake on a day-to-day basis. Each milliequivalent of these minerals will contribute 1 milliosmole. Carbohydrate and fat may be ignored when calculating renal solute load from dietary content, because, when fully metabolized, both carbohydrate and fat yield only carbon dioxide and water, neither of which significantly affects renal solute load. The relative effects of several dietary constituents on both osmolality and renal solute load are shown in Table 2-10. It is clear that the osmolality of the diet is not predictive of the renal solute load.

Although the renal solute load of the diet can be calculated in absolute terms, it takes on importance only when related to the water balance of specific infants (Table 2-12)* Let us assume that a hypothetical infant has an insensible water loss of 400 mL/day. Water output in the stool is 100 mL/day. If one liter of dietary

Renal solute load is an important consideration early in infancy or in infants with fluid-restricted diets.

Table 2-11

Table 2-12

---

*For simplicity in discussing the concept of renal solute load, 1 liter of milk and 1 liter of formula are assumed in the following examples to supply one liter of water, which they do not, since the solute reduces the amount of water per liter of milk or formula.

Table 2-11 Estimation of renal solute load (RSL)*

Protein—g	X	4
meq Sodium	X	1
meq Potassium	X	1
meq Chlorine	X	1
Σ = RSL		

Source: Ziegler, E. E.; and Fomon, S. J. 1971. Fluid intake, renal solute load, and water balance in infancy. *J. Pediatr.* 78:561–568.

*Estimate applies to full–term (not low–birth–weight) infants and to children receiving generous intakes of protein. Low–birth–weight infants retain a higher percentage of the potential solute in their diet and consequently this method overestimates actual renal solute load in these rapidly growing infants.

Table 2-12 Effect of diet on renal solute load

		Healthy	Decreased intake, otherwise healthy	Decreased intake and fever
Intake (mL)		1000	750	750
Insensible loss (mL)		400	400	550
Stool (mL)		100	100	100
Urine				
Volume (mL)		500	250	100
Concentration (milliosmole/liter) if diet is	human milk	162	243	608
	formula	220	330	825
	cow milk	440	660	1650

water is ingested, the amount of water remaining for the excretion of solute by the kidney is 500 mL. If this baby is being breast–fed, the liter of human milk consumed will potentially provide 81 milliosmoles of solute to be excreted. This solute will be diluted in the 500 mL remaining after insensible and intestinal losses of water. Consequently, the kidney will produce a urine with a concentration of 162 milliosmoles/liter. If the same infant is being fed a commercial infant formula with a renal solute load of 110 milliosmoles/liter, the urine concentration will be 220 milliosmoles/liter. If whole cow milk, with a renal solute load of 220 milliosmoles/liter, is being given, the urine concentration would be 440 milliosmoles/liter. None of these concentrations creates a particular stress for the infant kidney.

If the infant's intake is reduced to 750 mL, the potential solute load will be reduced by one-fourth. However, the concomitant reduction in the amount of water available for renal excretion will be disproportionately large, with water available decreasing from 500 mL to 250 mL. The urine concentration will increase to 243 milliosmoles/liter (human milk), 330 milliosmoles/liter (formula) and 660 milliosmoles/liter (cow milk). Thus far this example demonstrates clearly that a moderate reduction in dietary intake by a normal infant will lead to a disproportionate increase in the concentration of the urine that is excreted.

If the same infant reduces his intake because of an illness associated with fever, insensible losses will increase at the same time that volume of intake decreases. Using the same hypothetical infant, let us assume that fever increases insensible loss from 400 to 550 mL/day. If the dietary intake is 750 mL/day and stool losses do not change, only 100 mL of water will be available for the formation of urine. If this child is being breast-fed, the resulting urine concentration will be 608 milliosmoles/liter. The formula-fed infant will have to concentrate to 825 milliosmoles/liter. Although both of these urines are concentrated, they are still within the capacity of the immature kidney. If the infant were being fed whole cow milk, a urine concentration of 1650 milliosmoles/liter would be required. This is well beyond the concentrating ability of the infant kidney. Thus, additional water would be required. If this additional water were not provided, an osmotic diuresis would ensue, dehydrating the child. It is for this reason that cow milk must always be modified before it is fed to young human infants. Renal solute load has been markedly reduced in commercially marketed formulas. Human milk still provides the greatest margin of safety.

Substitution of strained baby foods for formula may have an effect similar to that of adding whole cow milk to the diet at an early age. Juices and fruits have average solute loads per 100 kcal that are lower than those of most formulas and similar to those of human milk. However, the solute loads of strained vegetables, meats, and high-meat dinners are two- to five-fold higher than even those of whole cow milk. The displacement of a large proportion of human milk or formula by solids, either at a very early

> A moderate reduction in dietary intake by a normal infant will lead to a disproportionate increase in the concentration of the urine that is excreted.

age or in older infants with fluid restriction, may create problems with free water and renal solute excretion.

Suggested Reading

Ad Hoc Committee to Review the Ten-State Nutrition Survey. 1975. Reflections of dietary studies with children in the Ten-State Nutrition Survey of 1968-1970. *Pediatrics* 56:320-326.

Cordano, A.; Baertl, J. M.; and Graham, G. G. 1964. Copper deficiency in infancy. *Pediatrics* 34:324-336.

Hambidge, K. M.; Hambidge, C.; Jacobs, M., et al. 1972. Low levels of zinc in hair, anorexia, poor growth, and hypogeusia in children. *Pediatr. Res.* 6:868-874.

Lebenthal, E. 1978. Use of modified food starches in infant nutrition. *Am. J. Dis. Child.* 132:850-852.

Moran, J. R.; and Greene, H. L. 1979. The B vitamins and vitamin C in human nutrition. *Am. J. Dis. Child.* 133:192-199, 308-314.

Olsen, R. E., editor. 1981. *Present knowledge in nutrition.* 5th ed. New York: The Nutrition Foundation, Inc.

Ziegler, E. E.; and Fomon, S. J. 1971. Fluid intake, renal solute load and water balance in infants. *J. Pediatr.* 78:561-568.

3 Breast-Feeding the Normal Infant

Contents

Trends in Breast-feeding **55**
Reasons to Breast-feed **56**
  Nutritional Adequacy **57**
  Resistance to Infection **60**
  Reduction of Allergy **61**
  Emotional Satisfaction **62**
  Bonding **63**
  Convenience **63**
  More Rapid Uterine Involution **63**
Contraindications to Breast-feeding **64**
  Breast Size **64**
  Unwilling Mother **64**
  Hepatitis B **65**
Physiology of Lactation **65**
  Milk Secretion **65**
  Milk Let-down **66**
Clinical Management of Breast-feeding **67**
  Prepartum Management **67**
  Initial Postpartum Management **68**
  Management Issues **69**
Maternal Medication and Breast-feeding **74**

Overview

Increasing numbers of mothers are breast–feeding their infants. Practitioners must be familiar with the benefits of breast–feeding and the situations in which it may be preferable not to breast–feed the infant. Management of breast–feeding should be based on the physiology of lactation and should begin before the birth of the baby. Many questions relating to routine management of breast–feeding are covered at the end of this chapter, including, in particular, the problem of maternal medication as it relates to breast–feeding.

TRENDS IN BREAST-FEEDING

Both the prevalence and duration of breast-feeding appear to be increasing. Recent data for the United States show that the number of infants being breast-fed at 1 week of age increased from 29% in 1955 to 45% in 1978. Between 1971 and 1978 the percentage of infants receiving breast milk at 2 months of age increased from about 14% to 35%. In 1978, according to survey data, nearly 21% of infants were still receiving some breast milk at 5 to 6 months of age. There seems to be a concerted effort among health professionals to encourage breast-feeding. Equally important in bringing about the increase, we suspect, have been groups of mothers, such as La Leche League, who have supported women wishing to nurse their infants. Whatever the reason for the increase, the practitioner will be called on progressively more often to offer sound advice on problems relating to breast-feeding.

The practitioner will be called upon progressively more often to offer sound advice on problems relating to breast-feeding.

The first decision to be made by the mother-to-be is whether or not to breast-feed. That this is a conscious decision shows how much infant nutrition has changed in the last 100 years. Most American women of childbearing age today were not breast-fed, nor did they grow up in homes where they saw siblings being nursed. Breast-feeding is no longer "second nature."

Table 3–1

Today, acceptable alternatives to breast-feeding are available, but in the "good old days" of 60 years ago the infant who was not breast-fed was at a considerable disadvantage in terms of morbidity and mortality (Table 3–1). Monthly mortality rates reported between 1915 and 1921 for eight American cities showed that through the first 12 months of life exclusively artificially fed infants were at higher risk of dying than were exclusively breast-fed infants. Mortality among artificially fed infants was six times higher at the third month of life and was still three-fold higher at 9 months of age. Although the two groups were probably not truly comparable in all other respects, there is no question about the hazards of bottle-feeding in poor, unsanitary environments

Table 3-1 Monthly mortality rates of infants in eight U.S. cities by mode of feeding (1915–1921)

Month of life	Exclusively breast-fed	Partly breast-fed	Exclusively artificially fed
1	16.9	36.4	54.7
2	5.8	14.7	24.6
3	3.7	12.9	21.2
4	3.4	9.0	19.2
5	3.3	5.7	18.1
6	2.1	5.9	17.7
7	1.9	4.0	14.1
8	2.9	3.3	11.3
9	3.2	2.9	10.7
10	3.8	2.3	9.3
11	2.4	2.5	6.0
12	4.4	2.7	6.4

Source: Woodbury, R. 1926. *Infant Mortality and Its Causes.* Baltimore: Williams & Wilkins.

lacking electric refrigeration. The problem of feeding infants whose mothers were unable to nurse them was often solved with a wet nurse. This solution created its own problems, as is well illustrated by the passage below taken from a turn-of-the century pediatrics textbook. In providing guidance on finding an appropriate wet nurse the author offered the following warning:

> . . . should be between 20 and 30 yrs, healthy, not fat, of good habits and character . . . Usually the woman comes from an unfavorable class . . . The change from poverty and hardship to ease or even luxury is hard for her to bear. She is liable to become lazy, to take insufficient exercise, to eat and drink unreasonably . . . She realizes the strength of her position, becomes dictatorial and insubordinate, and interferes with the discipline of the household. Commonly she has vicious habits and vicious associates and the influence upon the child is not for good.

REASONS TO BREAST-FEED

If a scientific basis for breast-feeding were needed, recent sophistication in nutritional biochemistry and immunology has provided one. The list of reasons to breast-feed seems to be increasing. It is worthwhile at this point to examine them in more detail.

Nutritional Adequacy

Milks of different animals vary considerably and appear to be suited specifically to the rates of addition of lean body mass and fat by different species.

The compositions of milks of different animals vary considerably and appear to be suited specifically to the rates of accretion of lean body mass and fat by different species. Although both cow milk and human milk contain about 67 calories per deciliter (20 calories per ounce), human milk contains only about 1.0–1.2 g protein per dL, or about 6% to 7% of its total calories as protein. Cow milk, in contrast, contains three times as much protein, about 18% to 20% of total calories. This higher protein intake seems well suited to the more rapid growth rate of the calf. Whale milk provides about 18% to 20% of its calories as protein but has a much greater caloric density—about 250 to 300 calories per dL (75 to 90 calories per ounce). Because of the differences in milk composition, the milks of virtually all other animals must be modified to some extent for them to be suitable for the more slowly growing human infant. The nutrient contents of human milk are the standards against which all other milks or formulas are measured. Some selected aspects of the composition of human milk are compared to those of cow milk and commercial infant formula in Table 3–2.

Table 3–2

The protein in human milk differs from that in cow milk in both quantity and quality.

Protein   Not only is the amount of protein in human milk less than that in cow milk, but the nature of protein is also different. Both human milk and cow milk contain casein and whey. The whey:casein ratio in human milk is 60:40, whereas the corresponding ratio in cow milk is 18:82. Both milks have an excess of essential amino acids relative to the requirements of the human infant, although recent data suggest that the taurine content of cow milk may be inadequate for the very small infant. Because taurine is present only in whey, the higher whey content of human milk may be desirable. Taurine is important in a number of biological functions including the conjugation of bile acids.

About 42% of the calories in human milk come from lactose.

Carbohydrate   The carbohydrate in both human milk and cow milk is lactose. Human milk contains approximately 7% lactose (weight per volume) or about 42% of total calories. This lactose concentration is higher than that of cow milk and is also higher than that of most of the commercially available infant formulas. The exact importance of lactose in the diet of the infant is unknown. That is, the nature of the biological advantage conferred on the infant by lactose in the diet is unclear. It is of interest, however, that lactose occurs naturally only in milk.

Table 3-2 Comparison of selected aspects of human milk and cow milk

Nutrient	Human milk	Cow milk	Infant formula*
Protein			
% kcal	6	21	9
Whey:casein ratio	60:40	18:82	18:82
Fat			
% kcal	56	50	50
% polyunsaturated fatty acids	9	4	49
Polyunsaturated:saturated (P:S) ratio	0.2:1	0.08:1	1.8:1
Linoleic acid—% kcal	3.8	1.1	20
Carbohydrate			
% kcal	38	29	41
Minerals			
Sodium—mEq/L	7	22	10
Potassium—mEq/L	13	35	17
Chloride—mEq/L	11	29	13
Calcium—mg/L	340	1170	550
Phosphorus—mg/L	140	920	460
Calcium:phosphorus	2.4:1	1.3:1	1.2:1
Iron—mg/L	0.5	0.5	12
Zinc—mg/L	1.2	3.9	4.2
Osmolality	280	270	278
Renal solute load	81	220	100

*Enfamil with Iron.

Fat The fat content of human milk varies somewhat but is generally about 3% to 3.5%, or a bit more than 50% of the total calories. The principal fatty acids in human milk are oleic and palmitic acids. The triglycerides in human milk are readily absorbed and digested, partly because there is a lipase secreted in human milk that is activated when it comes in contact with bile salts in the small intestine.

The importance of the high concentration of cholesterol in human milk is not known.

There is also a high concentration of cholesterol in human milk. The significance of the high content of this lipid is uncertain. Some investigators have speculated that cholesterol intake is important during the early stages of development of the human infant. While there is no proof of this hypothesis, the presence of large amounts of cholesterol in human milk should perhaps make us wary of removing virtually all cholesterol from the diets of newborn infants, as is effectively done in commercial formulas.

Minerals and renal solute load The mineral content of human milk is considerably lower than that of cow milk. The sodium content, for example, is less than one-third and the potassium content is less than one-half that found in cow milk. The amounts of all major minerals in human milk have been demonstrated to be fully adequate for normal growth of the full-term infant. The major advantage of the lower mineral content in human milk is the lower amount of solute that must be excreted by the kidney. The lower protein and mineral contents of human milk combine to give a renal solute load of approximately 80 milliosmole/liter. In comparison, the renal solute load for cow milk is approximately 220 milliosmoles/liter. Modified cow-milk formulas approach renal solute loads as low as that of human milk.

The low renal solute load of human milk gives an extra margin of safety to the infant, whose kidneys may be unable to concentrate maximally during the early weeks of life. As protein intakes and urea levels increase, concentrating ability improves, making renal solute load of less concern in older infants.

Of the minerals, iron is the only one whose adequacy in human milk is questioned.

Of the minerals, iron is the only one whose adequacy in human milk is questioned. Both human milk and cow milk contain approximately 0.5 mg iron per liter. Despite the seemingly similar contents of iron, it was noted clinically for years that although infants fed cow milk tended to become iron deficient, iron deficiency among breast-fed infants was rare. Recent evidence demonstrates that the bioavailability of iron from the two milks is markedly different. Only about 5% to 10% of the iron in cow milk is absorbed. In contrast, nearly 50% of iron in human milk is bioavailable. This high bioavailability seems to be a quality of the milk itself rather than a property of the infant's intestinal tract, because studies in which human milk has been fed to adults confirm an equally high absorption of iron. The relationships of human milk and cow milk to iron deficiency anemia are discussed more fully in Chapter 8.

Vitamins The adequacy of vitamins in human milk is still disputed. The fact that breast milk has supported the species for generations without the use of supplementary vitamins is, for some nutritionists, proof of the adequacy of the vitamins in breast milk. Other nutritionists cite the fact that vitamin deficiencies have been seen in breast-fed infants. Most nutritionists agree that human milk from a well-nourished mother is adequate in all vitamins with the possible exception of vitamin D. Assays of the lipid fraction of human milk have shown human milk to be deficient in this vitamin. More recent work has found a vitamin D sulphate in the aqueous fraction of human milk. The high concentration of this aqueous factor has been cited as evidence for the adequacy of vitamin D in human milk. Laboratory bioassays of vitamin D activity in human milk, however, suggest inadequacy. Good data for humans are lacking, although rickets does occur in breast-fed infants, again indicating possible inadequacy. Our own feeling is that vitamin D in human milk is probably not sufficient to meet the requirements of the infant who is not getting considerable exposure to sunlight. In northern and more temperate areas, especially in urban areas where air pollution is common, it is unwise to rely on the vitamin D content of human milk in combination with endogenous production to meet requirements.

It is unwise to rely on the vitamin D content of human milk in combination with endogenous production to meet requirements.

Resistance to Infection

Recent advances in the immunology and bio-chemistry of human milk have given a scientific basis for the long acknowledged effect of breast-feeding in reducing morbidity and mortality.

Table 3-3

Recent advances in the immunology and biochemistry of human milk have given a scientific basis for the long acknowledged effect of breast-feeding in reducing morbidity and mortality in the U.S. and less developed countries (Table 3-3). Human milk contains substantial numbers of macrophages as well as T-lymphocytes and B-lymphocytes. In addition to accomplishing phagocytosis, macrophages produce lactoferrin, an iron-binding protein that inhibits the growth of bacteria, notably staphylococcus and *Escherichia coli*, by depriving them of iron needed for growth. The function of T-lymphocytes in human milk is not completely clear, as the responses of these T-cells to certain stimuli do not parallel the responses to the same stimuli seen with the T-cells in plasma. The B-lymphocytes in human milk are thought to be responsible for the production of most of the immunoglobulins present in human milk. There is evidence that B-lymphocytes in the Peyer's patches of the mother's intestinal tract home to the breast after being sensitized by exposure to antigens—largely, presumably, the maternal intestinal flora. After migration to the breast, these cells produce secretory immunoglobulin A (IgA), the predominant immunoglobulin in human milk. To the extent that mother and infant share a common fecal flora, these antibodies offer some protection to the infant. For example, antibodies against rotavirus

Secretory IgA is the predominant immunoglobulin in human milk.

Table 3-3 Host resistance factors passed in human milk

Cellular

Macrophages

Phagocytosis

Production of lysozyme, lactoferrin, lactoperoxidase, and complement

Lymphocytes

B-cells: IgA, IgM, IgG

T-cells: Cellular immunity

Humoral

Immunoglobulins—especially IgA

Polysaccharide growth factor for lactobacillus

Antiviral and antibacterial lipid factors

C_3, C_4

Source: Modified from Pittard, W. B. 1979. Breast milk immunology. *Am. J. Dis. Child.* 133:83-87.

and antibodies able to neutralize the toxin produced by enterotoxigenic *E. coli* have been demonstrated in human milk.

Immunoglobulin concentrations are highest in colostrum, consumed by the infant in the first few days after birth. Their decreased concentration in milk is offset by the increased volume consumed. Concentrations of IgA, IgG, and IgM are relatively constant after the first week through at least six months of lactation, and the concentrations do not appear to vary with socioeconomic status.

The value of breast-feeding in reducing morbidity and mortality of infants raised in developing countries is generally agreed upon. The importance of breast-feeding in reducing morbidity and mortality in less hostile environments is still debated. Several studies have suggested that even in more developed countries with good sanitation, breast-feeding increases protection against a variety of infections. The methodology of the studies carried out to date precludes reaching a firm conclusion on this question, but well-designed studies in the future will probably document this advantage.

Reduction of Allergy

Since the early studies of Johnstone and Glaser in 1953 the usefulness of a cow-milk-free diet in the prevention of allergy has been

The permeability of the intestine to protein is known to be higher in the newborn than it is later in life.

debated. The permeability of the intestine to proteins is known to be higher in the newborn than it is in older humans, most likely because of relatively low secretory IgA levels early in life. This permeability allows the passage of macromolecules to which antibodies may be formed. Almost all children, by the age of 2 or 3 years, can be demonstrated to have antibodies to milk proteins circulating in plasma. The relationship of this phenomenon to milk allergy per se and atopy in general is unclear. A variety of reactions to the ingestion of cow milk have been reported. Whether there is an allergic basis for these reactions is, however, less certain. Although human milk and cow milk share certain proteins that theoretically could be sensitizing, reactions to the ingestion of human milk by the infant have not been reported. Foreign proteins can be secreted in milk, however, and the ingestion of cow-milk protein or egg protein by nursing mothers has been reported to cause reactions in some infants.

At the present time human milk seems to be the least allergenic diet for the human infant.

As new immunologic techniques are developed, the extent and nature of cow-milk hypersensitivity and the role of breast milk in preventing it will be better delineated. At the present time the most one can say is that human milk seems to be the least allergenic diet for the human infant. Whether breast-feeding prevents the development of allergic manifestations or merely delays them to a later age when other foreign proteins begin to be ingested cannot be said with certainty. This subject is discussed more fully in Chapter 9. From a practical point of view it would seem reasonable to suggest that infants born to families with a history of severe atopy be breast-fed for as long as is reasonably possible.

Emotional Satisfaction

Although most women derive emotional satisfaction from breast-feeding, this is not the case for all women.

Most women who choose to nurse their infants seem to derive a large measure of emotional satisfaction from breast-feeding. This is not the case for all women, however, especially for those who do not receive adequate support from family and medical personnel. If breast-feeding gets off to a bad start, if the infant is fussy and the mother interprets this as an inability to satisfy her infant, breast-feeding can become an unpleasant experience for all concerned. In addition, in our desire to encourage breast-feeding we should not lose sight of the fact that not all women want to nurse their infants. The decision not to breast-feed should be respected and no attempt should be made, as often seems to be done, to make the mother feel guilty for choosing to bottle-feed. Appropriate bottle-feeding can be a satisfying experience for infant, mother *and* father, and has permitted the healthy growth of many millions of infants.

Bonding

Maternal-infant bonding is frequently cited as a reason to encourage breast-feeding. Our current state of knowledge suggests that the management of a newborn infant and mother during the first ten to twelve hours of life may affect the emotional responses of each toward the other and thus affect the bonding process. Because the infant is in an alert state during the first several hours following delivery, this is an ideal time for maternal-infant interaction. In the case of the mother who is planning to breast-feed, this interaction may include suckling her infant at the breast. The decision to bottle-feed an infant, however, does not preclude an adequate interaction, and consequently, the desirability of bonding should not be used as an argument to induce women to breast-feed who would otherwise choose not to.

Convenience

Convenience is frequently cited as a reason to breast-feed.

Convenience is frequently cited as a reason to breast-feed, because adequate quantities of milk are nearly always immediately available. No doubt the freedom of not having to worry about formula preparation, bottles, nipples, and so on can be a great convenience. Mothers who are breast-feeding find they can eat a bit more and still not have to worry about weight gain. They can travel without taking along a lot of paraphernalia and can still be assured that food is available.

For many women, the feeling that they must hide somewhere to feed their infants may make breast-feeding both unsatisfying and inconvenient at times.

On the other hand, many women are uncomfortable nursing their infants in the presence of anyone but their immediate family. At home this means, in many instances, that the mother must leave the company of friends to feed her infant. Away from home, cultural taboos make it particularly difficult for women to nurse their infants. Many infants end up being nursed in restrooms. For many women the feeling that they must hide somewhere to feed their infants may make breast-feeding both unsatisfying and inconvenient at times. Finally, for the working mother breast-feeding may be a distinct inconvenience if not an impossibility. In encouraging women to breast-feed, one must keep in mind the relative nature of some of the advantages of breast-feeding.

More Rapid Uterine Involution

Presumably because of the recurrent secretion of oxytocin associated with milk let-down, nursing women experience a more rapid involution of the uterus following delivery. This is perhaps less a reason to encourage breast-feeding than a beneficial side effect of breast-feeding for the mother.

CONTRAINDICATIONS TO BREAST-FEEDING

Many of the "medical" reasons given either for not starting to breast-feed or, more often, for stopping breast-feeding are groundless when subjected to careful scrutiny; they represent convenience for the practitioner rather than sound medical advice.

There are few absolute contraindications to breast-feeding. Many of the "medical" reasons given either for not starting to breast-feed or, more often, for stopping breast-feeding are groundless when subjected to careful scrutiny; they represent convenience for the practitioner rather than sound medical advice. For example, many practitioners suggest that a mother taking any medication should not nurse her infant. As discussed later, infants can often continue to be breast-fed under these conditions if the physician is willing to ascertain the degree to which the medication does indeed enter breast milk. Inadequate milk production early in the course of breast-feeding frequently elicits a suggestion of bottle-feeding, rather than support and encouragement for further breast-feeding. Infants are frequently weaned from the breast because of mastitis. Here again, there is no absolute contraindication to continued nursing, certainly not from the unaffected breast. Milk can be expressed manually from the affected breast, and normal nursing can be resumed in a matter of a few days.

Breast Size

The ability to produce milk is not a function of breast size.

Mothers can be assured that the ability to produce milk is not a function of breast size. The effect of nursing on breast size is more difficult to ascertain. Oski (1968) surveyed 750 women six months after delivery or six months after weaning their infant from the breast. Only about 27% of women who breast-fed for two weeks or less noted any change in breast size. Of women who had nursed their infant for six months or more, about 48% noted a change. About half of the women who had nursed for six months or more reported a decrease from what breast size had been prior to pregnancy; 36% reported no change in size but a loss of tone. Corresponding figures for mothers who did not nurse their infants were 24% and 16%.

Unwilling Mother

The most valid contraindication to breast-feeding is the desire of the mother not to breast-feed.

In our opinion, the most valid contraindication to breast-feeding is the desire of the mother not to breast-feed. Many women, even when aware of the apparent benefits of breast-feeding, choose not to breast-feed for a variety of reasons that are valid for them. Their decision should be supported. Attempting to induce unwilling mothers to breast-feed through inducing guilt or through other mechanisms sets up a situation that is probably destined to failure and that may neglect the best interests of both the mother and her infant in the broader sense.

Hepatitis B

Women who are hepatitis-B-surface-antigen (Hb_SAg) positive may pass the hepatitis-B virus to their infants through milk. It is uncertain how frequently this occurs. Vertical transmission of Hb_SAg from mothers who are carriers to their infants by all routes has been reported in various studies to have occurred 0% to 63% of the time. Acute hepatitis B in the mother during the last trimester of pregnancy or during the first several months postpartum will result in transmission to the infant about 75% of the time. Women who are acutely infected with hepatitis B or who are known chronic carriers of the disease should refrain from nursing their infants. In both cases, even though bottle-fed, the infant should receive high-titer hepatitis-B immunoglobulin.

> Women who are acutely infected with hepatitis B or who are known chronic carriers of the disease should refrain from nursing their infants.

PHYSIOLOGY OF LACTATION

Two physiological mechanisms involved in lactation that bear directly on the clinical management of breast-feeding are milk secretion and milk let-down.

> Two physiological mechanisms involved in lactation that bear directly on the clinical management of breast-feeding are milk secretion and milk let-down.

Milk Secretion

Milk production is regulated by the hormone prolactin. Prolactin is released from the anterior pituitary in an amount proportional to the amount of nipple stimulation. This mechanism allows the infant to control the amount of milk being produced. The infant who is larger or hungrier will suck more, thereby causing increased production of milk.

Several drugs are known to increase prolactin levels. One of these, chlorpromazine, is occasionally used to increase milk production during the initiation of nursing. This approach is not generally required or recommended, although it may be useful in special circumstances.

There are several implications of the hormonal control of milk secretion. First, a woman need not have been pregnant in order for sucking to induce the release of prolactin. Because of this, women who adopt infants and wish to nurse can begin to lactate after a number of weeks of nipple stimulation. Second, the direct relationship between sucking stimulation and milk production suggests that demand feeding might be preferable to a rigid schedule during the initiation of breast-feeding. In fact, studies of Bantu babies as well as of infants in more industrialized nations have suggested that infants fed on demand tend to be bigger at the end of 10 to 14 days than those fed on a rigid three-hour to four-hour schedule. In one study mothers who fed on demand also complained of less nipple soreness and were more likely to be nursing their infants successfully at the end of one month.

Milk Let-down

Milk let-down or milk ejection is probably equally as important as milk secretion in successful breast-feeding. The anticipation of nursing her infant or the sounds of the infant crying will cause the mother to experience milk let-down. Signs of milk let-down are milk dripping from the breasts, both before and during nursing, and uterine cramps. This reflex is mediated through a neurohumoral mechanism that causes the release of oxytocin from the posterior pituitary. Oxytocin causes the contraction of myoepithelial cells in the breast, pushing milk into the larger ducts and thereby making it available to the sucking infant.

The let-down reflex is mediated through a neuro-humoral mechanism that causes the release of oxytocin from the posterior pituitary.

Attention to both the physical and emotional comfort of the mother during the time that she is nursing her infant is essential if breast-feeding is to be successful. Just as several physiological and physical stimuli can cause the release of oxytocin, several unpleasant stimuli can inhibit its release. More than 30 years ago Newton and Newton (1948) studied the effect of harassment of the mother during nursing on the amount of milk obtained by the infant. When mothers were distracted with mildly painful stimuli, the average amount of milk obtained by infants at each feeding decreased nearly 2 ounces. When oxytocin was injected in the presence of the same distractions, the amount of milk obtained returned to control levels. There is a significant correlation between the lack of milk ejection symptoms in mothers and the inability to nurse infants successfully. Anxiety, the fear of failure, the fear of interruption, self-conciousness, or a general lack of support can certainly contribute to an inhibition of milk let-down. Similarly, painful or cracked nipples and the anticipation of pain on nursing can also lead to inhibition. If milk let-down does not occur effectively and the infant is not satisfied, the hungry infant may continue to cry, convincing the mother that she is inadequate, thereby setting up a vicious cycle. Oxytocin may be useful during a period of several days to interrupt the vicious cycle. Nasal administration of oxytocin has been effective in promoting milk let-down. However, oxytocin therapy should never be used for prolonged periods of time.

Successful nursing relates closely to symptoms of milk let-down.

CLINICAL MANAGEMENT OF BREAST-FEEDING

Management of breast-feeding should begin well before the birth of the infant. Mothers who are contemplating breast-feeding will have many questions that the practitioner must be prepared to answer.

Prepartum Management

The decision to breast-feed or bottle-feed is often made by the mother in conjunction with her obstetrician during prepartum care. Not infrequently, however, the decision is not made until the birth of the infant, when a tired, sometimes groggy mother is asked how she plans to feed her infant. Since the pediatrician or primary care practitioner will be responsible for the nutritional care of the newborn, it is important that, whenever possible, he or she meet with the mother prior to delivery to give anticipatory guidance. However, many women do not choose a physician to care for the infant until after the baby's birth. Also, in large hospitals and clinics referral to pediatric care is made only after delivery. The physician can overcome these problems to some degree by establishing a good working relationship with the obstetricians in the area and by letting mothers already in the practice know that he or she likes to talk with expectant mothers well before delivery.

The mother who is convinced that she will breast-feed successfully usually is successful.

The practitioner should accomplish three main tasks during the prenatal visit. The first is to make the mother aware of the relative advantages of breast-feeding. The second is to allay the anxiety surrounding the fear of failure, especially for the mother having her first child. Nothing succeeds in breast-feeding like the expectation of success. Studies have shown that the mother who is convinced that she will breast-feed successfully usually is successful. We suggest that an expectant mother contemplating breast-feeding talk with a number of women who have successfully breast-fed infants. In this way the expectant mother can learn that there are a variety of ways to nurse an infant successfully. Some mothers will have fed on demand for many months, whereas others will have developed a more structured feeding pattern after the first three to four weeks to allow them more freedom of movement. Once the expectant mother realizes that there is practically no wrong way to nurse an infant, much of the anxiety associated with the decision will be removed. In addition, there are several good books available for mothers who wish to nurse, and there are groups such as La Leche League that can be very supportive.

Third, the mother should be instructed in ways to prepare her nipples for the initiation of breast-feeding. Many women go through no preparation prior to delivery, and within several days the sucking of an avidly nursing infant creates sore or cracked nipples. During the last three to four weeks of pregnancy, some form of nipple stimulation should be initiated in order to toughen the skin. Gentle massaging with a bath towel or a soft bath brush or manual or oral stimulation should be done on a daily basis. Women with inverted or retracted nipples should begin to elongate them gradually day by day.

Initial Postpartum Management

Breast-feeding may be begun whenever both mother and infant appear to be ready. In many instances this may be immediately postpartum when the mother is first holding her infant. For other mothers, especially those who have had a difficult delivery or whose infants are sluggish at birth, the first feeding is better delayed for a number of hours. Breast-feeding is best carried out in a calm, quiet atmosphere in which the mother does not fear interruption. For this reason, the delivery or postpartum recovery room is usually not the ideal place to start. Many hospitals have birthing rooms, which resemble bedrooms, for uncomplicated deliveries; such rooms are ideal for beginning nursing.

Most infants should be fed on demand, at least for the first three to four weeks.

We suggest that most infants be fed on demand, at least for the first three to four weeks. Initially the infant should be nursed for five minutes at each breast, alternating the breast used to initiate the feeding. On the second and third days, the length of nursing can be increased to from 10 to 15 minutes at each breast. Mothers should be instructed in nipple care. This means washing with plain water rather than with soap and avoiding petrolatum and ointments such as A and D because they may cause irritation. The most important aspects of nipple care are simple cleanliness and keeping the nipples dry.

The mother breast-feeding her first child requires a great deal of support during these first few days. It is extremely important that hospital nurses and aides assigned to care for nursing women be interested in supporting breast-feeding. They should also have a common base of knowledge concerning breast-feeding. Mothers may be confused when, for example, on one shift they are told that tea will help their milk to come in but on the next shift are told that they need to drink plenty of milk to make milk. Education of the paraprofessional staff in the physiologic and emotional aspects of breast-feeding is paramount.

Education of the paraprofessional staff in the physiologic and emotional aspects of breast-feeding is paramount.

Breast-feeding is more likely to be successful if both the mother and the new father have realistic expectations about the course of events during the first few days. The normal weight lost by the infant during the first week may be interpreted by a new breast-feeding mother as being the result of inadequate milk supply. In addition, since many women are now being discharged from hospital 48 to 72 hours after giving birth, most are going home before adequate milk production has been established. It is now incumbent on the primary care practitioner, the office nurse, and the father to provide the support that might have been given in the past by the nursing staff or by grandmothers and extended family.

A final initial concern is the nutritional management of the mother who is breast-feeding. Much of the weight gained during pregnancy serves to store energy in preparation for lactation. Depending on the adequacy of fat stored, the average nursing mother requires approximately 500 calories per day more than she would need if not nursing. Protein, calcium, and phosphorus requirements also increase, as do the requirements for many of the vitamins and trace minerals. Data from dietary surveys carried out in the United States suggest that the diets of most American women are generous in both protein and energy. Thus the nursing mother probably need not make any qualitative changes in her diet. She will, however, require increased quantities of food. This requirement can best be assessed by observing both her milk output, as evidenced by the growth of her infant, and the changes in her own weight.

Management Issues

Several questions regarding nutrition and other factors may arise during the extended management of infants who are breast-feeding. We will address a number of these issues.

Need for vitamin or mineral supplements As a general rule, no supplements are required for the mother as long as she is eating a well-balanced diet. However, there may be specific instances in which supplementation is desirable. For example, the vegetarian mother should be supplemented with additional vitamin B_{12}, especially if she has not been taking it previously. Iron supplementation may also be desirable for the vegetarian mother. Vitamin and mineral supplementation for the mother must be addressed on a case-by-case basis.

As discussed previously, there is some controversy about the need for vitamin and mineral supplementation for the breast-fed infant. We suggest that all breast-fed infants be supplemented with vitamin D. This is usually most easily accomplished by the use of a preparation containing vitamins A, C, and D. Although vitamins A and C are present in sufficient quantities in breast milk, the usual supplementation dose is not enough to cause concern for possible hypervitaminosis A.

In general, mineral contents of breast milk are sufficient for the growing infant. Even those infants exclusively breast-fed for six or more months are rarely found to be iron deficient. Fluoride, however, does not cross into human milk even when the mother's diet is being supplemented. Consequently, it is desirable to supplement the nursing infant with fluoride. Whether this supplementation is best started in the first month of life is debated. The Committee on Nutrition of the American Academy of Pediatrics (1979) has suggested that breastfed infants receive supplementation in the amount of 0.25 mg fluoride per day beginning shortly after birth.

Fluoride does not cross into human milk, even when the mother's diet is being supplemented.

Need for additional water   Rarely does the breast-fed infant need additional water. The low renal solute load of human milk provides a wide margin of safety for infants. Breast milk will meet the fluid requirements of even those infants with a low-grade fever and with a slight decrease in intake. Although high environmental temperatures increase insensible water losses, the healthy baby who is nursing regularly will not require additional water.

Stool pattern   The stools of infants are especially sensitive to dietary influences. Changes in stools in response to changes in diet are most likely mediated through changes in the fecal flora. The lower protein and higher lactose content of human milk favor the establishment of a fecal flora with a predominance of lactobacilli and bifidobacilli. The higher protein intakes from formulas are associated with a change to a more putrefactive flora with a predominance of *E. coli.*

Jaundice in the breast-fed infant   Hyperbilirubinemia seen in the breast-fed infant may be divided into two types. The normal elevation of bilirubin during the first week of life may be accentuated in the breast-fed infant. Years ago, early feeding was noted to decrease the peak bilirubin concentration achieved during the first week in life. This decrease was initially attributed to caloric intake. However, later it was shown that the feeding of water achieved the same decrease. The decrease in bilirubin is now thought to be mediated through a more rapid passage of meconium, which decreases the amount of bilirubin available for enterohepatic recirculation. The lower volume of intake by breast-fed infants

The normal elevation of bilirubin during the first week of life may be accentuated in the breast-fed infant.

during the first several days probably results in a slower clearance of meconium, thereby accentuating hyperbilirubinemia.

A late unconjugated hyperbilirubinemia is seen in a small number of breast-fed infants. This rise in bilirubin has been attributed to an inhibition of glucuronyl transferase by pregnanediol, a metabolite of progesterone transmitted in the milk of some mothers. The milk of these mothers has also been reported recently to have an increased concentration of free fatty acids, which may also affect bilirubin conjugation. Cessation of breast-feeding for 36 to 48 hours results in a marked decrease in the serum bilirubin. Breast-feeding can then be resumed. As long as serum bilirubin levels are not excessive, this form of jaundice is not a contraindication to resuming breast-feeding.

Supplemental formula feeding   Because milk production is directly proportional to nipple stimulation, decreased sucking at the breast will result in decreased milk production. Thus, for the infant of a mother who is initiating lactation, any bottle-feeding during the first four to six weeks is contraindicated. Most women go through a period during the first several weeks when their milk supply seems inadequate. Although it is tempting at this time to give a supplementary bottle, this response will tend to exacerbate the milk inadequacy. The practitioner should provide support for the mother at this time and encourage her to put the baby at the breast more frequently. Once lactation is well established and the infant is several months old, there is no harm in an occasional bottle-feeding. Popular wisdom suggests that once the baby has had a feeding from an artificial nipple it will never go back to the breast. The experience of many mothers belies such a conclusion. For the mother who is concerned that missing a feeding will decrease her milk supply, we suggest that she pump her breast or manually express the milk into a bottle to be used for the feeding while she is away from the infant.

For the infant of a mother who is initiating lactation, any bottle-feeding during the first four to six weeks is contraindicated.

Once lactation is well established, there is no harm in an occasional bottle-feeding.

Storage of human milk   If simple precautions are followed, human milk can be stored. Cleanliness is a must. Some authorities feel that manual expression results in less contamination than the use of a pump. Discarding the initial 5–10 mL expressed will also reduce the number of bacteria in the milk collected. Large quantities of milk should not be stored for prolonged periods of time. If a woman plans to be away for one or two feedings, there is no reason why milk cannot be pumped or expressed into a sterile bottle and stored for 6 to 8 hours in the refrigerator. Storage for longer than 18–24 hours requires pasteurization or freezing.

Contraception and nursing Although it is well documented that lactation prolongs postpartum amenorrhea, breast-feeding should not be relied on to provide adequate contraception. The evidence on the safety of oral contraceptives during nursing is somewhat conflicting. Use of oral contraceptives may decrease milk supply. In addition, many of the steroid hormones in oral contraceptives may be passed in the milk. There are reports of short-term effects of these hormones on infants. The long-term effects are not completely known. As a general rule, mothers who plan to breast-feed their infants should plan to rely on some other form of contraception, such as an IUD.

Adequacy of intake Breast-feeding should remove the need of the mother to preoccupy herself with the volumes of milk taken by the infant. If an infant is wetting its diapers regularly, is sleeping two to three hours between feedings, is generally content, and is gaining weight at a reasonable rate, the mother can be assured that her milk supply is adequate. Attempting to assess intake by weighing babies before and after feedings, especially when done at home, only serves to increase the mother's anxiety and, more often than not, will lead to the false conclusion that the milk supply is inadequate.

If an infant is gaining weight at a reasonable rate, the mother can be assured that her milk supply is adequate.

Duration of nutritional adequacy We recently saw a young child who, because of suspected milk allergy, had been maintained on a diet in which human milk provided 90% or more of all intake for the first 2½ years of life. The child had grown normally along the 50th percentile and was not anemic. This attests to the continuing nutritional quality of human milk if the quantity is sufficient.

Most women who are healthy can nurse their infants without supplemental feeding for at least the first six months of life. A recently published study looked at a group of La Leche League mothers and determined retrospectively the growth of infants who had been exclusively breast-fed for longer periods of time. When compared to the 50th percentile of the NCHS standard, there was no difference in the rate of growth of exclusively breast-fed infants up to 9 months of age. If a woman wishes to continue exclusively breast-feeding and her child's increases in length and weight are satisfactory, there is no reason she should not do so. Every infant, however, will at some time outgrow its mother's milk supply. This may occur earlier than 6 or 7 months in some cases. A progressive slowing of weight gain and linear growth will signal the need for supplementary foods, but this does not mean that the infant must be weaned from the breast. For the infant beyond 4 or 5 months, the addition of solid foods should be considered.

Most women who are healthy can nurse their infants exclusively for at least the first six months of life.

Many authorities suggest that infants not be fed whole cow milk before the age of 12 months. Therefore, it is desirable that breast-feeding mothers continue to nurse for as long as possible even when there is a need for additional foods to supplement the diet.

Weaning should be a gradual process, whatever age is chosen. It is best accomplished by switching one feeding at a time to the bottle or, for the older infant, to the cup. Additional feedings are dropped gradually, according to the mother's desire. The evening feeding is usually the last to be dropped. Weaning is quite easy for some mothers and infants and quite difficult for others.

Factors affecting milk composition Milk output and composition are affected by a variety of factors, including maternal nutritional status, maternal diet, stage of lactation, time of day, and time during an individual feeding. Both the quality and, especially, the quantity of milk of severely malnourished women is diminished. However, malnutrition of the degree required to cause these alterations is seldom encountered in the United States.

Maternal diet affects milk composition. Recent studies have suggested that the increased use of polyunsaturated vegetable oils in the American diet has caused a shift toward fatty acids of higher chain length in the milk of American mothers. Linoleic acid content of human milk can be altered markedly by dietary intake.

The stage of lactation also affects milk composition. The nitrogen content of human milk decreases progressively during the first four to six weeks, being relatively stable thereafter. Lactose content increases slightly during prolonged lactation. Data on changes in fat content are conflicting.

Finally, it should be noted that the composition of milk changes during feeding. In particular, the fat content of milk at the end of the feeding (hind milk) is two to three times higher than in foremilk, causing some nutritionists to speculate that this bolus of fat at the end of the feeding provides a satiety factor for the infant.

Maternal medication As a general rule, it should be assumed that all medications cross into breast milk to some degree. While there are distinct exceptions to this rule, it is easier to start with this assumption. The presence or absence of drugs in milk is of less concern than the amount that is present. The quantity of any medication entering breast milk will depend on the degree to which it is protein-bound in plasma, the pH of the plasma, and whether or not the drug is alkaline or acidic. Drugs that are weakly basic, such as caffeine, are not ionized at plasma pH and pass more readily into breast milk than do drugs that are weakly acidic, such as aspirin and phenobarbital, which are ionized. There is now a large body of literature reporting the concentrations of drugs in breast milk to be expected when mothers are consuming therapeutic dosages. In the last section of this chapter is a list of the

Milk output and composition are affected by maternal nutritional status, maternal diet, stage of lactation, time of day, and time during an individual feeding.

It should be assumed that all medications cross into breast milk to some degree.

more commonly prescribed drugs, the relative degree to which they pass into human milk, and the potential side effects to the infant. As is obvious from Table 3–4, maternal medication need not be a contraindication to breast-feeding in most instances. The decision of whether or not an infant should continue to be breast-fed by a women taking medication should be made on a case-by-case basis. If the mother is taking a medication that absolutely contraindicates breast-feeding, consideration should be given to changing her medication to a suitable substitute.

Isotope scans Whether or not an infant should be breast-fed after the mother has undergone isotopic scans can be a difficult question to answer since it depends on both the physical and the biologic half-lives of the isotope administered. For example, the use of a ^{131}I-labelled albumin would contraindicate breast-feeding for a longer period of time than would the use of the same iodine isotope for a thyroid scan. From a practical point of view, the safest approach is to have the mother continue to pump her breasts and to count the radioactivity in her milk intermittently. Nursing may be resumed when counts return to background levels.

MATERNAL MEDICATION AND BREAST-FEEDING

Maternal medication need not be an absolute contraindication to breastfeeding. Although it is preferable that the mother receive no medication at all, this is frequently not possible. Few drugs are absolute contraindications to nursing. The most commonly encountered situation is the mother on a medication known to be excreted in milk in low concentration. Management of this situation requires a knowledge of the potential side effects of the drug, especially as it affects the neonate. A drug may be acceptable in one situation and not in another. For example, jaundiced infants or infants with glucose-6-phosphate dehydrogenase (G-6-PD) deficiency ("primaquine sensitivity") should not be nursed by a mother on sulfonamides, a medication that would not preclude breast-feeding other infants. Risks to the infant from maternal medication can be minimized in some instances by using an alternative drug or by monitoring the infant. In most instances the risk to the infant will be low. Whether the risk is acceptable is a judgment to be made by the practitioner and the parents.

Table 3–4 lists commonly prescribed maternal medications and a tabulation of (1) whether or not they are excreted in milk, (2) what the perceived side effects are for the infant, and (3)

Few drugs are absolute contraindications to nursing.

Table 3–4

Table 3-4 Maternal medication and breast-feeding

Drug	Excreted in milk?	Potential side effects	Breast-feeding acceptable?
Alcohol	Yes	Generally few	If used in moderate amounts
Aloe	Yes	Catharsis	Conflicting opinions
Amphetamines	No	—	Yes
Ampicillin	Yes	Generally none	Yes
Aspirin	Yes	Platelet dysfunction	If used in low doses as analgesic
Atropine	Yes	Atropine intoxication	No; said to inhibit lactation
Bishydroxycoumarin	Yes	Anticoagulation	Generally felt to be safe; monitor infant with mother
Caffeine	Yes	Wakefulness	Generally felt to be safe if used in moderation
Cascara	Yes	Catharsis	Drug should be avoided if possible
Cephalexin	No	—	Yes
Chloral hydrate	Yes	—	Yes
Chloramphenicol	Yes	Possible marrow suppression	Not recommended
Chlordiazepoxide	Yes	—	In usual therapeutic dose
Chlorothiazide	Yes	—	Probably so, but manfacturer suggests opposite
Chlorpromazine	Yes	?	Yes
Codeine	Yes	—	Yes
Contraceptives—oral	Yes	Decreased milk production	Drug should be avoided if possible
Cortisone	Yes	Poorly studied	Probably not, based on animal data
Cyclamates	Yes	—	Yes
Diazepam	Yes	Lethargy, weight loss, jaundice	No
Diphenhydramine	Yes	—	When used in usual therapeutic dosage
Diphenylhydantoin	Yes	—	Questionable
Ergot	Yes	Vomiting, diarrhea	No
Erythromycin	Yes*	—	In usual therapeutic doses
Furosemide	No	—	Yes
Guanethidine	Yes	—	Yes
Heroin	Yes	None to date	Appears to be safe; other factors may contraindicate
Hydrochlorothiazide	Yes	None to date	Probably so; manufacturer suggests opposite
Iodides	Yes	May affect thyroid	Felt to be contraindicated

Table 3-4 Maternal medication and breast-feeding (continued)

Drug	Excreted in milk?	Potential side effects	Breast-feeding acceptable?
Isoniazid	Yes*	CNS, hepatic	Maternal TB may be contraindication
Kanamycin	Yes	Renal, auditory	Probably; measure drug concentration in milk
Lincomycin	Yes	—	Yes
Liothyronine	No	—	Yes
Lithium	Yes*	Lithium toxicity	Not recommended
Mandelic acid	Yes	—	Yes
Meperidine	Yes	—	Yes
Meprobamate	Yes*	—	Probably not
Methadone	?	—	Yes
Methyldopa	Yes	?	Questionable
Metronidazole	Yes*	—	Dose to infant not considered significant
Morphine	Yes	—	Yes
Nalidixic acid	Yes	One case of hemolytic anemia attributed to nalidixic acid	Generally felt to be safe
Nicotine	Yes	—	If abstention from cigarettes impossible, safe to 15–20 cigarettes per day
Nitrofurantoin	Yes	—	Yes
Novobiocin	Yes	—	Yes, if not jaundiced
Oxacillin	No	—	Yes
Penicillin	Yes	Possible sensitivity	Probably so
Phenobarbital	Yes	—	Yes, in usual dosage
Phenolphthalein	Yes	—	Yes
Primidone	Yes	Somnolence	Probably not
Prochlorperazine	Yes	—	Yes
Propantheline	No	—	Yes
Propranolol	No	—	Yes
Propylthiouracil	Yes*	Goiter, agranulocytosis	No
Primethamine	Yes	—	Limited data, apparently safe
Reserpine	Yes	Nasal stuffiness, lethargy, diarrhea	Probably not
Rhubarb	Yes	—	Yes
Senna	Yes	Diarrhea	Yes, in low doses
Spironolactone	No	—	Yes
Streptomycin	Yes	—	Generally felt to be contraindicated

Table 3-4 Maternal medication and breast-feeding (continued)

Drug	Excreted in milk?	Potential side effects	Breast-feeding acceptable?
Sulfisoxazole	Yes*	Kernicterus; hemolysis in sensitive individuals	Avoid during first two weeks or if jaundiced
Tetracycline	Yes	Possible tooth discoloration	Debated, no data
Thioridazine	Yes	—	Yes
Thyroid	Yes	—	Yes
Tolbutamide	Yes	—	Yes
Trifluoperazine	Yes	—	Yes
Warfarin	Yes	Anticoagulation	Generally felt to be safe; monitor infant with mother
Other compounds			
DDT	Yes	Intoxication	Levels generally found in human milk not a contraindication
Gallium $^{131}I, ^{125}I$	Yes	Irradiation	No; biological half-lives vary; count milk samples until counts return to background level, then resume nursing
PCBs	Yes	—	Levels generally found in human milk not a contraindication.
Telepaque	Yes	—	Yes

Sources: Hervada, A. R.; Feit, E.; and Sagraves, R. 1978. Drugs in breast milk. *Perinatal Care* 2:19-25; O'Brien, T. E. 1974. Excretion of drugs in human milk. *Am. J. Hosp. Pharm.* 31:844-854; Vorherr, H. 1974. Drug excretion in breast milk. *Postgraduate Medicine* 56:97-104.

*Indicates that drug concentration in milk is equal to or greater than that in maternal plasma.

Only those drugs not excreted into human milk can be considered absolutely safe.

whether nursing is generally considered safe when the mother is medicated with the drug in question. Only those drugs not excreted into human milk can be considered absolutely safe. For all others, the judgement that continued nursing is acceptable assumes that usual therapeutic doses are being used and indicates that past reports have not documented untoward effects on the infant. In all instances, the infant must be monitored closely for potential problems. Any unexplained signs or symptoms should be cause for an interruption of nursing, at least temporarily. Whenever doubt exists about the relationship of the drug to the infant's symptoms, determination of the concentration of the drug in the milk and in the infant is desirable. Using this information, the practitioner can decide whether the drug in question in the dose being used is safe.

Suggested Reading

Committee on Nutrition, American Academy of Pediatrics. 1979. Fluoride supplementation: revised dosage schedule. *Pediatrics* 63:150–152.

Hambraeus, L. 1977. Proprietary milk versus human breast milk in infant feeding. *Ped. Clin. N. Amer.* 24:17–36.

Lawrence, R. A. 1980. *Breast-feeding: A guide for the medical professor.* St. Louis: C. V. Mosby Co.

Lönnerdal, B.; Forsum, E.; Gebre-Medhin, M.; and Hambraeus, L. 1976. Breast-milk composition in Ethiopian and Swedish mothers. II. Lactose, nitrogen, and protein contents. *Am. J. Clin. Nutr.* 29: 1134–1141.

Martinez, G. A.; and Nalezienski, J. P. 1979. The recent trend in breast-feeding. *Pediatrics* 64:686–692.

Newton, M. and Newton, N. R. 1948. The let-down reflex in human lactation. *J. Pediatr.* 33:698–704.

O'Brien, T. E. 1974. Excretion of drugs in human milk. *Am. J. Hosp. Pharm.* 31:844–854.

Olds, S. W.; and Eiger, M. S. 1976. *The complete book of breast-feeding.* New York: Workman Publishing Co.

Oski, F. A. 1968. Program, American Pediatric Society, p. 58. Cited in McMillan, J. A.; Nieberg, P. I.; and Oski, F. A. 1977. *The whole pediatrician catalogue.* Philadelphia: W. B. Saunders Co., p. 62.

4 Formula-Feeding the Normal Infant

Contents

Uses of Infant Formulas   80
Cow-Milk Formulas   80
   Evaporated-Milk Formulas   81
   Modified Cow-Milk Formulas   83
Skim Milk   85
Goat Milk   86
Soy-Based Formulas   87
   Indications   87
   Composition   88
   Cautions   88
Choice of Formula   90
Management of Bottle-feeding   91
   Intakes by Formula-fed Infants   91
   Growth of Formula-fed Infants   92
   Vitamin and Mineral Supplementation   93
   Sterilization   93
   Duration of Formula-feeding   95
   Additional Topics   96

Overview

Many generations of infants have done well on formula-feeding and the majority of American infants are still fed cow-milk formulas. Cow milk must be modified before it is fed to infants. Evaporated-milk formulas have been supplemented by commercially prepared formulas. There are few differences among the commercially marketed standard infant formulas. Soy formulas are fed in increasing amounts, primarily because of suspected secondary lactose intolerance. A variety of questions relating to bottle-feeding are covered at the conclusion of the chapter.

USES OF INFANT FORMULAS

Despite the increasing prevalence of breast-feeding, the majority of infants in the United States are still raised on infant formula. Formulas based on modified cow milk are used initially in the majority of formula-fed infants. The development of lactose-free formulas based on soy protein has provided the physician with an alternative means of feeding the infant who is apparently intolerant to cow-milk protein or to lactose. These formulas have become increasingly popular and now constitute nearly 20% of infant-formula sales. In addition to the modified-cow-milk formulas and soy formulas used in the nutrition of normal infants, there are now a variety of infant formulas in which the source of protein, fat, or carbohydrate has been altered. Such formulas are indicated for the treatment of specific types of malabsorption and are covered in detail in Chapter 11.

COW-MILK FORMULAS

The nutritional requirements and growth rates of the human infant differ considerably from those of the calf. Understandably, then, the milk of each species has evolved differently to meet these different nutritional requirements. Some of the major differences between human milk and cow milk were discussed in Chapter 3 (see Table 3–2). Many human infants have probably been fed unmodified cow milk and have thrived. Ideally, however, cow milk must be modified before it is suitable for the human infant. Cow milk provides more than three times the protein of human milk. The mineral content is also proportionately greater. Both the protein and mineral intakes from whole cow milk far exceed the requirement of the growing infant, and the excesses serve only to increase the renal solute load.

Cow milk must be modified before it is suitable for the human infant.

A major concern about using unmodified cow milk for infant feeding is the possibility of inducing iron deficiency anemia.

Ingestion of whole cow milk has been shown to cause intestinal blood loss in a substantial percentage of infants with iron deficiency anemia.

Ingestion of whole cow milk has been shown to cause intestinal blood loss in a substantial percentage of infants with severe iron deficiency anemia. Bovine serum albumin is passed in cow milk and apparently damages the intestinal tracts of some young infants. The intestinal blood loss does not occur if the milk has been boiled or evaporated. Iron-deficiency anemia is discussed fully in Chapter 8. It is now generally agreed that cow milk should be altered in some fashion before it is fed to infants. The simplest modification was the early use of an evaporated milk formula with additional carbohydrate. With the current sophistication of the infant-formula industry, formulas based on cow milk are now produced that parallel much more closely the composition of human milk.

Evaporated-Milk Formulas

Evaporated milk is cow milk that has been homogenized, sterilized, and concentrated. When evaporated milk is reconstituted one-to-one with water, the composition of the original milk is obtained. Evaporated milk should not be confused with condensed milk, to which large quantities of sugar are added prior to evaporation.

The renal solute load of evaporated-milk formula is still considerably above that of human milk or of the commercially produced formulas.

Other than reducing the risk of intestinal blood loss, the use of evaporated milk reconstituted one-to-one offers little advantage over the use of whole cow milk. Traditionally, evaporated milk has been diluted with water in a ratio of approximately 2:3, and additional carbohydrate has been added. Corn syrup has most frequently been used.* The major effect of these modifications is a 33% reduction in protein intake. The addition of nonprotein energy in the form of corn syrup solids reduces the percentage of energy supplied by protein in the formula from 21% to 16%. The use of additional water also reduces the absolute protein and mineral contents per 100 mL of formula by about 16%. Taken together these changes diminish the renal solute load from approximately 220 milliosmoles/liter to 180 milliosmoles/liter. Even with this modification, the renal solute load of evaporated-milk formula is still considerably above that of human milk or of the commercially produced formulas. The percentage of total calories supplied by fat in this formula is also reduced, but the fat source remains the same and is considerably higher in less well-absorbed saturated fatty acids than is human milk or commercial infant formula.

---

*One 13-oz can of evaporated milk is added to 17 oz of water; 2 tablespoons of corn syrup are added.

Table 4-1

Several generations of infants have been raised on modified evaporated-milk formulas, which attests to the adequacy of these formulas. Perhaps the major advantage of evaporated-milk formula over commercial formula in the past was the relative cost. The cost of the ingredients used to prepare an evaporated-milk formula is compared with the costs of several commercially available formulas in Table 4-1. One of the problems in calculating these costs is accounting for the time required to prepare the formulas. In addition, the cost of adding vitamins and iron to evaporated milk must be included. Currently many lower income families, for whom absolute differences in cost would be most important, are covered under the Supplemental Food Program for Women, Infants, and Children (WIC programs) and have commercial infant formula provided at very low or no cost, which tends to make the cost argument moot.

The biggest disadvantage to the traditional evaporated-milk formulas is the potential for errors in preparation. The substitution of salt for sugar in formula preparation has led to severe hypernatremia in infants. Another disadvantage is that fat absorption is

Table 4-1   Relative cost per liter of milk and various formulas

Diet	Cost/L	Additional vitamins or iron, if needed	Total cost
Whole cow milk	$0.49	$0.05	$0.64
EVM 2:3 + 5% DM* (2 parts evaporated milk to 3 parts water + 5% dextrin maltose (DM)	0.55	0.05	0.60
Commercial modified cow-milk formula—liquid concentrate†	1.01	—	1.01
Commercial modified cow-milk formula—ready-to-feed†	1.25	—	1.25
Soy formula—concentrate†	0.77	—	0.77

*Assumes cost of one can of evaporated milk ($0.48) and 2 tablespoons of Karo syrup ($0.05).

†Costs are averages of three commercial brands in Baltimore and Chicago areas (1980).

less efficient when cow milk or its derivatives are fed in early infancy. Finally, the nuisance of having to prepare the formula may lead to an inappropriately early switch to whole cow milk. For these reasons we recommend the use of commercial infant formula for mothers who choose not to breast-feed their infants.

Modified Cow-Milk Formulas

The standard for composition of all commercial infant formulas is the nutrient content of human milk.

Composition The commercial infant formulas based on cow milk are frequently referred to as "maternalized" or "humanized" milk formulas. The rationale for the composition of all commercial infant formulas in the United States is the nutrient content of human milk. Rather than start with whole or evaporated milk and modify it by adding other nutrients, as is done when an evaporated-milk formula is prepared, the formula manufacturers begin with components isolated from cow milk and reconstruct a "milk" similar in composition to human milk. The compositions of four of the major milk formulas in the United States are shown in Table 4–2. All four formulas provide 9% of energy as protein. This is 50% higher than the 6% of energy from protein in human milk and provides a margin of safety to compensate for any inferiority in protein quality. Fat provides 48% to 50% of energy. Although the sources of oil differ among the three formulas, all three provide all of their dietary fat from vegetable oils; they differ strikingly from human milk in that they contain essentially no cholesterol. The cholesterol content of human milk is relatively high, as was pointed out earlier. The carbohydrate in all four formulas is lactose. Sodium, potassium, and chloride contents have been adjusted to approximate concentrations in human milk, although calcium and phosphorus contents are slightly higher. Vitamin and mineral contents have been adjusted upward in some instances to assure that all formulas in amounts usually consumed provide the recommended dietary allowance for all nutrients. All four formulas have osmolalities and renal solute loads comparable to that of human milk.

Table 4–2

There are differences among the milk-based formulas, particularly in the sources of protein and fat.

Differences among brands Table 4–2 shows that there are differences among the four formulas, particularly in the sources of protein and fat. Enfamil and Similac use nonfat-milk protein with a whey:casein ratio of 18:82. SMA and Similac PM 60/40, on the other hand, add demineralized whey to adjust this ratio to 60:40. This tends to increase the content of taurine in the formula, a change that would be important nutritionally if taurine were essential for the human infant. The question of whether it is

Table 4-2 Proximate composition of several milk-based infant formulas

Nutritional characteristic	Formula			
	Enfamil (Mead Johnson Nutritional Div.)	Similac (Ross Laboratories)	SMA (Wyeth Laboratories)	PM 60:40 (Ross Laboratories) 0.68 Kcal/ml
Kcal distribution (%)				
Protein	9	9	9	9
Fat	50	48	48	50
Carbohydrates	41	43	43	41
Source				
Protein	Nonfat milk	Nonfat milk	Nonfat milk with whey added	Nonfat milk with whey added
(whey:casein ratio)	(18:82)	(18:82)	(60:40)	(60:40)
Fat	Soy oil 80% Coconut oil 20%	Soy oil 60% Coconut oil 40%	Oleo, coconut, oleic (safflower), and soybean oils	Coconut oil 50% Corn oil 50%
Carbohydrates	Lactose	Lactose	Lactose	Lactose
Sodium (meq/L)	10	11	7	7
Potassium (meq/L)	17	20	14	15
Chloride (meq/L)	13	15	10	14
Calcium (mg/L)	550	510	444	400
Phosphorus (mg/L)	460	390	330	200
Calcium:phosphorus	1.2:1	1.3:1	1.3:1	2:1
Magnesium (mg/L)	48	41	53	42
Copper (mg/L)	0.6	0.6	0.47	0.42
Iodine ($\mu g/L$)	69	100	69	42
Iron (mg/L)	12	12	12.6	2.6
Zinc (mg/L)	4.2	5	3.7	4.0
Vitamin A (IU/L)	1675	2500	2642	2500
Vitamin D (IU/L)	420	400	444	400
Vitamin E (IU/L)	12.7	17	9.5	15
Vitamin C (mg/L)	54	55	58	55
Vitamin B_1 (mg/L)	0.5	0.65	0.71	0.65
Vitamin B_2 (mg/L)	0.6	1	1.05	1.0
Niacin (Eq/L)	8.4	7	10.0	7.3
Vitamin B_6 (mg/L)	0.4	0.4	0.42	0.3
Vitamin B_{12} ($\mu g/L$)	2	1.5	1.05	1.5
Folate ($\mu g/L$)	107	100	52.8	50
Renal solute load (milliosmoles/L) *	100	108	91	102
Osmolality (milliosmoles/L)	278	290	300	260

*Estimates calculated using the method of Ziegler and Fomon (1971).

essential remains unsettled. The differences in the sources of fat in the formulas have not been demonstrated to have nutritional significance.

All four formulas have been marketed for many years and each has been the sole source of nutrition for thousands of growing infants. For this reason, the formulas are presumed adequate. It must be admitted, however, that because formulas such as these are reconstructed from milk components and other ingredients, the possibility of error always exists. Indeed, there have been several instances in the past when major errors in formula production have resulted in severe illness for the infants consuming them. In addition, the long-term effects of infant-formula diet are not known. For example, it is too soon to tell whether the complete removal of cholesterol from the infant's diet at an early stage in development will prove to have been beneficial or, perhaps, harmful. These comments should not be construed to mean that commercial formulas are unsafe or nutritionally unsound. They are not, however, human milk.

SKIM MILK

All of the potential problems of feeding whole cow milk to an infant are magnified when skim milk is fed.

All of the potential problems of feeding whole cow milk to an infant are magnified when skim milk is fed. Skim milk is virtually devoid of fat, which normally provides 50% of the energy in whole cow milk. The removal of fat makes skim milk a hypocaloric food for infants, with an energy density of 10 calories/ounce (0.33 kcal/mL). In addition, skim milk is deficient in essential fatty acids. The removal of fat also markedly alters the distribution of calories in the diet. Skim milk provides nearly 40% of its calories as protein. When skim milk is consumed in sufficient volume to meet the energy requirements of the infant, the protein intake becomes exceedingly high.

Neither skim milk nor 2% milk is considered adequate foods for infants. However, Fomon et al (1977) carried out a study in which a group of healthy term infants were fed skim milk for 56 days, beginning at 112 days of age. Interestingly enough, these infants grew in length at a rate comparable to a control group fed a commercially available formula. Weight gain, however, was inferior, and at the end of the three-month period, the infants fed skim milk tended to be long and lean. Fomon and coworkers have emphasized that the normal rates of linear growth observed in this study do not attest to the adequacy or desirability of using skim milk in infant feeding. We see no place for skim milk in the diets of infants during the first year of life, even for those infants who appear to be becoming obese. For obese infants there are other more appropriate dietary manipulations available to slow weight gain.

Ross Laboratories markets a formula to be used during the second part of the first year as a transition from standard formula to whole cow milk. This formula, Advance, has a reduced energy density (0.53 kcal/mL, 16 kcal/oz). Protein provides 20% of calories. There is little apparent nutritional advantage to this formula over standard formula, except for those infants who are exceedingly overweight and for whom a reduction in overall intake is desirable.

GOAT MILK

Relatively little goat milk is drunk in the United States. The use of goat milk in infant nutrition has been confined primarily to those infants with suspected allergy to cow milk. In the past it was not uncommon to see children who were intolerant to cow milk switched to a goat-milk formula. Nevertheless, there is little or no evidence to corroborate the contention that the caseins and whey in goat milk are less allergenic than those in cow milk. There is, however, a difference in the fatty acid composition of the two milks that might make the fat in goat milk somewhat more absorbable. With the advent of soy formula fewer and fewer children have been switched to goat milk as a response to suspected milk intolerance.

There is little or no evidence to corroborate the contention that the caseins and whey in goat milk are less allergenic than those in cow milk.

Goat milk parallels cow milk in composition in most respects. The protein concentration and the energy density are similar. However, there are some notable differences between the two milks. The sodium content of goat milk is less than that of cow milk. At the same time the other minerals, potassium in particular, are slightly higher. Because of the high protein and mineral contents, goat milk must be modified in the same fashion as cow milk before it is suitable for human infants.

It is very important to remember that the folic acid content of goat milk is low.

From a clinical point of view it is very important to remember that the folic acid content of goat milk is low. Goat milk contains about 6 μg of folic acid per liter, well below the 50 μg/liter found in human milk and cow milk. It is virtually impossible to provide adequate amounts of folic acid (RDA: 30 μg/day) with goat milk. Numerous cases of severe megaloblastic anemia have been reported in infants and children consuming most of their calories as goat milk. All children fed goat milk should receive a vitamin supplement that assures an intake of 50 μg of folic acid per day.

SOY-BASED FORMULAS

Since their introduction some 30 years ago, soy formulas have gained wide acceptance in the management of a variety of feeding problems in infancy.

Indications

There are three principal areas in which the use of a soy-based formula has been thought to offer some advantage over the use of cow-milk formulas: the prevention and treatment of allergy to cow milk, the management of colic, vomiting, and other minor feeding disorders in infancy, and the management of lactose intolerance in infancy.

Since the studies of Glaser and Johnstone in the early 1950s, soy formulas have been thought to offer some advantage in the prevention and treatment of allergy in general and of allergy to cow milk specifically. These studies were biased in their patient selection, however, a problem acknowledged at the time by the authors. More recent studies suggest that soy protein is every bit as antigenic as cow milk protein (Eastham et al, 1978). The absorption of whole proteins that may serve as antigens occurs primarily during the early months of life. After this period, the intestinal tract is better able to exclude foreign proteins. Consequently, some of the apparent hypoallergenicity of soy formulas may relate to the fact that many infants, if not breast-fed, are started in cow-milk formulas, changing to soy-based formulas only later, when they are less likely to be allergic. One can only speculate about whether the apparent benefits of soy formula in allergy would disappear if large groups of infants were fed soy-based formulas from birth. It is clear that the best way to minimize the risk of allergy from the intestinal absorption of whole proteins is by breast-feeding for a minimum of three months, preferably longer (see Chapter 3).

Soy formulas are often prescribed for infants with colic or vomiting. Many of these infants have been tried on two or three of the cow-milk formulas before being changed to soy. In some instances, the change to soy seems beneficial; in others, the problems fail to resolve. The evidence that colic or spitting up usually relates to the formula being fed is not impressive. In most instances, the resolution of the condition is probably unrelated to any formula change, yet the formula that the child is consuming at the time of resolution is given credit. It has been suggested that colic may be related to lactose intolerance, but there are no studies confirming this.

Marginal notes:

Soy protein is every bit as antigenic as cow-milk protein.

The evidence that colic or spitting up usually relates to the formula being fed is not impressive.

Following diarrhea, lactose intolerance due to transient loss of intestinal lactase is a well-recognized phenomenon in infants and children. Because the soy formulas contain no lactose, they are frequently prescribed following episodes of diarrhea, on the presumption that the infant may be lactose intolerant. When the child does well, the parents and physician are often reluctant to change the child back to a lactose-containing diet. Such a course may be overly cautious in many instances. However, there would seem to be no nutritional problem with continuing to use a soy-based formula, although some children may be branded as lactose intolerant when in fact they could drink formula or, later in life, milk without problems.

Composition

Table 4–3

The composition of the soy-based formulas commonly available in the United States are shown in Table 4–3. These formulas are blends of individual ingredients. The distribution of energy among protein, fat, and carbohydrate varies little among the formulas. The source of protein in all is soy-protein isolate. Because soy protein is deficient in methionine, the amino acid is added. The sources of fat and carbohydrate vary somewhat among the formulas, but we see little reason to choose among them on this basis.

Cautions

Numerous studies have demonstrated the nutritional adequacy of soy-based formulas when properly constituted. A recent occurrence with two soy formulas, however, has pointed up the potential for error in the manufacture of infant formulas. During 1979 a large number of infants were forced to have a hypochloremic alkalosis resembling Bartter's syndrome. After this syndrome was ruled out, further investigation revealed that all the infants so affected had been consuming one of two soy-based formulas, Neo-Mullsoy and CHO-Free. The chloride contents of these two formulas were found to be inadequate and were thought to account for the marked electrolyte derangement. Both products were later reformulated and have since been withdrawn from the market. Particular caution must be exercised when unexplained symptoms appear in an infant who is receiving all or nearly all of its nutrients from a single formula. Although the formula itself could be faulty in such a case, it is equally likely that improper preparation or use by parents might account for the problem.

Particular caution must be exercised when unexplained symptoms appear in an infant who is receiving all or nearly all of its nutrients from a single formula. Although the formula itself could be faulty in such a case, it is equally likely that improper preparation or use by the parents might account for the problem.

Table 4-3 Proximate composition of several soy-based infant formulas

Nutritional characteristic	Formula				
	Isomil (Ross Laboratories)	ProSobee (Mead Johnson Nutritional Division)	Nursoy (Wyeth Laboratories)	i-Soyalac (Loma Linda Foods)	Soyalac (Loma Linda Foods)
Kcal distribution (%)					
Protein	12	12	13	12	12
Fat	48	48	47	49	49
Carbohydrates	40	40	40	39	39
Source					
Protein	Soy protein isolate (SPI + L-methionine	SPI + L-methionine	SPI + L-methionine	SPI	Soy protein
Fat	Soybean 60% and coconut 40% oils	Soybean and coconut oils	Oleo, coconut, oleic (safflower) and soybean oils	Soybean oil	Soybean oil
Carbohydrates	Sucrose 50% and corn syrup 50%	Corn syrup solids	Sucrose	Sucrose, modified tapioca starch	Corn syrup, soybeans and sucrose
Sodium (meq/L)	13	13	8.6	14.5	15.0
Potassium (meq/L)	18	21	18.6	20.0	18.6
Chloride (meq/L)	15	16	10.3	14.7	10.9
Calcium (mg/L)	700	630	624	625	625
Phosphorus (mg/L)	500	500	437	417	417
Calcium.phosphorus	1.4:1	1.3:1	1.4:1	1.5:1	1.5:1
Magnesium (mg/L)	50	74	65	62	73
Copper (mg/L)	0.5	0.6	0.45	0.5	0.5
Iodine (μg/L)	0.15	69	67.6	47	47
Iron (mg/L)	12	12	12	12.5	12.5
Zinc (mg/L)	5	5.3	3.6	5.2	5.2
Vitamin A (IU/L)	2500	2090	2600	2083	2083
Vitamin D (IU/L)	400	420	416	417	417
Vitamin E (IU/L)	17	10.7	9.4	15.6	15.6
Vitamin C (mg/L)	55	54	57	62.5	62.5
Vitamin B_1 (mg/L)	0.4	0.5	0.70	0.52	0.52
Vitamin B_2 (mg/L)	0.6	0.6	1.0	0.6	0.6
Niacin (Eq/L)	9	8.4	9.9	8.3	8.3
Vitamin B_6 (mg/L)	0.4	0.4	0.4	0.4	0.4
Vitamin B_{12} (μg/L)	3	2	2.1	2.1	2.1
Folate (μg/L)	100	107	52	104	104
Renal solute load (milliosmoles/L)*	126	130	123	130	125
Osmolality (milliosmoles/L)	250	200	266	280	210

*Estimates calculated using the method of Fomon and Ziegler (1971).

CHOICE OF FORMULA

For the infant who is not going to be breast-fed, it makes most sense to use a milk-based, lactose-containing formula that parallels human milk in its composition.

Because infant formula will be the sole source of nutrients for many infants for prolonged periods of time, the choice of formula should be made primarily for nutritional reasons. However, it must be recognized that there are many formulas on the market and that the choice among them is, unfortunately, usually made for nonnutritional reasons. In general, for the infant who is not going to be breast-fed, it makes the most sense to use a milk-based, lactose-containing formula that parallels human milk in its composition. Although the whey:casein ratio of SMA is theoretically superior to that of Enfamil and Similac, clinical data supporting this difference in the term infant are lacking. All three formulas have animal protein, which has a higher percentage of its amino acids as essential amino acids than does soy protein. The other primary difference between the milk-based formulas and the soy formulas is the presence of lactose. The importance of lactose in the diet is uncertain, but preliminary data for human infants suggest that lactose enhances the absorption of calcium as has been demonstrated in animal studies. Consequently, at our present state of knowledge, unless lactose intolerance is documented, a milk-based lactose-containing formula makes most sense. In documented lactose intolerance or when intolerance to milk protein has been demonstrated, any of the well-established commercial soy-based formulas is an adequate nutritional alternative and is probably the best choice based on cost. The question of whether to use soy formula for the infant with a strong family history of allergy is discussed fully in Chapter 9.

Given the nutritional equivalency of most of the formulas marketed, parents and physicians will usually choose a formula for other than nutritional reasons. Pediatricians and primary care practitioners should be aware of the effect that hospital policy regarding formula has on the subsequent choice of formulas by parents. The economic pressures of operating a formula room have convinced many hospitals to accept one commercial formula as the "house" formula. This formula is supplied at low or no cost by the manufacturer because a parent exposed to one type of formula in the hospital is likely to continue to use the same brand at home. The hospital implicitly endorses the nutritional value of the product when it supplies formula to the mother. Some hospitals attempt to minimize such unintentional endorsement by rotating the house formula or by parent education programs.

In some instances formula choice will be dictated by cost and availability. This is particularly true for women who are receiving formula through WIC programs. The choice of formula on this basis is perfectly appropriate.

Finally, some parents will prefer to use one formula over another because of past experience. A mother may say that one product was "too strong" for her previous infant, whereas another formula caused no problem. As long as the formula chosen is nutritionally adequate, there is no reason to try to change the parents' preference.

MANAGEMENT OF BOTTLE-FEEDING

Issues in the management of bottle-feeding include gauging of proper intake, differences in growth, nutritional supplements, sterilization, and duration of formula-feeding.

Intakes by Formula-fed Infants

Whereas the milk supply of the breast-fed infant is regulated by the infant's sucking, the task of gauging the proper intake for the bottle-fed infant falls to the mother. The mother's regulation of and preoccupation with the intake of the bottle-fed infant is a major difference between breast-feeding and bottle-feeding. Ideally, the infant should be fed "ad lib" so that the infant is able to regulate his or her own intake. The end point for ad lib feeding will vary considerably, depending on how the infant is fed. There is a time during the feeding at which the bottle could be withdrawn and the infant would be content. If allowed to suck uninterrupted, however, the infant would take perhaps ½ to 1 oz more. Feeding should be stopped after this. The overanxious parent will often coax the infant to take an additional ½ to 1 oz. Depending on who is feeding the infant, the intake per feeding might vary as much as several ounces. Many infants, even when fed ad lib, do not take the same amount of formula at all feedings. Although this should not be surprising, it is very upsetting to many inexperienced mothers.

The range of intakes for normal bottle-fed infants is quite wide. The data of Fomon and his coworkers (1971) show clearly that the volumes and calorie intakes by healthy, normally growing infants vary from infant to infant by as much as 40% during the first month of life (Table 4–4). By the age of 3 months, the range has narrowed somewhat, although the variation between the 10th and 90th percentiles is still nearly 25%. Data from children followed through the first three years of life by Beal (1970) show that this wide variability in normal intakes is not unique to infants.

The mother's regulation of and preoccupation with the intake of the bottle-fed infant is a major difference between breast-feeding and bottle-feeding.

Table 4–4

Table 4–4 Energy intakes of bottle-fed infants*

Sex and weight percentile	Energy intake by age—kcal/kg/day		
	8–13 days	42–55 days	84–111 days
Male			
10th	82	91	81
50th	111	108	96
90th	142	133	106
Female			
10th	82	83	82
50th	113	108	94
90th	143	125	109

Source: Fomon, S. J., et al. 1971. Food consumption and growth of normal infants fed milk-based formulas. *Acta. Paediatr. Scand.* (Suppl. 223).

*All infants were fed ad libitum with formula providing 0.67 kcal/dL (20 kcal/oz). To calculate volume intakes in mL, multiply energy intake by 1.5.

Parents whose infants' intakes fall at the low end of the scale are often concerned. As long as an infant is growing normally and has adequate fluid intake as indicated by random urine specific gravities, there is no need for concern.

The time-honored method for establishing the optimal intake for a bottle-fed infant is to begin with 3 or 4 oz of formula at each feeding. The infant is allowed to feed until voluntary intake stops. No further formula should be given. If all 3–4 oz are consumed, an extra ½ oz is put into the bottle for the next feeding. Parents should be advised that ideally the infant should be leaving a small amount of formula at the end of each feeding. This indicates that the infant is getting all he or she wants but that the parents are not force feeding.

> Parents should be advised that ideally the infant should be leaving a small amount of formula at the end of each feeding.

Growth of Formula-fed Infants

Despite all attempts not to overfeed the bottle-fed infant, the growth and weight gain of bottle-fed infants suggests that they probably receive more food than their breast-fed counterparts. Bottle-fed infants tend to double their birth weight more rapidly than breast-fed infants do. It is impossible to say whether this

> Bottle-fed infants tend to double their birth weight sooner than breast-fed infants do.

more rapid weight gain reflects an increased intake of formula by the bottle-fed infant or the earlier introduction of solid foods. With the current trend toward withholding solid foods until the age of 4 to 6 months, this question may soon be resolved.

Vitamin and Mineral Supplementation

Formulas based on evaporated milk will supply insufficient quantities of vitamins C and D unless the milk used is fortified with these vitamins. Consequently, a multivitamin preparation for infants should be used daily for infants being raised on this type of formula. The necessity of supplementing folic acid to goat milk has already been mentioned. It is clear from Tables 4-2 and 4-3 that the commercial milk-based and soy-based infant formulas supply vitamins and minerals (with the exception of fluoride) in adequate concentrations to meet the Recommended Dietary Allowance when these formulas are consumed in quantities sufficient to provide most of the child's protein and energy intake.

It is important that a source of iron be assured for all infants. The easiest way to do so is through the use of an iron-fortified formula. There has been some concern among both practitioners and parents that the iron in the formula may cause symptoms. However, several double-blind studies have shown no difference between iron-fortified and unfortified formulas in this regard.

The fluoride content of city water supplies varies considerably from one part of the country to another. For this reason, formula manufacturers add no fluoride to their product. Fluoride should be supplemented using a sliding scale based on the fluoride concentration of the local water supply. The recommendations for supplementation from the Committee on Nutrition of the American Academy of Pediatrics are shown in Table 4-5. Fluoride reduces the likelihood of developing dental caries in two ways. Its major effect is through its incorporation into the enamel of developing teeth. In addition, fluoride appears to effect a beneficial change in tooth architecture. Because enamel formation in permanent teeth begins as early as 3 to 5 months of age, a source of fluoride should be assured at this age and should be continued until the age of 12 to 14 years, when the enamel of the third molars is complete.

Sterilization

In the past, sterilization of bottles, nipples, and formula was considered essential. More recently, attitudes toward sterilization have relaxed. It is difficult to give a hard and fast rule concerning the necessity of sterilization. Human milk is certainly not sterile,

There has been some concern among both practitioners and parents that the iron in the formula may cause symptoms. However, several double-blind studies have shown no difference between iron-fortified and unfortified formulas in this regard.

Fluoride should be supplemented using a sliding scale based on the fluoride content of the local water supply.

Table 4-5

Table 4–5 Recommended supplemental dosage of fluoride (mg/day)

Age of child	Fluoride in drinking water (ppm)		
	<0.3	0.3–0.7	>0.7
2 wk–2 yr	0.25	0	0
2–3 yr	0.50	0.25	0
3–16 yr	1.00	0.50	0

Source: American Academy of Pediatrics, Committee on Nutrition. 1979. Fluoride supplementation: revised dosage schedule. *Pediatrics* 63:150–152. Copyright American Academy of Pediatrics.

and there is no reason to think that the infant cannot tolerate the ingestion of small numbers of bacteria. The improper preparation or storage of formula, however, may result in exposure of the infant to far greater numbers of potentially pathogenic organisms. The need for sterilization is probably greatest in the homes in which it is least likely to be carried out.

> The need for sterilization is probably greatest in the homes in which it is least likely to be carried out.

Two standard methods of sterilization have been used in home preparation of infant feedings. One begins with the sterilization of bottles, nipples, and all ingredients to be used; the formula is then prepared sterilely. The other method starts with clean utensils and ingredients; following the preparation of the formula and the filling of the bottles, both are sterilized together. Refrigeration after either method is essential. Both methods are time consuming. A study some years ago showed that the majority of mothers stop sterilizing formula within the first three months, regardless of the advice of their physicians.

> The majority of mothers stop sterilizing formula within the first three months, regardless of the advice of their physicians.

Sterilization is probably not necessary in most environments if some simple precautions are taken. Formula should not be prepared in large batches. If more than a single feeding is prepared, storage in a refrigerator is a must. More and more mothers are using liquid concentrate, which they simply dilute with water one-to-one. It is suggested that bottles and nipples be washed in a dishwasher, if available, or that an individual bottle and nipple be washed immediately prior to preparing formula. The formula is then prepared in the bottle in which it is to be given and is fed shortly thereafter. Some mothers feel uneasy about using water directly from the tap. In these cases, water may be boiled and stored in the refrigerator for use in formula preparation.

Duration of Formula-Feeding

Opinions about the length of time that formula should be fed before the change to whole cow milk have varied considerably in the last several decades; the subject continues to be somewhat controversial. Until very recently, there had been a trend toward a progressively shorter duration of formula-feeding. However, with the tendency to encourage more and more prolonged breast-feeding, there is also a trend toward more prolonged use of infant formula. Most pediatric nutritionists agree that a minimum of six months of formula-feeding is desirable. Many feel that formula should be continued throughout the first year of life.

Most pediatric nutritionists agree that a minimum of six months of formula-feeding is desirable. Many feel that formula should be continued throughout the first year of life.

The basis for recommending 12 months is the desire to minimize the risk of iron deficiency anemia. In theory, more prolonged consumption of formula should help to ensure this in two ways. As previously mentioned, whole cow milk is known to induce intestinal blood loss in some infants. This phenomenon appears to be most pronounced during the first six months of life, but it is also seen in infants 6 to 12 months old with severe or rapidly developing iron deficiency anemia. The true prevalence of the phenomenon in the general population is unknown. Advocates of prolonged use of infant formula suggest that it is prudent to avoid whole cow milk and thereby any risk of intestinal blood loss. In addition, the introduction of solid foods to the infant's diet is being postponed to progressively later ages. This delays the introduction of iron-fortified cereals as well as meats and other sources of iron. The continued use of an iron-fortified formula assures an adequate iron intake for the infant whose diet is entirely "milk" of one form or another. Iron fortification of the diet is discussed more fully in Chapter 8.

Many practitioners feel that such prolonged use of infant formula is unnecessary. In encouraging the change to whole cow milk, they cite considerations such as cost and ease for the mother, and they note that many of the infants they have cared for have had whole cow milk introduced between 6 and 12 months of age without encountering significant problems with anemia. While we concur that ideally formula should be continued throughout the first year of life, it is difficult to be dogmatic about this. Many mothers with young infants will have already raised several children who started whole milk at 6 months of age or less. These mothers will be difficult to convince that delaying whole cow milk in their most recent offspring is really necessary. In these cases the practitioner should be aware that the change to whole milk possibly predisposes the infant to the development of iron deficiency, and he or she should screen for this problem during subsequent follow-up.

Additional Topics

Iron-fortified formula In the infant who is not breast-fed, iron-fortified formula is the best source of iron for the first six months of life. Except in the rare instance of congenital hemolytic anemia, there is no advantage to using an unfortified formula. Unless there is a compelling reason to do otherwise, iron-fortified formula should be used.

Warming of formula Although it has been traditional to warm formula prior to feeding, this is not necessary. It has been shown that infants can be fed formula taken directly from the refrigerator with no ill effects. This evidence runs counter to the convictions of many mothers (and pediatricians). If the formula is to be warmed, it is important that it not be overheated. Placing the bottle in a pan of tepid water for a few minutes warms it somewhat and avoids the danger of inadvertently feeding the infant excessively hot liquid.

Additional fluids Does the bottle-fed infant need additional fluids? The answer to this question is almost always no. The commercial infant formulas available have a low renal solute load and when consumed in normal quantities provide more than adequate fluid for the infant. If formula intake is reduced markedly, especially if reduction is associated with any circumstance tending to increase the infant's insensible water losses, then additional free water may be appropriate. The circumstances in which additional fluid should be offered to the bottle-fed infant are the same as those for the breast-fed infant.

Fruit juices In the past fruit juices were introduced early primarily to provide vitamin C. Commercial infant formulas are fortified with vitamin C, and unless the formula is overzealously sterilized, thereby destroying ascorbic acid, there is no need for additional vitamin C. There is no reason, however, not to introduce fruit juices after the age of 2 to 3 months. Juice may be a good alternative to formula for the infant who is gaining weight too rapidly. Many parents dilute juice initially. There is no reason not to do this.

Freshly squeezed citrus fruit juices are occasionally associated with an irritation of the skin around the mouth. This irritation is not a manifestation of allergy in most cases; it results from an excessively high concentration of peel oil in the home-squeezed juice. Peel-oil concentrations are controlled in the commercial production of all juices.

Regurgitation Many parents and practitioners have noticed that bottle-fed infants seem to have more problems with burping and regurgitation. This probably results from excessive air swallowing during bottle-feeding. In the breast-fed infant, sucking is only partially responsible for the delivery of milk to the infant; the milk ejection reflex also plays a major role. The bottle-fed infant must rely entirely on sucking. Also, the rubber nipple does not elongate to the same extent as the human nipple. Both of these factors predispose the infant to air swallowing. In addition, some parents do not exercise proper caution in assuring that the nipple is always filled with formula, occasionally allowing the infant to suck air directly from the bottle.

Formula intolerance As mentioned previously, colic, spitting up, restlessness, and a variety of other nonspecific symptoms have all been attributed to formula intolerance. Many instances of these symptoms may be due to immaturity of the infant's intestinal tract or may have nothing to do with feeding whatsoever. Formula intolerance certainly does exist. We have seen infants in the nursery who have developed proctitis after several feedings with modified-cow-milk formulas. Resolution occurred after switching to breast milk or soy formula. Intolerance to soy protein has also been reported on many occasions. Well-defined intolerances are rare, however. In most instances, the practice of changing formulas because of presumed intolerance probably succeeds by allowing the problem time to resolve itself spontaneously as the infant matures. At the present time there is nothing more sophisticated to recommend for apparent formula intolerance.

Feeding cereal from the bottle The practice of adding cereal directly to formula and feeding it through the nipple probably derived from the difficulty of spoon-feeding any semi-solid food to an infant during the early months of life when the protrusion reflex of the tongue is still prominent. As will be discussed in Chapter 5, the addition of cereal is probably best delayed until it can be given easily by spoon. Adding cereal to formula for young infants is not recommended, because the hole in the nipple has to be considerably enlarged to allow easy flow of the mixture. The rapid flow of formula that may result can cause aspiration.

Nursing bottle caries The practice of putting older infants to bed with a bottle as a pacifier should be avoided, as it leads to prolonged bathing of the teeth in formula or juice. This increases the likelihood of development of caries.

Introduction of the cup   The age at which the cup is introduced varies considerably from infant to infant and from mother to mother. Many mothers who breast-feed their children will wean them directly to a cup after the age of 7 to 8 months. Delaying the introduction of the cup to 12 months of age or longer seems equally valid. By this age many infants readily give up the bottle in favor of the cup. Others use a cup at mealtime but still prefer a bottle prior to going to bed in the evening. There should be no problem with this practice as long as care is taken to prevent nursing bottle caries.

Suggested Reading

American Academy of Pediatrics, Committee on Nutrition 1976. Commentary of breastfeeding and infant formulas, including proposed standards for formulas. *Pediatrics* 57:278–285.

American Academy of Pediatrics, Committee on Nutrition 1979. Fluoride supplementation: revised dosage schedule. *Pediatrics* 63:150–152.

Beal, V. A. 1970. Nutritional intake. In: McCammon, R. W. (editor) *Human growth and development.* Charles C. Thomas Co. Springfield, Ill.

Eastham, E. J.; Lichanco, T.; Grady, M. I.; and Walker, W. A. 1978. Antigenicity of infant formulas: role of immature intestine on protein permeability. *J. Pediatr* 93:561–564.

Fomon, S. J.; Filer, L. J., Jr.; and Ziegler, E. E. 1977. Skim milk in infant feeding. *Acta Paediatr. Scand.* 66:17–30.

Fomon, S. J.; Thomas, L. N.; Filer, L. J., Jr., et al. 1971. Food consumption and growth of normal infants fed milk based formulas. *Acta Paediatr. Scand.*, Supplement 223:1–24.

Neumann, C. G.; and Alpaugh, M. 1976. Birthweight doubling: a fresh look. *Pediatrics* 57:469–473.

Saarinen, U. M.; Pelkonen, P., and Siimes, M. A. 1979. Serum immunoglobulin A in healthy infants. An accelerated postnatal increase in formula-fed infants compared to breast-fed infants. *J. Pediatr.* 95:410–412.

Ziegler, E. E.; and Fomon, S. J. 1971. Fluid intake, renal solute load and water balance in infants. *J. Pediatr.* 78:561–568.

5 Solid Foods

Contents

When to Introduce Solids 100
  When Are Solid Foods Tolerated? 101
  When Are Solid Foods Nutritionally Required? 102
  Other Reasons for Starting Solids 103
Sequence of the Addition of Solid Foods 104
  Infant Cereals 105
  Fruits 107
  Vegetables 108
  Meats 109
  Other Foods 109
Additives in Commercial Baby Foods 109
  Salt 110
  Sugar 110
  Modified Starch 110
  Other Additives 111
Homemade Baby Food 111
Foods Generally Not Fed to Young Infants 112
  Allergens 113
  Foods Causing Flatulence 113
  Nitrates in Foods 113
  Honey 114

Additional Issues Concerning the Feeding of Solid Foods   114

Junior Foods   114

Heating of Strained Foods   115

Transition to Table Foods   115

Serving Size   115

Overview

Although the digestive capacity to handle solid foods is adequate shortly after birth, there is no benefit to the early introduction of solids. Waiting until the infant is developmentally ready at 4 to 6 months of age offers several advantages. The nutrient content of commercial baby foods and the methods and cautions that apply to making baby foods at home are covered in this chapter; particular subjects such as salt, sugar, and modified starches are also addressed. Certain foods are not advised for young infants, including potential allergens, foods high in nitrates, and honey.

WHEN TO INTRODUCE SOLIDS

During the first year of life a transition is made from a diet in which milk or formula provides all nutrients to one in which progressively larger amounts of the infant's nutritional needs are met by semi-solid and solid foods. Because many of the foods initially introduced are not truly solid, the German word *beikost* is sometimes used to refer to these foods as a group. In this chapter "solid" food will be used to refer to the entire gamut of puréed and semi-solid foods used to accomplish the change between an all-milk diet and one in which the infant consumes table foods with the rest of the family.

The two primary questions to be answered in regard to solid foods are when to add them to the diet and in what order. The answer to the first question has changed considerably over the years. At the turn of the century, pediatrics textbooks suggested that a particularly robust infant could be given small amounts of zweibach as the initial solid food around the end of the first year. During the last 20 years, however, many infants were begun on cereal as early as 3 weeks of age. More recently there has been a reverse trend toward progressively later introduction of solid foods. In arriving at a decision about when to add solid foods, the practitioner must balance several factors: the necessity of meeting the infant's nutrient requirements, the infant's stage of development, and the social pressures on parents and from parents to achieve what is perceived as a "landmark" in the infant's life. For an infant of any age, the practitioner must consider whether the infant's digestive system is able to tolerate the solids that will be

In arriving at a decision about when to add solid foods, the practitioner must balance several factors: the necessity of meeting the infant's nutrient requirements, the infant's stage of development, and the social pressures on parents and from parents to achieve what is perceived as a "landmark" in the infant's life.

added to the diet, whether milk or formula is still adequate as the sole food, and which solid foods are required to meet the nutritional requirements of the infant.

When Are Solid Foods Tolerated?

Initially, the infant receives all of its nutrients in fluid form; this is primarily because the infant is unable to chew or to swallow solid foods easily, rather than because of any deficiencies of intestinal digestive function. The breast-fed or formula-fed infant is already digesting and absorbing whole protein, long-chain triglycerides and cholesterol, and disaccharides. Although digestion and absorption of protein, fat, and carbohydrates improve somewhat during the first two to three months following birth, these processes are relatively efficient even in the neonate. When solid foods are added to the diet, complexity of dietary carbohydrate increases, as a variable amount of polysaccharide is substituted for disaccharide. Vegetable protein, somewhat less digestible than animal protein, is also added to the diet. The level of pancreatic amylase, the enzyme required for the initial hydrolysis of starch, is low at birth. This level increases during the first few months of life. It is uncertain when the capacity to digest starch reaches adult levels. Feeding of starch from wheat and rice does not result in excessive energy losses in the stool, indicating that most of the starch is digested and absorbed. It has been argued, however, that not all of the starch ingested is, in fact, absorbed in the small intestine, an indeterminant amount perhaps being fermented in the large intestine.

Other than the addition of complex carbohydrate to the diet, the addition of solid foods poses no particular additional stress on the developing intestinal tract. Experience during the past 20 years with thousands of infants suggests that there is clinical tolerance to the addition of solid foods at 2 to 3 weeks of age or even earlier. One practitioner (Sackett, 1956) has published his experience with the early introduction of solid foods, aiming for the achievement of three meals a day containing a variety of cereals, meats, fruits, and vegetables before the age of 3 weeks. Such experience attests to the tolerance and resilience of young infants. Efficiency of digestion of solid foods introduced at these early ages is not equal to the efficiency that will be attained later; the infant's ability to tolerate solid foods does not necessarily make their early addition desirable.

When solid foods are added to the diet, complexity of dietary carbohydrates increases, as a variable amount of polysaccharide is substituted for disaccharide.

Efficiency of digestion of solid foods introduced at these early ages is not equal to the efficiency that will be attained later; the infant's ability to tolerate solid foods does not necessarily make their early addition desirable.

When Are Solid Foods Nutritionally Required?

When the addition of solid food at any particular age is advocated, nutritional reasons are frequently advanced in support of the decision. In truth, it is difficult, on a purely nutritional basis, to arrive at an ideal age for the addition of solid foods.

Usefulness of solids as an iron source   Some proponents of the early introduction of solids have suggested that they are a good source of additional iron. However, with the advent of iron-fortified formulas, the formula-fed infant's need for other iron-containing foods is nil. The question of the adequacy of dietary iron is more complex in the case of the breast-fed infant. The low concentration of iron in human milk is offset to a large degree by its high bio-availability. Cereals, usually the first solid foods fed, contain a variety of compounds that decrease the absorption of nonheme iron. For this reason, the addition of cereal to the diet of the breast-fed infant alters the absorption of iron from human milk. Although the point is still argued, human milk is probably an adequate source of iron for the exclusively breast-fed infant through 6 to 8 months. In those instances in which additional iron is required, it can be supplied as ferrous sulfate without requiring a marked change in diet.

With the advent of iron-fortified formulas, the formula-fed infant's need for other iron-containing foods is nil.

Supplementing breast-feeding   A valid reason for the addition of solids to the diet of the breast-fed infant is to offset a possible insufficiency of milk as the infant and his requirements for all nutrients grow. Both experience with exclusively breast-fed infants and data on the amount of milk produced by healthy mothers show that at some point the breast-fed infant will outgrow its milk supply. The age at which this begins to occur has been controversial. Some suggest that either solid foods or supplemental formula should be given to the breast-fed infant at the age of 3 to 4 months. A recent retrospective study of healthy American infants suggests that exclusive breast-feeding to the age of 8 or 9 months is usually accompanied by excellent growth and weight gain. Unquestionably, some exclusively breast-fed infants will begin to fall off their growth curve before the age of 6 months, while others may be doing well at 1 year. The decision to supplement must be individualized. If growth has been adequate for the first 5 to 6 months, it is preferable to supplement with solids rather than with formula, especially in unsanitary environments, where the use of bottles and nipples poses additional problems.

Additional considerations From the nutritional perspective, meeting the young infant's nutrient requirements with a mixture of liquid and solid foods rather than with milk or formula exclusively is not detrimental to the child's health. The claim that the early addition of solid foods is particularly beneficial is equally difficult to support. When dry infant cereals are prepared with water, the energy density of the resulting mixture is generally less than that of milk or formula. When mixed with milk, the energy density nearly doubles. On the average, the substitution of baby foods for formula will probably decrease the total energy and protein intakes rather than increase it. However, experience suggests that the addition of solid foods to the infant's diet is rarely accompanied by a concomitant decrease in milk or formula intake. The practical effect of introducing solid foods is usually an increase in total nutrient intakes. Infants who are fed more gain weight more rapidly. It is not certain whether excessively rapid weight gain in infancy is related to obesity in later life; the subject is discussed more fully in Chapter 13.

> The practical effect of introducing solid foods is usually an increase in total nutrient intakes.

Other Reasons for Starting Solids

Although nutritional considerations give relatively little guidance in choosing the optimal age for the introduction of solids, there may be other reasons on which to base the decision.

Sleeping through the night Many parents believe that the introduction of cereal, especially at the last feeding of the evening, will cause the infant to sleep through the night. Several studies of this possible relationship have reached the same conclusion: Solid foods in the diet have no effect on the age at which an infant begins to sleep through the night.

> Solid foods in the diet have no effect on the age at which an infant begins to sleep through the night.

Development of taste The development of taste is sometimes suggested as a reason for not delaying the introduction of solid foods for too long. One also hears occasionally that postponing exposure to different textures will result in problems. These claims seem to be unsubstantiated. There are no data to suggest that infants who are exclusively breast-fed or bottle-fed during most of the first year are any less likely to acquire a taste for a wide variety of foods later in life than infants who are introduced to solid foods much earlier.

Developmental readiness The excessively early introduction of solids may set up a situation full of frustration for both mother and infant. Fomon and his colleagues (1979) suggested that the addition of solid foods to the diet should relate primarily to the infant's ability to participate actively in the feeding process and to the ease with which he or she can accept into the mouth and swallow semi-solid and puréed foods. This approach is entirely reasonable. The newborn infant rejects the nipple or any other object placed directly in its mouth. When the nipple is placed on the infant's cheek, the routing reflex causes the infant to open its mouth and take the nipple. The protrusion reflex that prevents the infant from accepting a nipple directly into its mouth also makes it difficult to feed solids. Most parents who begin to feed their infants cereal at an early age find that only by stroking the cheek with the spoon are they able to get the cereal back far enough into the mouth so that the infant does not spit most of it out. Trying to spoon-feed an infant who is too young is frustrating for the parents and potentially dangerous for the infant.

The protrusion reflex disappears between 3 and 4 months of age. During this time and a bit later, the infant is achieving progressively better head control. Good head control and the neuromuscular maturity of the oral cavity make it far easier for the infant to begin to accept food from a spoon. Developmentally, then, most infants will be ready to accept solid foods between the ages of 5 and 6 months. Given the lack of any nutritional imperative for the introduction of solid foods at an earlier age, 4 to 6 months, depending on the individual infant, appears to be a reasonable lower age limit for the introduction of solid foods. At the same time, for the mother who is content with breast-feeding or bottle-feeding exclusively and whose infant is growing normally, there is no reason why solid foods need to be introduced at this age.

> Good head control and the neuromuscular maturity of the oral cavity make it far easier for the infant to begin to accept food from a spoon.

SEQUENCE OF THE ADDITION OF SOLID FOODS

In the United States cereal has traditionally been the first solid food introduced into the infant's diet. This choice probably stemmed from the ease of preparing a pap or pablum in the days before commercial baby foods were available. Cereals have generally been followed by fruits, then vegetables, and finally meats. There is no compelling nutritional reason to follow this sequence. One could argue that the earlier addition of meats rather than cereals to the diet of the breast-fed infant would be preferable in terms of iron absorption. Depending on their ethnic backgrounds, some parents may choose to add solids in an order other than the traditional one. Within reason, this is perfectly acceptable.

As a rule, new foods should be introduced one at a time. This facilitates the recognition of specific food intolerance. In accordance with this principle, single-grain cereals should be introduced before mixed and high-protein cereals. The choice of which fruits or vegetables to introduce is best made taking into account the likes and dislikes of the family. Since feeding should be a happy social occasion, many practitioners suggest that parents introduce fruits and vegetables that they enjoy themselves. The ultimate goal is to provide small quantities of a variety of foods at each meal to accustom the older infant to the variety of foods that will be served when he or she eats from the table with the family.

The introduction of solid foods provides an opportunity for the practitioner to begin to educate the new mother in principles of nutrition. Nutritional requirements for adults are considerably less stringent than those for children. Most young couples will have been eating primarily according to habit. With the birth of a baby, additional attention to the tenets of good nutrition is desirable. The choice of the amount and type of solid food added to the diet will have implications for protein intake and renal solute load. In addition, the effects of adding a particular type of cereal, fruit, or vegetable may differ depending on whether or not the infant is being breast-fed or bottle-fed.

The introduction of solid foods provides an opportunity for the practitioner to begin to educate the new mother in principles of nutrition.

Infant Cereals

Composition Three single-grain infant cereals are currently on the market: rice, oats, and barley. Mixed cereals are made of wheat, oats, corn, and (depending on the manufacturer) barley and soy. High-protein cereals made from the same grains are also marketed. Most cereals are fortified with B vitamins. Iron, generally in the form of electrolytically reduced iron, is also added by all three major manufacturers.

Table 5-1

The contents of selected nutrients for five commonly used dry cereals are shown in Table 5-1. Dry cereals in general provide between 3.6 and 3.9 kcal/g. This information is helpful to the nutritionist but gives little guidance to the practitioner or mother, since the cereal will be mixed with either formula or milk prior to feeding. Anderson and Fomon (1971) found that the ratio of diluent to dry cereal varied somewhat with the age of the child but was approximately six parts of water to one part of cereal on a weight basis. Mothers were found always to mix cereal with

Table 5-1 Approximate contents of selected nutrients in infant cereals

Food type	Nutrients*							
	Energy (kcal/ 100 g)	Protein (% kcal)	Ca (mg/100 kcal)	Ca:P ratio	Sodium (mEq/ 100 kcal)	Potassium (mEq/ 100 kcal)	Iron (mg/ 100 kcal)	Renal solute load† (milli-osmoles/100 kcal)
Jar (wet)								
Rice with applesauce and bananas	71	8.2	45	—	0.6	1.8	7.1	8.8
Oatmeal with applesauce and bananas	64	9.4	19	—	0.2	2.7	8.0	9.1
Mixed with applesauce and bananas	78	6.7	3.3	—	0.2	2.4	6.1	8.4
Dry								
Rice	382	8.0	222	1.6:1	0.4	1.7	12.5	10.6
Barley	383	13.9	194	1.2:1	0.4	2.4	12.5	17.3
Oatmeal	377	16.4	199	1.1:1	0.4	2.7	12.7	20.1
Mixed	381	16.7	195	1.2:1	0.4	3.2	12.5	20.8
High-protein	372	40.3	171	1.1:1	0.4	10.7	12.9	51.9

*Values given are averages of information supplied by Beech-Nut and Gerber.
†Estimated by the method of Ziegler and Fomon, 1971. *J. Pediatr.* 78:561–568.

Dry cereals mixed with formula provide 40%-50% more calories than wet (jar) cereals.

either milk or formula, never with water. The resulting energy density of this mixture was approximately 1.1 kcal/g. Jar (wet) cereals have a lower energy density, about 0.64 to 0.78 kcal/g.

The range of protein contents in cereals is quite wide. Rice, traditionally the first cereal introduced, provides between 7% and 8% of energy as protein. Barley, oatmeal, and standard mixed cereals provide 13% to 17% protein kcal. These cereals can be added one at a time to give variety. High-protein cereals provide nearly 40% of energy as protein. Consumption of foods this high in protein by infants is undesirable and unnecessary, partly because of the potential effect of high-protein cereals on renal solute load.

The quality of the protein in cereals is less than that in human milk or formula. The higher protein content of all cereals except rice tends to offset this. The excess of essential amino acids in milk or formula compensates for the relative deficiencies of essential amino acids in the cereals. Digestibility of cereal proteins is somewhat less than that of milk proteins.

All dry infant cereals are supplemented with calcium and phosphorus. Concentrations of these minerals are in the range of those of breast milk. The calcium:phosphorus ratios range from about 1:1 to 2:1. When the cereals are mixed with water, sodium and potassium intakes from cereals are actually less per 100 calories than are those from infant formula.

The addition of cereal to the diet of a young infant poses a potential problem regarding water balance. Because infant cereals are generally mixed with milk or formula, the potential renal solute load of the dry cereal is added to the solute load of the milk or formula. This means that the milk or formula being fed must contain enough free water for the infant to excrete the additional solute generated from the dry cereal. Because most of the cereals have protein contents between 7% and 17% of calories and are relatively low is electrolyte content, the estimated renal solute load per 100 kcal approaches that of human milk and is less than that of infant formula. However, the high protein content of the high-protein cereals will have a significant effect on renal solute to be excreted. Table 5-2 shows the effect of adding dry cereal to the diet of a 4 kg infant consuming 110 kcal/kg/day as infant formula. An increase of energy intake of 10% or 20% as rice cereal causes little change in renal solute load. In contrast, high-protein cereal markedly increases the potential renal solute load. While it is likely that the healthy infant can handle an increase of this magnitude, there are circumstances in which such a change is not well tolerated (see Chapter 2).

Table 5-2

High-protein cereal markedly increases the potential renal solute load.

Fruits

A variety of individual strained fruits (applesauce, peaches, and pears) as well as mixed fruits are commercially available. Most fruits contain minimal amounts of protein, supplying most of their energy in the form of carbohydrate. Some manufacturers add small amounts of additional carbohydrate in the form of corn syrup and modified starch. The energy density of fruits ranges from approximately .4 kcal/g for applesauce up to .8 kcal/g for certain fruits mixed with tapioca (Table 5-3). Fruits are low in electrolyte content. Most are fortified with ascorbic acid and are good sources of this vitamin.

Table 5-3

Table 5-2 Effect on renal solute load of adding cereal to the diet

A 4 kg infant is consuming 110 kcal/kg/day as infant formula:

Total energy intake = 440 kcal/day

Total volume intake = 660 mL/day

Renal solute = 139 milliosmoles/day

Energy intake is increased with dry cereal:

10% increase with	Additional RSL	Percent change
Rice	4.4 milliosmoles	3
High-protein	23.0 milliosmoles	16.5
20% increase with		
Rice	8.8 milliosmoles	6
High-protein	46.0 milliosmoles	33

Table 5-3 Ranges of energy and protein contents of strained baby foods

Food	Energy (kcal/100 g)	Protein (% kcal)
Fruits	45–82	0–5
Vegetables	25–71	5–31
Meats	89–134	48–60
Egg yolks	195	20
Dinners	41–86	9–22
High-meat dinners	72–111	22–29
Desserts	68–93	0–13

Vegetables

There are eight to ten strained vegetables currently on the market in pure form. In addition, several forms of mixed vegetables in strained form are available. The energy density of strained vegetables varies from about .25 to .7 kcal/g (Table 5-3), making them a slightly less dense source of energy than fruits. Their protein content on the other hand is higher than that of fruit, and it varies among vegetables. Carrots, for example, provide approximately 11% of energy as protein, whereas green beans provide nearly 21%.

Depending on the manufacturer, nonfat milk or milk solids and wheat flour may be added during the manufacturing of strained vegetables. This is an important factor to consider for infants who may need to be on a milk-free or gluten-free diet.

Meats

Meats are a high-density source of energy, usually containing more than 1 kcal/g (Table 5–3). Although mothers frequently complain about the amount of water that is added during the preparation of strained meats, it would be undesirable to have these foods any more calorically concentrated than they are. Meats are obviously a good source of high-quality protein, providing about 50% of total calories as protein. Their high protein content makes them undesirable for the feeding of small infants because of the effect on renal solute load. In the past the addition of meat to the diet was considered an important means of increasing iron intake. With the high bioavailability of iron in human milk and the fortification of infant formulas and cereal, this is less a consideration now than it was in the past.

Other Foods

In addition to the traditional cereals, fruits, vegetables, and meats, a variety of other products such as meat dinners, soups, desserts, and yogurts are available. Once the infant has been introduced to several individual foods, the additional products can be introduced for variety if the mother wishes. The nutrient contents of individual products in the same general category may be significantly different. Complete product information with nutritive values and lists of ingredients are available from all of the major baby food manufacturers upon request. These pamphlets are extremely useful when trying to plan diets that are milk-free, lactose-free, gluten-free, or egg-free. (See Appendix A.)

ADDITIVES IN COMMERCIAL BABY FOODS

Parents are frequently concerned about salt, sugar, modified starch, and other food additives in the baby foods that they buy. The use of these ingredients in baby foods has changed considerably over the past decade.

Salt

In the early 1970s baby food manufacturers were criticized for the large amounts of salt added to their products. Salt was being added primarily to appeal to parents rather than to infants. There was concern among pediatricians and nutritionists about whether the ingestion of excessively large amounts of salt in infancy might determine a pattern of salt consumption throughout life that could play a role in the development of essential hypertension.

A marked decrease in added salt was effected by all manufacturers early in the 1970s. More recently all three manufacturers have virtually eliminated added salt from baby foods. There is no reason to add salt, because solid foods fed in reasonable variety will provide more sodium per 100 kcal than does human milk. Consumption of strained foods by infants 4 and 7 months of age has been shown not to be influenced by whether or not salt is added (Fomon et al 1970). It is important that parents be made aware that salt is not added to most baby foods and that additional salt will not improve their infant's appetite for these foods. Many parents will taste the foods they are about to feed to their infants and will reflexly reach for the salt shaker.

It is important that parents be made aware that salt is not added to most baby foods and that additional salt will not improve their infant's appetite for these foods.

Sugar

Many consumers have been concerned about the amount of sucrose added in the past to commercial baby foods. There seems to be little nutritional justification for this concern, especially because most infants consuming these foods do not yet have teeth and are not at risk for dental caries. Nevertheless, current manufacturing practice is to use as little additional sugar as possible in the production of juices, fruits, and desserts. In general, this obligates the manufacturer to require higher natural sugar content of fruits, especially those that tend to be tart. This may or may not increase the ultimate cost of these baby foods to the consumer. Addition of some sugar during processing is not harmful. As pointed out in Chapter 2, the concern for "empty calories" is unwarranted.

Modified Starch

Modified starches are used in the preparation of some vegetables, meat dinners, and desserts. Modified starches are naturally occurring starches that have been changed chemically to increase cross-linking. They are used in commercial baby foods to maintain smooth texture and to prevent the separation of water during storage. The safety of modified starches for infants has been studied extensively by the Committee on Nutrition of the American Academy of Pediatrics. The Committee has concluded that modified starches of the types and in the quantities used are safe for infants.

Other Additives

Food additives, such as nitrates and monosodium glutamate that are frequently used in the manufacture of canned foods for adult consumption are not added to baby foods. Preservation of baby food is accomplished by sterilization during the manufacturing process. After thorough consideration of all aspects of commercial baby foods, there is no reason to think that they are not a safe source of nutrients for infants.

HOMEMADE BABY FOOD

For a variety of reasons, many women prefer to make their own strained foods. Two methods seem to be most widely used. A small baby-food grinder currently on the market allows the mother to purée small portions of the foods that she is already cooking for the rest of the family. Other women prefer to use a blender or food processor to purée small amounts of the family's food or to prepare a larger batch of food specifically for the infant.

Baby foods need not be sterile, but it is important that the mother be careful not to contaminate the food during preparation. This is generally not a major problem if a small amount of food is being prepared for a single meal. A greater danger arises when larger quantities of food are prepared in advance for storage and subsequent use. If puréed foods are to be stored for more than 16 to 24 hours it is suggested that they be put in small plastic bags or in ice trays and that they be frozen. This greatly retards multiplication of bacteria; individual servings can be thawed when needed. The same caveat regarding the storage of homemade baby foods applies to prolonged storage of commercial baby foods once they have been opened, especially if the mother feeds the infant from the jar itself.

Mothers who plan to prepare their own baby foods should also be cautioned regarding the use of seasonings. A recent study in the Pittsburgh area showed that many mothers seasoned the foods they were cooking before removing a portion for their infant (Table 5-4). Nearly all others added some seasoning to the infant's food separately. When the sodium content of 70 samples of baby food made by these mothers was analyzed, the mean amount of

Margin notes:

Food additives, such as nitrates and monosodium glutamate, that are frequently used in the manufacture of canned foods for adult consumption are not added to baby foods.

Baby foods need not be sterile, but is is important that the mother be careful not to contaminate the food during preparation.

Table 5-4

Table 5-4 Sodium content of unprocessed and home-prepared foods

Food	Mean sodium content		Added sodium (mg/100 g)
	Unprepared (mg/100 g)	Home-prepared (mg/100 g)	
Peas	2	145	143
Corn	1	215	214
Squash	1	45	44
Carrots	47	135	88
Green beans	7	197	190
Poultry	62	242	180
Beef	60	156	96
Rice	7	344	337
White potato	4	219	215
Miscellaneous	30	175	145
Mean	22	183	165

Source: Adapted from Kerr, C. M., Jr.; Reisinger, K. S.; and Plankey, F. W. 1978. Sodium concentration of homemade baby foods. *Pediatrics* 62: 331–335. Copyright American Academy of Pediatrics.

added salt was approximately 65% higher than the maximum suggested by the Food and Nutrition Board of the National Academy of Sciences; it was ten times that found in baby foods that were being commercially manufactured with no added salt.

Mothers who wish to prepare their own baby foods should consider cooking with no added salt, seasoning the portion to be fed to the family only after the baby's portion has been separated.

Mothers who wish to prepare their own baby foods should consider cooking with no added salt, seasoning the portion to be fed to the family only after the baby's portion has been separated. They should also be aware that many canned products for adult use, as well as some frozen foods, contain considerable amounts of added sodium. This is true, for example, of many of the canned soups that are available and that are frequently fed to infants.

FOODS GENERALLY NOT FED TO YOUNG INFANTS

A number of foods are traditionally not added to the diet of infants in the first year of life. The basis for withholding some of these foods seems to be sound. In other cases, it is difficult to ascertain why the custom arose.

Allergens

Some foods are considered to be more allergenic than most during the first year of life. Whole eggs and products containing egg white, such as ice cream, have been avoided in an effort not to expose the infant to egg white. Chocolate has also been avoided. We are not aware of data indicating that these foods are particularly more allergenic than others for infants. With the trend toward prolonged exclusive breast-feeding or bottle-feeding, the introduction of these foods in natural sequence should cause no problem.

Many parents note a rash around the mouth of their infant after feeding freshly squeezed citrus juices and mistakenly conclude that the infant is allergic to citrus fruits or citric acid. Actually the rash is caused by peel oils, which can be quite irritating to the skin, even in adults, but which are an important constituent of the flavor of citrus fruits. Infants who have difficulty with home-squeezed juices may do well on commercially prepared juices because they are produced with a narrow range of acceptable peel-oil concentrations.

Peel oils can be quite irritating to the skin, even in adults, but they are an important constituent of the flavor of citrus fruits.

Foods Causing Flatulence

Some foods, such as onions, broad beans, cabbage, and broccoli, have a reputation for producing flatulence or for being hard to digest. These foods are generally not available in strained form from commercial manufacturers but may be added to the diet by mothers who prepare their own foods or add table foods at an early age. We can give no hard and fast rule about the advisability of using these foods during the first year. Although the addition of small amounts may be tolerated, there is no nutritional reason to include them in the diet and they are probably best avoided during the first 12-15 months.

Nitrates in Food

Certain vegetables, such as spinach, carrots, and beets, have high concentrations of nitrates. The consumption of nitrates per se causes no problems. Home preparation of these vegetables with subsequent storage, however, allows for the conversion of nitrates to nitrites, ingestion of which has been associated with methemoglobinemia in infants. This disorder has occurred after home preparation of carrot soup, carrot juice, and spinach purée. It is not certain whether home preparation of puréed forms of these foods poses a major risk. All of the vegetables implicated in the production of methemoglobinemia after home preparation are currently marketed by commercial baby-food companies. Tests of these commercial products have shown no problem with the concentrations of nitrite. If home-prepared purées are to be fed, we suggest that they be used fresh with no subsequent storage.

Honey

Honey was formerly an ingredient in many commercial baby foods. Because of its appeal to many people as a "natural" food, it is likely that it could find its way into the diets of many infants whose mothers choose to prepare their own baby foods. Late in the 1970s an increased number of cases of infant botulism alerted us to the potential danger of honey for infants. Botulism in the adult results from consumption of contaminated food in which there is preformed toxin. Ingestion of spores from *Clostridium botulinum* by the adult causes no problems as the intestinal environment prevents toxin production. The intestinal milieu of the infant, however, may not destroy the spores, allowing for colonization and subsequent production of toxin. To date, honey has been the only food implicated in the production of infant botulism in this manner. It is possible that other foods will be identified in the future. Current recommendations suggest that infants not be fed honey before 1 year of age.

ADDITIONAL ISSUES CONCERNING THE FEEDING OF SOLID FOODS

The practitioner should be able to provide parents with information and advice about baby foods and about making the transition from strained foods to table foods. In general, the child's appetite and ability to handle and chew food should determine the types of foods provided at various developmental stages.

Junior Foods

Some junior foods are the same as puréed foods only in larger jars. Other junior foods differ from strained foods in texture. Rather than being a homogenous purée, many junior foods have small pieces that must be chewed somewhat. The nutrient contents of junior foods differ very little from those of the corresponding strained food. Junior foods can be started at any time that the infant has teeth, generally about 7 to 8 months of age. The age at which infants accept the more coarse textures of junior foods is highly variable. Despite an adequate ability to chew and swallow, many infants will resist junior foods until the end of the first year or even later. There is no compelling reason to switch from strained foods to junior foods other than to achieve the smooth transition to table foods.

Heating of Strained Foods

Foods that have been warmed slightly are generally more appealing, even if not more nutritious. Foods that come directly from a jar at room temperature can be served as is or can be warmed by placing the jar in warm water. Foods that have been stored in the refrigerator may be warmed to remove the chill. The temperature at which the bottle-fed infant will tolerate solid foods depends largely on the habits previously established with regard to warming of formula.

Transition to Table Foods

Some mothers report that their infants are eating from the table by 1 year of age. Others continue to feed commercially prepared baby foods well into the second year. Mothers will generally make this switch when they think that their infants are ready. Parents need to be made aware that certain foods—peanuts and potato chips, for example—are not appropriate for infants and small children because of their potential for aspiration. Some parents question whether fish can safely be fed to infants and small children. While commercially prepared fish cakes and fish sticks are generally bone-free and present no problem, fish filets can contain small bones and must be prepared with great care if they are to be fed to infants and small children.

Serving Size

Strained baby foods are generally marketed in 3½ to 4½ oz jars. Some junior foods, such as meats and meat dinners, come in similar sizes. Others, including many vegetables and desserts, are sold in 7½ to 7¾ oz jars. The manufacturers generally list one jar as the appropriate serving size, but in reality the infant's appetite is the best guide to the appropriate quantity. If mothers have breast-fed their infants or have not been accustomed to forcing additional formula by bottle, and if the introduction of solid foods has been delayed until an age at which the infant can participate somewhat, the infant's appetite will be the best guide. Studies published more than 50 years ago documented the ability of infants less than a year old to select a diet completely adequate both in quantity and quality when presented with a variety of foods. The infants studied frequently went on "jags" in which they would eat a single food in large quantity for several days in preference to other foods. Parents should understand that the rejection by an infant of a particular new food or a food that was previously well accepted rarely indicates a permanent dislike.

Suggested Reading

American Academy of Pediatrics, Committee on Nutrition. 1974. Salt intake and eating patterns of infants and children in relation to blood pressure. *Pediatrics* 53:115–121.

Anderson, T. A.; and Fomon, S. J. 1971. Commercially prepared infant cereals: Nutritional considerations. *J. Pediatr.* 78:788–793.

Andrew, E. M.; Clancy, K. L.; and Katz, M. G. 1980. Infant feeding practices of families belonging to a prepaid group practice health care plan. *Pediatrics* 65:978–988.

Beal, V. A. 1969. Termination of night feeding in infancy. *J. Pediatr.* 75:690–692.

Fomon, S. J. 1975. What are infants fed in the United States? *Pediatrics* 56:350–353.

Fomon, S. J.; and Anderson, T. A., editors. 1972. *Practices of low income families in feeding infants and small children with particular attention to cultural subgroups.* Rockville, Md.: U. S. Department of Health, Education and Welfare, Public Health Service, Health Services and Mental Health Administration, Maternal and Child Health Service. DHEW Publ. No. (HSM) 72–5606.

Fomon, S. J.; Filer, L. J.; Anderson, T. A.; and Ziegler, E. E. 1979. Recommendations for feeding normal infants. *Pediatrics* 63:52–59.

Fomon, S. J.; Thomas, L. N.; and Filer, L. J., Jr. 1970. Acceptance of unsalted strained foods by normal infants. *J. Pediatr.* 76: 242–246.

Kerr, C. M., Jr.; Reisinger, K. S.; and Plankey, F. W. 1978. Sodium concentration of homemade baby foods. *Pediatrics* 62:331–335.

Sackett, W. W. 1956. Use of solid foods early in infancy. *GP* 14: 98–102.

6 Feeding of the Preschool Child, Older Child, and Adolescent

Contents

Feeding the Preschool Child 118
  RDA 118
  Parental Concerns 119
  Role of the Practitioner 120
Children's Attitudes Toward Food 121
  Family Influences 121
  Role of Television Advertising 121
Nutritional Status of Preschool Children 123
Preadolescent Children 124
Nutritional Requirements of Adolescents 124
  Energy and Protein Requirements 124
  Vitamin and Mineral Requirements 126
  Factors Affecting Food Intake 127
"Junk Food" 129
  Nutritional Value 129
  Appropriate Place in the Diet 130

Overview

The preschool period is characterized by excessive parental concern about food intake, which normally decreases after the rapid growth of infancy slows. During the preschool years children develop their attitudes toward food, primarily from their mothers. Television also plays a role in developing food attitudes. Later, the pubertal growth spurt imposes increased requirements for nutrients, iron in particular. The teenager is attracted to a variety of fast foods, many of which are termed "junk food." On closer scrutiny most of these foods are nutritionally valuable in the diet in appropriate amounts.

FEEDING THE PRESCHOOL CHILD

For several reasons, the period between infancy and adolescence is one with relatively few nutritional problems. During early infancy rapid growth imposes high nutrient requirements that can be met with a relatively narrow variety of foods. By the end of the first year the velocity of linear growth and weight gain has slowed dramatically, decreasing further toward the end of the second year. This slower rate of growth is accompanied by a proportionate decrease in nutrient requirements. At the same time, the older child is able to eat and digest a much wider variety of foods. The combination of relatively lower nutrient requirements and broader food choice makes it easier to feed preschool and older children than it to feed the infant.

The combination of relatively lower nutrient requirements and broader food choice makes it easier to feed preschool and older children than it is to feed the infant.

RDA

The Recommended Dietary Allowances for protein, energy, and other nutrients for children between the ages of 1 and 10 years are found in Tables 2-2, 2-7, and 2-9. As previously indicated, these can be useful guidelines in assessing the diets of children, but many children are completely healthy even though they consume diets that fail to meet these allowances. Most parents are aware of the value of a balanced diet that includes foods from a variety of food groups. By the time the child is 1 to 1½ years of age, most of his or her intake will be from table foods. Breakfasts and dinners will tend to parallel those eaten by the rest of the family. Lunch may be prepared especially for the child if he or she is at home alone with the mother at lunchtime. In general, however, the child's diet will largely resemble the diet of the rest of the family, differing only in quantity. Typical menus for preschool children vary widely, depending on the ethnic background and socioeconomic status of the family. Nutrient values of some foods for a preschool child are shown in Table 6-1. Within broad limits, those diets that are satisfactory for older children and adults will be qualitatively acceptable for younger children. There is no need for routine vitamin supplements for this age group. Those studies that have suggested deficiencies in the dietary intakes of certain nutrients

Table 6-1

Within broad limits, those diets that are satisfactory for older children and adults will be qualitatively acceptable for younger children.

Table 6-1 Comparison of selected nutrients in three glasses of milk and a peanut-butter-and-jelly sandwich

Nutrient	Cow milk (750 mL)	Peanut-butter-and-jelly sandwich*
Energy (kcal)	517	525
Protein (g)	24.7	14.0
(% kcal)	19.1	10.6
Fat (g)	27.7	16.9
Carbohydrates (g)	36.0	61.3
Calcium (mg)	937	80
Phosphorus (mg)	720	199
Iron (mg)	0.75	2.7

Source: Graham, G. G. Feeding trials in children. 1971. In Stewart, G. F., and Willey, C. L., editors. *Proceedings of Third International Congress of Food Science and Technology, 1970.* Chicago: Institute of Food Technologists, pp. 358–364.

*Assumes 2 slices bread, 10 g butter, 32 g peanut butter, and 35 g jelly.

have generally keyed on the amount eaten rather than on the distribution of foods within various food groups. We do not find it useful for the practitioner to dwell on the basic four food groups or to provide a series of suitable, typical menus for children, because it is unlikely that the practitioner will be successful in altering the family's food habits.

Parental Concerns

Not surprisingly, the marked slowing of the growth rate that occurs toward the second year of life is associated with a marked decrease in appetite. The infant who has been an avid breast-feeder or who has consumed an entire bottle following seemingly large quantities of cereals, vegetables, and fruits, begins to dawdle in the high chair, often being more interested in playing with finger foods than in eating them. This eating pattern, which often begins as early as 12 to 15 months, continues to concern parents for a number of years. The discrepancy between the child's appetite and actual food

The discrepancy between the child's appetite and actual food consumption and the parents' expectation of what the child should eat to remain healthy creates the major nutritional problem in the preschool years.

consumption and the parents' expectation of what the child should eat to remain healthy creates the major nutritional problem in the preschool years.

In a study done more than ten years ago, Eppright and coworkers (1969) looked at the eating behavior of more than 3000 children and the concern expressed about this behavior by their mothers. Some interesting figures emerged, figures that confirm trends familiar to anyone caring for large numbers of children. Of mothers with 1-year-old children, 10% felt that their child ate too little food, while 28% of mothers with children between 3 and 4 years of age expressed anxiety about the same problem. Among the problems listed by mothers of 2- to 3-year-old children were the following: the child's food choice was too limited (40%), the child dawdled while eating (37%), the child ate too few fruits and vegetables (27%), and the child drank too little milk (20%). Many of these figures were higher among mothers of older children. No more than 5% to 6% of mothers expressed concern that their child was eating too much at any age.

Role of the Practitioner

The practitioner must try to bring parental expectations about eating more in line with reality.

Perhaps the most important role that the primary care practitioner can play in the nutrition of preschool and older children is to try to bring parental expectations more closely into line with reality. In doing this, the practitioner should keep in mind the social and cultural background of the family. In some families in which food is or was previously scarce, wasting food may be very difficult to tolerate. In other families, serving a large meal may be a traditional way for the mother to express love for her family. Many parents put unduly large portions of food on their children's plates and are then disappointed when much of the food is left uneaten. For the healthy child who is growing adequately, appetite is the best guide to food intake. Just as appetite among adults varies from season to season, day to day, and meal to meal, variation in appetite among younger children is normal and should be expected.

The approach to feeding taken by many parents probably creates some of the problems about which they complain.

The approach to feeding taken by many parents probably creates some of the problems about which they complain. From early infancy, a child's eating is a social interaction, first with its mother alone and later in the larger context of the family. Excessive parental concern with nutrient intakes may be disruptive and may overshadow the other important aspects of mealtime. The parents' use of food at times other than meals may also contribute to these problems. One study found that nearly 25% of mothers used food as a reward, while 10% of mothers used deprivation of favorite foods as punishment. Food was used to pacify an unruly child by nearly 30% of mothers. The use of foods in these ways between meals may contribute to problems during mealtimes.

In the study mentioned above, mothers were asked how they dealt with the dawdling, poor food intake, and so on, of their children. To their credit, nearly half of the mothers questioned said that they tended to ignore this kind of behavior. Another 15% said they would reason with the child or coax him or her to eat the food, a similar percentage would force the child to eat the food, and slightly more mothers would punish the child if his or her consumption did not meet their expectations.

CHILDREN'S ATTITUDES TOWARD FOOD

The attitudes that children have toward food in general and toward specific foods develop slowly over a number of years. As the child gets older, he or she begins to have some input into the diet selected either in a direct fashion or through others, primarily the mother.

Family Influences

In most families the mother is the principal influence on food selection. The factors on which she bases her selection as determined in one study are shown in Table 6-2. The food likes and dislikes of the husband, those of the family as a whole, and cost are the most important factors influencing her choice. It appears that the younger the child, the less input he or she has in choosing the foods that are served. Obviously, this varies somewhat from meal to meal. Up to the age of 6 only 2%-4% of children were found to have much say about what was served for dinner (Table 6-3). Children appear to have maximum input about what they eat for breakfast or at snack time. Even so, only about one-third of children have significant input in these areas.

Table 6-2

Table 6-3

Role of Television Advertising

One of the areas that is of increasing concern to parents and practitioners is the effect of television advertising on children in the realm of nutrition and, in particular, advertising of breakfast cereals. Recent studies indicate that the average young child watches between 3 and 4 hours of television per day on weekdays and nearly 3 hours of television on a typical Saturday morning. Manufacturers of breakfast cereals and toys seem to be the principal advertisers at the times that young children watch

Table 6-2 Factors strongly affecting meal-planning choices
for preschool children

Factors	Percent of mothers listing factor
Husband's likes	81
Likes of other family members	72
Food cost	68
Child's likes	58
Preparation time	48
Family health problems 33	33

Source: Eppright, E. S.; Fox, H. S.; Fryer, B. A., et al. 1969. Eating behavior of preschool children. *J. Nutr. Ed.* 1:16–19. (Summer). Published with permission from Society for Nutrition Education.

Table 6-3 Percentage of children allowed to make decisions about
which foods are eaten, by age and meal

Meal	Age					
	1–1½ yr	1½–2 yr	2–3 yr	3–4 yr	4–5 yr	5–6 yr
Breakfast	4.7	6.0	16.9	28.0	27.1	33.0
Noon meal	3.9	2.3	7.1	8.4	12.7	12.6
Evening meal	3.2	0	3.6	2.5	3.3	1.8
Snacks	5.7	10.6	22.3	25.5	27.2	36.5

Source: Eppright, E. S.; Fox, H. S.; Fryer, B. A., et al. 1969. Eating behavior of preschool children. *J. Nutr. Ed.* 1:16–19. (Summer). Published with permission from Society for Nutrition Education.

television. It is unlikely that the advertisers would be willing to spend the sums of money that they do if their advertisements were not to some extent effective.*

---

*None of this is meant to suggest that cereals do not have a role to play in providing a good breakfast.

Television is a potent force, but food habits are still sanctioned in the family, primarily by the mother.

Children's response to television advertisements are affected by several variables. One variable, in particular, is the child's attitude toward advertisements in general. As children get older they develop an increasing distrust of products advertised on television. The amount of time that the child watches television alone as compared with time spent viewing with a parent also appears to be important in shaping attitudes toward advertisements. In addition, it has been suggested that the frequency with which the child actually goes shopping with the mother will directly influence whether or not the child's desires are actually translated into food purchases. Mothers have reported that younger children are more likely to make requests for specific foods than are older children. Although this fact could be interpreted to mean that older children are less susceptible to food advertisements on television or that the child has stopped asking for many foods because he has learned that the mother will not respond, it could also mean that the mother of the older child has already been "trained" to purchase certain foods that the child desires. Although one should not underestimate the potential effect of food advertising on children's food habits, most studies agree that the mother is the primary person who sanctions food habits. By comparison, doctors, teachers, and other health professionals have been found to have relatively little influence. Most children internalize their mothers' views on which foods are acceptable and unacceptable, and because, in most families, the mother is the final arbiter of food purchases, there is no reason that television advertising must have a negative effect on children's diets.

NUTRITIONAL STATUS OF PRESCHOOL CHILDREN

The nutritional status of preschool children in the United States, in general, is exceptionally good. Not surprisingly, both height and weight of children in this age group correlate to some degree with socioeconomic status. However, as was pointed out in Chapter 2, the 3rd and 97th percentiles for protein intake (% protein kcal) are about the same across a wide range of family incomes, suggesting it is not differences in the overall quality of the diet that cause the correlation. Probably, the amount of food eaten is more important. Children from families of higher socioeconomic classes tend to be heavier and taller, but this does not imply that those who are shorter and weigh less are necessarily undernourished. The main nutritional problem among American children continues to be obesity, and the problem is increasing. Significant undernutrition

The main nutritional problem among American children continues to be obesity, and the problem is increasing.

in the preschool age group is an isolated finding, often associated with significant underlying disease or complex social problems.

PREADOLESCENT CHILDREN

During the years immediately before the pubertal growth spurt in both boys and girls, the rate of linear growth decreases slightly while the rate of weight gain increases. The net effect is a slight increase in total body fatness just prior to puberty. Nutrient requirements on a by-weight basis decrease slightly during these years. A wide variety of diets can meet these nutrient requirements easily. Overt nutritional problems, except in association with chronic underlying disease, are rare. Food habits are relatively well established. The child is eating an increasing proportion of meals away from home, either at school or with the families of friends. The energy, protein, and micronutrient requirements for preadolescent children are outlined in Tables 2-2, 2-7, and 2-9.

Preadolescent American children are relatively free of nutritional problems.

NUTRITIONAL REQUIREMENTS OF ADOLESCENTS

Nutrient requirements increase dramatically during adolescence. At no other time in life are the absolute needs for protein and energy higher in the male or, with the exception of pregnancy and lactation, in the female. The pubertal growth spurt begins between the ages of 10 and 12 years in girls and between 12 and 14 years in boys. The girl who was previously growing about 5.5 cm per year increases in height at the rate of 9 cm per year. The rate of weight gain increases from 2.5 kg to nearly 7.5 kg per year. Even greater changes occur in boys. For males, overall growth during adolescence contributes about 15% to final height and nearly 50% to final weight.

At no other time in life are the absolute needs for protein and energy higher in the male or, with the exception of pregnancy and lactation, in the female, than during adolescence.

Energy and Protein Requirements

There is a broad range of recommended intake of energy for both boys and girls during adolescence. Between 2000 and 3700 calories are recommended for boys between the ages of 11 and 14 years. The corresponding recommendation for girls is 1500 to 3000 calories. These recommended intake ranges are so broad because of (1) the normal variation in energy requirements among individuals of the same size, and (2) the four-year age span involved. For most children this is about the period of time during which

Figure 6-1

The practitioner must use size and stage of development, rather than chronological age, in assessing dietary intake requirements of adolescents.

Table 6-4

the growth rate in both height and weight increases rapidly and then slows down. Figure 6-1 shows velocities of height gain for five individual boys going through their pubertal growth spurt. It is clear that the general nutritional recommendations for 12- to 13-year-old boys must cover the requirements for boys growing at maximum velocity as well as the requirements for those who have not yet entered puberty. Therefore, the practitioner must use size and stage of development, rather than chronological age, in assessing the dietary intake requirements of adolescents.

Although the new Recommended Dietary Allowances give ranges for suggested energy intakes, no corresponding range is given for protein. Table 6-4 shows the percentages of energy that would be supplied from protein at the higher and lower recommended energy intakes for both boys and girls consuming the RDA for protein. Using Table 6-4, we find the recommended protein intakes very low at the higher intakes of energy. It is reasonable to assume that when the higher intakes of energy are required for rapid growth, protein intakes should also be increased. During puberty, adolescents

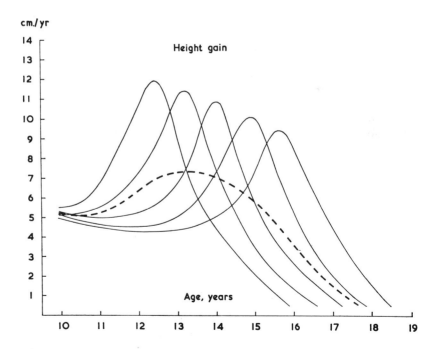

Figure 6-1 Growth velocity curves of five boys during puberty. *Source:* Tanner, J. M.; Whitehouse, R. H.; and Takaishi, M. 1966. Standards from birth to maturity for height, weight, height velocity and weight velocity: British children, 1965. Richard H. Dobbs and Douglas Gairgird, editors. *Arch. Dis. Child.* 41:454–471.

Table 6-4 Recommended energy and protein intakes during adolescence

Category	Age (years)	Weight (kg)	(lb)	Height (cm)	(in.)	Energy needs* (kcal)	Protein (g)	(% kcal)†	(Range % kcal)†
Males	11–14	45	99	157	62	2700 (2000–3700)	45	6.7	(9.0–4.9)
	15–18	66	145	176	69	2800 (2100–3900)	56	8.0	(10.7–5.7)
Females	11–14	46	101	157	62	2200 (1500–3000)	46	8.4	(12.3–6.1)
	15–18	55	120	163	64	2100 (1200–3000)	46	8.8	(15.3–6.1)

Source: Recommended Dietary Allowances, 9th ed. 1980. Reproduced with the permission of the National Academy of Sciences, Washington, D.C.

*Energy allowances for children through age 18 are based on median energy intakes of children these ages followed in longitudinal growth studies. The values in parenthesis are 10th and 90th percentiles of energy intake, to indicate the range of energy consumption among children of these ages.

†Calculated from Recommended Dietary Allowances using the median figure and the extremes for energy needs.

may eat extraordinarily large quantities of food. Because the diet consumed is relatively well balanced, increases in energy intake are virtually always accompanied by adequate increases in protein intake.

Vitamin and Mineral Requirements

The recommendations for most vitamins and minerals are higher for the adolescent than for preadolescent children. The exceptions are those for vitamins B_1, B_{12}, and D. The recommended intake of vitamin B_{12} increases during childhood but has reached its maximum before the age of onset of puberty. The requirement for vitamin D is constant from infancy to adulthood, at which time it decreases somewhat. As discussed in Chapter 2, the requirement for most vitamins and minerals will depend on total protein and energy intake and growth rate.

Because of the large increases in food intake during adolescence, there is usually no problem in meeting the increased vitamin and mineral requirements accompanying the growth spurt. The increased consumption of a qualitatively adequate diet will supply vitamins and minerals in proper proportions. Routine vitamin and mineral supplements are not required, with the possible exception of supplemental iron.

The increase in red-cell mass and muscle mass that occurs in both boys and girls during the adolescent growth spurt increases the dietary iron requirement the same amount for both sexes. As was pointed out earlier, the iron density (mg Fe/1000 kcal) of most diets is relatively constant. Because, on the average, adolescent boys consume up to 30% more calories than adolescent girls, boys are more likely to meet their iron requirements by diet alone. The adolescent girl who restricts her intake somewhat because of concerns about her weight and body image may have difficulty meeting her iron requirement during this period of time. This need not be the case if the diet provides adequate sources of heme iron—that is, meat. As growth velocity slows in boys, the requirement for iron decreases again to a preadolescent level. At the time of menarche in girls, iron requirements for menstruation supplant those for growth. For this reason, there is no decrease in the iron requirement for teenage girls following puberty. The decrease in dietary intake that occurs following the cessation of growth in the girl makes it more difficult to meet iron needs from diet alone. There are also problems in meeting iron requirements of children being raised as vegetarians; these are discussed in Chapter 7.

Because, on the average, adolescent boys consume up to 30% more calories than adolescent girls, boys are more likely to meet their iron requirements by diet alone.

Factors Affecting Food Intake

The marked changes in physical appearance that occur during puberty are accompanied by marked changes in mental attitude. With the acquisition of secondary sex characteristics, a reappraisal of self-image occurs. In addition to the adjustments occurring within the individual there is a gradual and often turbulent redefinition of roles and relationships with both parents and peers. A full treatment of the difficulties of the adolescent and the difficulties of caring for the adolescent are beyond the scope of this discussion. Both peer pressure and change in self-image do, however, affect the amounts and kinds of foods that adolescents will eat.

Both peer pressure and change in self-image affect the amounts and kinds of foods that adolescents will eat.

The eating habits of teenagers are unquestionably erratic. Breakfast may often be missed. Snacking is a way of life. Many of the popular snack foods—pizza and hamburgers, for example—are clearly nutritious. Soft drinks and candy are less so but probably pose their biggest threat to dental rather than to overall health. Of perhaps greatest concern is the amount of dieting among teenagers, boys for athletics such as wrestling and, more frequently, girls for general body image.

Dwyer and her coworkers (1969) studied the attitudes of Boston high school seniors toward their weight and overall

Table 6-5

appearance. Both boys and girls were asked what they actually weighed. They were also asked what their proper weight should be—that is, what they thought they ought to weigh for health reasons. Finally, each subject was asked to give a desired weight— that is, what he or she would like to weigh, if possible. Table 6-5 summarizes the responses. On the average, girls reported their weight to be about 4 lb higher than what they thought their proper weight for health should be. When responses from girls were grouped by body fatness of the individuals, only girls in the lean category had expressed a desired weight higher than their reported weight, and this difference was about 1½ lb. The trend was opposite in boys. On the average, most boys thought they should weigh and wanted to weigh more than they actually did. Only boys classified as obese had any desire to lose weight. Both boys and girls were shown silhouette drawings of different body types and were asked to indicate which silhouette was most masculine and which was most feminine. Girls had a much narrower view of which female body type connoted femininity than did boys. Similarly, boys had a narrower view than girls did of which body type connoted masculinity. Although this study did not address food preferences or intakes, it is clear from other experience that satisfaction or, more frequently, dissatisfaction with one's weight and overall appearance is a potent factor in food selection by teenagers. Perhaps the teenage girl who develops anorexia nervosa may simply be manifesting in an extreme way a feeling that is nearly universal among adolescent girls. (Anorexia nervosa is discussed in Chapter 10.)

Satisfaction or, more frequently, dissatisfaction with one's weight and overall appearance is a potent factor in food selection by teenagers.

Table 6-5 Attitudes toward weight by high-school seniors*

Characteristics	Girls	Boys
Age (yr)	17.4 ± 0.4	17.6 ± 0.6
Stature (cm)	162.6 ± 6.0	175.6 ± 6.6
Weight (kg)	57.4 ± 9.0	69.9 ± 11.8
Proper weight (kg)	52.4 ± 4.8	72.1 ± 8.7
Desired weight (kg)	53.9 ± 4.9	71.5 ± 7.5

Source: Dwyer, J. T.; Feldman, J. J.; Seltzer, C. C., et al. 1969. Adolescent attitudes toward weight and appearance. *J. Nutr. Ed.* 1:14-19 (Fall). Published with the permission from Society for Nutrition Education.

*Students were asked what they weighed ("weight"), what they thought they should weigh ("Proper weight") and what they would like to weigh ("Desired weight").

"JUNK FOOD"

The term "junk food" has many different connotations. For some people it is synonomous with "empty calories." For others it is equated with hamburgers, french fries, and milkshakes, especially if bought at a fast-food franchise. As a rule the term "junk food" is used to refer to any food that an individual does not consider nutritious. The unfortunate use of this term probably results in many foods that are perfectly acceptable in reasonable quantity and proportion being branded as unacceptable. Since most of the foods in question are foods consumed with great relish by teenagers, so-called junk food becomes a source of conflict between adolescents and their parents. For this reason, some comments concerning this kind of food are in order.

The term "junk food" is used to refer to any food that an individual does not consider nutritious. The unfortunate use of this term probably results in many foods that are perfectly acceptable in reasonable quantity and proportion being branded as unacceptable.

Nutritional Value

The nutritional value of foods served in franchised fast-food restaurants is frequently questioned, and it is to these foods that the term "junk food" is most frequently applied. There is no question that Americans are eating more and more meals away from home. It has been estimated that 50% of the food dollar in 1980 was captured by the food-service industry. About 20% of this share belonged to fast-food franchises. Some of the concerns expressed about the nutritional value of these foods involve questions of protein adequacy, fat content, and the adequacy of amounts of certain vitamins, notably vitamins A and C. It is worthwhile to examine these concerns one by one.

Nutrient analyses are not available for all fast-food chains. In some instances where nutrient information is available, it has been calculated from food composition tables based on usual serving size. For our analysis we have used data provided by an independent food-testing laboratory that was contracted to sample and analyze foods from one fast-food franchise in seven different locations around the United States (Table 6-6).

Table 6-6

The concern that protein intake from these foods is inadequate seems unfounded. The average hamburger or cheeseburger contains about 420 calories, between 20% and 25% of these being provided by protein, most of which is animal protein. When sample meals such as hamburger, french fries, and milkshake were fed to rats, the PER value was approximately 2.4, compared with a casein reference of 2.5.

Whether or not fat intake is excessive depends greatly on the types of food chosen. A sample calculation of a quarter-pound hamburger with french fries and a chocolate milkshake shows that

Table 6-6 Selected nutrients in a meal made up of a Quarter Pounder®, french fries, and a chocolate shake

Food item	Energy (kcal)	Protein (% kcal)	Fat (% kcal)	Carbohydrate (% kcal)	Iron (% RDA)	Calcium (% RDA)	Vitamin C (% RDA)
Quarter Pounder® hamburger	424	23	46	31	23	6	—
French fries	220	5	47	48	3	—	21
Chocolate shake	383	10	21	69	5	33	5
Total	1027	14	37	49	31	39	26

Source: Raltech Scientific Services (formerly WARF Institute, Inc.) 1980. *Nutritional analysis of food served at McDonald's restaurants.* McDonald's System, Inc. Reprinted courtesy of McDonald's Corporation.

approximately 37% of the 1027 calories consumed would be supplied by fat. This fat intake is not excessive. The concern about vitamin A intake is well-founded. None of the usual foods eaten contain large amounts of preformed retinol or carotenes. Vitamin C content, however, appears to be adequate. Potatoes are quantitatively a good source of vitamin C. A regular order of french fries provides approximately 21% of the USRDA for ascorbic acid and twice as much as is needed on a daily basis to prevent scurvy.

Perhaps the most compelling criticism of fast-food franchises is the narrow variety of food choices that they offer. Recently some franchises have begun to introduce salad bars, which at least offer patrons the opportunity to improve the vitamin content of meals eaten there. It is unlikely, however, that teenage boys will flock to the salad bar.

Few unfranchised restaurants are able to provide information on nutrient contents of the foods they serve. Probably much of the food served in fast-food franchises is no less nutritious than that served in other restaurants. It is quite likely that a meal eaten at a fast-food franchise would be superior to the "meal" that many teenagers would prepare at home, left to their own devices. A number of school lunch programs around the country have begun to use fast-food franchises with great success. Their use is based on the premise that the least nutritious meal is the one left uneaten.

The least nutritious meal is the one left uneaten.

Appropriate Place in the Diet

In most instances, there is no nutritional justification for the term "junk food." While there is a valid concern for the narrow variety of foods chosen by teenagers eating in fast-food restaurants, this narrow choice is more a function of the adolescent than of the foods offered. Consuming several meals a week outside the home in fast-food restaurants should present no nutritional problem to the teenager who has a reasonable diet at home.

Suggested Reading

Clancy-Hepburn, K.; Hickey, A. A.; and Nevill, G. 1974. Children's behavior responses to TV food advertisements. *J. Nutr. Ed.* 6:93–96.

Dwyer, J. T.; Feldman, J. J.; Seltzer, C. C.; and Mayer, J. 1969. Adolescent attitudes toward weight and appearance. *J. Nutr. Ed.* 1:14–19 (Fall).

Eppright, E. S.; Fox, H. M.; Fryer, B. A., et al. 1969. Eating behavior of preschool children. *J. Nutr. Ed.* 1:16–19 (Summer).

Hinton, M. A.; Eppright, E. S.; Chadderdon, H.; and Wolnis, L. 1963. Eating behavior and dietary intake of girls 12–14 years old. *J. Am. Diet. Assn.* 43:223–227.

Litman, T. J.; Cooney, J. P.; and Stief, R. 1964. The views of Minnesota schoolchildren on food. *J. Am. Diet. Assn.* 45:433–440.

Raltech Scientific Services, Inc. 1980. *Nutritional analysis of food served at McDonald's restaurants.* Oakbrook, Ill. McDonald's Corporation.

Young, E. A.; Brennan, E. H.; and Irving, G. L. 1978. Perspectives on fast foods. *Dietetic Currents* 5:23–30.

7 Vegetarianism in Children

Contents

Factors Affecting Vegetarianism   133

Types of Vegetarianism   134

Lacto-ovovegetarians   134

Lactovegetarians   134

Pure Vegetarians   134

Nutritional Problems in Vegetarianism   135

Energy, Protein, and Growth   136

Vitamin Intake   139

Mineral Intake   141

Zen Macrobiotics   143

Dietary Regimens and Their Adequacy   143

Nutritional Problems in Zen Macrobiotic Children   144

Management of the Vegetarian Child   145

Dealing with Parental Beliefs   146

Specific Dietary Recommendations   146

Natural Foods, Organic Foods, and Megavitamins   147

Natural Foods   147

Organic Foods   148

Megavitamin Therapy   149

Overview

Vegetarianism is compatible with good nutrition, though there are more problems for the growing child than for the vegetarian adult. Energy intakes *and growth may be a problem because of the bulkiness and low fat content of the diet. There are often inadequacies of vitamin B_{12} and vitamin D in vegetarian diets. Zen macrobiotics in its most strict forms permits too narrow a range of foods to allow adequate nutrition, particularly in children but even in adults. Managing vegetarian children requires a knowledge of the principles of good nutrition and an acceptance of the parents' decision to raise their child as a vegetarian. Natural and organic foods often play a role in these diets and the practitioner should be familiar with them.*

FACTORS AFFECTING VEGETARIANISM

Primary care practitioners and nutritionists are in agreement that the number of adults, and consequently their children, who are following vegetarian regimens is increasing. It is impossible to estimate how many people will adopt vegetarianism. There is no question that the increased number of reports of complications associated with improper vegetarian diets is increasing. Food habits are difficult to change. Vegetarians have made a conscious commitment to alter their diets. It is paradoxical that those seemingly most interested in nutrition are not infrequently subject to the complications of improper diet.

Vegetarianism and good nutrition are not incompatible. Because the vegetarian's range of food choices is narrower and because vegetarianism involves the proscription of high-quality animal protein and the quantities of fat that accompany it, assuring an adequate diet is more difficult for the vegetarian than for the omnivore. Caring for the vegetarian child presents a particular challenge for the practitioner. Until the pubertal growth spurt, the younger the child, the higher the nutrient requirements associated with growth. The smaller capacity of the child's intestinal tract makes it more difficult to meet many of these needs with the low energy density and reduced digestibility of foods of vegetable origins. In practical terms, the practitioner will often be dealing with a set of young parents for whom vegetarianism may be only one of many precepts that depart from tradition. Their views on non-nutritional health-related matters may require the practitioner to alter his or her approach to a variety of problems associated with the general care of children. It is important to realize that these views are sincerely held and that vegetarianism is a more difficult but nevertheless normal way of nourishing a child.

Vegetarian parents may have a variety of unorthodox views on health care practices that affect their child's well-being.

TYPES OF VEGETARIANISM

Vegetarian diets are usually classified according to the strictness with which animal foods are excluded from the diet.

Lacto-ovovegetarians

Lacto-ovovegetarians generally eat no flesh of any kind but are not adverse to drinking milk or eating eggs. Although the range of animal foods accepted by the lacto-ovovegetarian is quite narrow, in a strict nutritional sense this person has a mixed diet. The nutritional problems associated with more strict vegetarianism are virtually unheard of in lacto-ovovegetarians who eat a reasonable amount of milk, cheese, or eggs.

The nutritional problems associated with more strict vegetarianism are virtually unheard of in lacto-ovovegetarians who eat a reasonable amount of milk, cheese, or eggs.

Lactovegetarians

Some vegetarians proscribe eggs in addition to meat. These are *lactovegetarians*. Lactovegetarians are also relatively free of nutritional problems. A careful inquiry into the foods eaten by many children in nonvegetarian families would probably lead one to conclude that many American children are for all intents and purposes lactovegetarians or lacto-ovovegetarians who occasionally eat a small amount of meat.

Pure Vegetarians

Pure vegetarians will eat only foods of vegetable origin. Pure vegetarians are sometimes referred to as *vegans*. The term vegan is probably better reserved for a subset of pure vegetarians that carries its proscription of the use of animal products beyond the realm of nutrition per se. Veganism is a philosophy that rejects, wherever possible, the use of any product of animal origin. Synthetic fibers, for example, are used in place of wool for sweaters. Imitation leather is used for shoes, purses, and other such articles. A vegan society exists in Britain; we are not aware of a similar organization in the United States.

Although classification of vegetarian diets by type is useful in approaching vegetarianism from a nutritional point of view, it is imperfect in that many vegetarians do not fall strictly into one category or another. Many vegetarians do not distinguish in their own minds among lacto-ovovegetarianism, lactovegetarianism, and pure vegetarianism. For this reason, the simple declaration that the child is being raised as a vegetarian does not provide complete information. In addition, some vegetarians will eat, for example,

Many vegetarians do not fall strictly into one category or another.

fish and chicken but not red meats. They may or may not drink milk. This variety is easily explained; most people do not decide to become lactovegetarian or lacto-ovovegetarian. Depending on the reasons for espousing vegetarianism, they usually begin by cutting red meat out of the diet. Frequently there follows an evolution to stricter forms of vegetarianism. As a practical matter, then, the practitioner must be willing to invest some time initially to learn the food habits of the vegetarian family, and he or she should be aware of the need to update this information from time to time to be certain that foods that were previously eaten have not been removed from the diet.

The practitioner must be willing to invest some time initially to learn the food habits of the vegetarian family, and he or she should be aware of the need to update this information.

NUTRITIONAL PROBLEMS IN VEGETARIANISM

This section deals with both theoretical and reported nutritional problems in vegetarian children. Because of the rarity of nutritional problems among children and adults with even a modest intake of animal protein, discussion will be directed primarily at the problems encountered in pure vegetarianism. As might be imagined, the infant who is breast-fed has relatively few problems during the early months of life, with the possible exception of vitamin B_{12} deficiency, which is treated later in this chapter. Clinical problems become apparent in vegetarian children, as with most children showing nutritional problems, shortly after weaning, when lower density, relatively indigestible foods are substituted for high-density human milk. Occasionally excessively prolonged exclusive breast-feeding may result in problems, but these are no different in vegetarian than in nonvegetarian children. The problems of vegetarian children can be categorized as those surrounding the adequacy of energy and protein intakes and their effect on growth, those involving the adequacy of vitamin nutriture, and those related to mineral, especially iron, nutrition (Table 7-1).

Table 7-1

Table 7-1 Potential dietary problems in vegetarian children

Dietary factors that may be inadequate	Cause of inadequacy
Energy	Bulk, indigestibility, low fat content
Protein	Indigestibility, amino acid imbalance
Vitamin B_{12}	No known vegetable sources
Vitamin D	Endogenous production not sufficient
Iron	Possibly lower intake, decreased bioavailability

Energy, Protein, and Growth

Energy intake The importance of adequate energy intake in the efficient utilization of all nutrients was stressed in Chapter 2. Based on the increasing prevalence of obesity among younger children in the United States, we can conclude that energy is rarely the limiting factor in the nutritional health of American children. Meeting the energy requirement of a vegetarian child, however, is made difficult by the bulk of the diet, its relative indigestibility, and its generally low fat content.

Vegetarian diets tend to be bulky; that is, their energy density is relatively low. The values for the energy density of strained fruits and vegetables given in Table 5-4 are similar to those for the fresh products. In addition, many of the foods of the vegetarian diet, such as rice and other cereals, physically occupy a large amount of space relative to the energy they contain. This makes them extremely filling. The young child, and even the adult, will generally reach a point of satiety before energy requirements have been met by these foods.

The problem of bulkiness is compounded by the relatively lower digestibility of vegetable products. The cellulose in vegetables is indigestible by humans. In addition, many of the starches may be incompletely digested, especially by younger infants. An emphasis on "natural" foods by many vegetarians frequently results in the feeding of whole-grain and undermilled products, which are even less digestible.

The consumption of animal protein is normally accompanied by consumption of large amounts of fat. Because of its high energy density (9 kcal/g), fat is an important energy source. All vegetarian diets will be low in fat intake unless a specific effort is made to counteract this by using vegetable oils and other separated fats. Although essential-fatty-acid deficiency has not been reported to be a problem among vegetarian children, their relatively low fat intakes make it more difficult to provide adequate dietary energy.

Protein intake Practitioners not knowledgeable in nutrition often voice concern about the adequacy of protein intake in vegetarian diets. The protein content of a number of common foods is shown in Table 7-2. Notice that meat is at the top of the list but that human milk is at the bottom. The quantity of protein in the diet of vegetarians is generally not a problem. However, protein quality is a potential problem. The relative deficiency of at least one essential amino acid in all vegetable proteins was discussed in Chapter 2. For example, cereals (rice, wheat, barley, and so on) are relatively deficient in lysine but are good sources of methionine. Legumes,

---

Margin notes:

Bulk, low fat content, and indigestibility make it hard for vegetarians to meet dietary energy requirements.

All vegetarian diets will be low in fat intake unless a specific effort is made to counteract this by using vegetable oils and other separated fats.

Table 7-2

The quantity of protein in the diet of vegetarians is generally not a problem. However, protein quality is a potential problem.

Table 7-2 Protein content of selected foods of animal and vegetable origin

Food	Protein (% of total kcal)
Beef	68
Egg	30
Legumes	20-25
Cow milk	20
Wheat	10-15
Potato	6-9
Rice	7-8
Human milk	6

Table 7-3 Complementarity of vegetable proteins

Food	Amino acid level	
	Methionine	Lysine
Legumes	low	high
Cereals	high	low

Table 7-3

Relative indigestibility of vegetable foods reduces vegetable protein availability as much as or more than it does energy availability.

quantitatively a good source of vegetable protein, provide adequate amounts of lysine but are deficient in methionine (Table 7-3). As long as cereals and legumes complement each other in the diet, overall amino acid balance should not be a problem.

Relative digestibility of vegetable foods reduces vegetable protein availability as much as or more than it does energy availability. Depending on the cereal and the degree to which it is processed, children digest cereal protein only 70% to 90% as efficiently as animal protein. The limited data available to date suggest that nitrogen absorption from legumes may fall at the lower end of this 70% to 90% range, depending on processing or preparation. The lower quality of vegetable protein, coupled with its relative indigestibility, means that protein intakes must be quantitatively higher if protein requirements are to be met. Whereas 8% of total energy as animal protein is sufficient for nearly all children, pure vegetarians need to take in 11% or 12% of total energy as vegetable protein. The currently marketed soy-based formulas, for example, all contain 11% or more of energy as protein. Because the soy protein isolates used in these formulas are highly digestible and are supplemented with methionine to improve quality, soy-based formulas provide more than enough protein.

Growth Few comprehensive studies of the growth of vegetarian children exist. Those data that have been published are sometimes difficult to interpret because data for lactovegetarians and lacto-ovovegetarians are mixed with those for pure vegetarians. The general impression that one gains from such studies and from experience, however, is that vegetarian children tend to grow more slowly than omnivorous children. While it is conceivable that this slower growth might result from micronutrient deficiency, the lack of specific signs of such deficiencies points instead to an inadequacy of either energy or protein or both. Adults who become vegetarians frequently report substantial weight loss during the changeover to a vegetarian diet. The poor growth of vegetarian children may be a parallel phenomenon related to low energy intake. Some data have suggested that the addition of animal protein to the diet of vegetarian children produces more rapid growth. Because an increase in energy intake must have accompanied this change, one cannot be certain whether it was the protein per se or the additional energy that caused the improvement.

From a clinical point of view, the difficult problem is not to determine whether energy deficiency or protein deficiency is primarily responsible for a slower growth rate but to decide at what point intervention becomes necessary. In the section on the assessment of nutritional status (see Chapter 1), we stressed the fact that growth curves are a statistical representation of the growth of children and do not necessarily carry health significance for an individual child. Consequently, the fact that a vegetarian child might be tracking the 3rd or 10th percentile is not incontrovertible evidence that the diet is inadequate. In this regard, it is important to differentiate conceptually between adequate growth and maximal growth. While it is unlikely that most younger vegetarian children will be growing at the maximal rate achievable with a mixed diet, their growth rate may be entirely acceptable to both the parents and the physician. Such is usually the case when the child has relatively normal height but is lean. On the other hand, the short child who is growing steadily may be of concern to the practitioner, although the parents may not share this concern. The practitioner should make the parents aware that growth of most vegetarian children, especially during late infancy and the toddler years, is

Vegetarian children tend to grow more slowly than omnivorous children.

The difficult problem is not to determine whether energy deficiency or protein deficiency is primarily responsible for a slower growth rate but to decide at what point intervention becomes necessary.

less than maximal. Whether catch-up growth occurs later in childhood has not been studied.

Vitamin Intake

Fruits and vegetables are generally perceived as good sources of vitamins. Citrus fruits are known for their content of vitamin C. Cereals, especially when fortified, are good sources of the B vitamins. Although retinol (vitamin A) is found only in foods of animal origin, the carotenes are vegetable counterparts with vitamin A activity. Thus most vitamins will be available in more than adequate quantities in vegetarian diets. There are two striking exceptions, however. Both vitamin B_{12} and vitamin D requirements are difficult, if not impossible, to meet in pure vegetarian diets.

Vitamin B_{12} As mentioned previously, there are no vegetable sources of vitamin B_{12}. Although there is some evidence that vitamin B_{12} can be synthesized by bacteria in the colon and it has been suggested that the vitamin B_{12} intake of vegetarians living in unsanitary environments may be larger than would be suggested, due to bacterial contamination of their food supply, the quantitative importance of these sources is questionable. Vitamin B_{12} is effectively stored in liver and muscle, making meat a good source of the vitamin. Egg yolk contains moderate amounts of B_{12}, while fluid milk has somewhat less B_{12} than most meats. Vegetarians frequently rely on brewer's yeast as a source of B_{12}. Most brewer's yeast sold in health food stores is fortified with B_{12}. However, brewer's yeast alone is not a reliable source of the vitamin.

There is a very effective enterohepatic recirculation of vitamin B_{12}. As a result, a vitamin-B_{12}-deficient diet can be consumed for years without apparent problems if stores were adequate previously. This is probably the reason that most adults in the United States do not experience problems for some time after they convert to vegetarianism.

Vitamin B_{12} levels in breast milk are similar to those in maternal plasma. Consequently, the infant who is breast-fed by a pure-vegetarian mother may be at risk for developing vitamin B_{12} deficiency. If the mother has only recently begun to follow vegetarian principles, she is likely to have adequate vitamin B_{12} stores. If, however, she has been a vegetarian for many years and has shunned vitamin supplements, she will probably produce milk low in vitamin B_{12} content. Nursing is one of the factors known to increase the overt manifestations of vitamin B_{12} deficiency in women with marginal vitamin B_{12} status. Ideally, all nursing mothers should be supplemented with vitamin B_{12}. If any question

A vitamin-B_{12}-deficient diet can be consumed for years without apparent problems if stores were adequate previously.

The infant who is breast-fed by a pure-vegetarian mother may be at risk for developing vitamin B_{12} deficiency.

of vitamin B_{12} inadequacy remains, the infant should be supplemented as well.

The older vegetarian child is also at risk for vitamin B_{12} deficiency. Unlike the adult who has switched from an omnivorous to a vegetarian diet, the vegetarian child may have received no animal protein, with the possible exception of human milk, since birth. We would expect the lack of previous animal protein, coupled with the requirements attendant to growth, to make the child particularly vulnerable. Interestingly, although there are many studies documenting the poor vitamin B_{12} status of vegetarian adults, there are no data for children. Nor are there large numbers of case reports of documented vitamin B_{12} deficiency in vegetarian children. It may be that vitamin B_{12} deficiency is going unrecognized, or the lack of apparent problems may reflect a willingness of parents to give vitamin supplements to vegetarian children.

Vitamin D and rickets   Although vitamin D is not found to any extent in vegetable foods, the potential for endogenous production of vitamin D makes it theoretically possible for the vegetarian child to maintain an adequate vitamin D status in the absence of exogenous intake. Practice differs considerably from theory. Although sunlight in tropical areas might be sufficient to maintain adequate vitamin D production in light-skinned children, in more temperate areas and for children with darker skin, exposure to sunlight is inadequate for sufficient vitamin D production. This is especially true in urban areas where smog further filters out ultraviolet radiation. In a survey of nonvegetarian children in Greece, which is at about the same latitude as Washington, D. C., 15% of infants examined during late winter and early spring had biochemical evidence of rickets. None had been receiving supplements of vitamin D. The disease was not found to be less prevalent in children who had had considerable exposure to sunlight. One survey of vitamin D intakes by vegetarian children in Boston documented that 15% of children were receiving less than 100 IU of vitamin D per day. Many of the children whose intakes did approach the RDA of 400 IU were being given vitamin supplements, and some were lactovegetarians.

Increasing numbers of cases of overt rickets in vegetarian children are being reported in the pediatric literature. Most frequently affected are black inner-city children whose parents are following vegetarian diets out of religious conviction. Typically, cases of rickets are identified because of fractures, bowing of the legs, or other classical skeletal deformities. More serious

> Some exogenous supply of vitamin D is needed for almost all vegetarian children.

> Increasing numbers of cases of overt rickets in vegetarian children are being reported.

manifestations such as tetany and overt convulsions have also been the presenting problem in some cases.

The infant of vegetarian parents should be supplemented with vitamin D from the very beginning. As was discussed in Chapter 3, the vitamin D activity in the aqueous fraction of human milk cannot be relied upon to meet the infant's vitamin D requirements. For the older child, if a commercial vitamin-D-fortified soy-based formula is used to provide a substantial proportion of the child's protein and energy needs, vitamin D intake may be adequate without additional supplementation. The formula is likely to be the only source of vitamin D, however, and as a progressively larger percentage of dietary requirements are met from solid foods, another source of exogenous vitamin D must be assured. For this reason, the prudent approach is to supplement all vegetarian children with a preparation containing vitamin D.

The prudent approach is to supplement all vegetarian children with a preparation containing vitamin D.

Mineral Intake

Calcium and iron intakes are the two principal areas of concern in the mineral nutriture of the vegetarian. Virtually all of the other major minerals are present in adequate quantities in vegetable sources.

Table 7–4

Calcium   Most people find it difficult to name a dietary source of calcium other than milk. As shown in Table 7–4, a variety of green vegetables, such as kale, spinach, and turnip greens, contain large amounts of calcium. They also contain substantial quantities of fiber, phytate, and oxalate, all of which may form insoluble complexes with calcium, thereby decreasing its bioavailability. Although some studies have suggested that low calcium intake may be a problem in vegetarians, most nutritionists feel that calcium intakes will be adequate to meet requirements as long as vitamin D status is normal.

Iron   Like calcium intake, iron nutriture must be thought of in terms of both quantity and bioavailability. Iron intake for most individuals varies with energy intake, because the iron density (mg/1000 kcal) of the diet is relatively constant. The iron content of several vegetable foods is shown in Table 7–4. In general, the iron density of vegetarian diets is not substantially lower than that of omnivore diets. Because of the bulkiness of vegetarian diets, however, the decreased energy intake by vegetarian children will be accompanied by a decrease in iron intake. Added to this is the fact that the iron consumed will be in a less bioavailable form. Iron from animal

The decreased energy intake by vegetarian children will be accompanied by a decrease in iron intake, and the iron consumed will be in a less bioavailable form.

Table 7-4 Calcium and iron content of selected foods

Food source	Mineral content (mg per 100 g food source)	
	Calcium	Iron
Egg	54	2.3
Milk		
Cow	137	0.05
Human	27	0.05
Almonds	234	4.7
Greens		
Collard	250	1.5
Turnip	246	1.8
Kale	249	2.7
Lentils	79	6.8
Raisins	62	3.5
Seaweed (kelp)	1093	—
Sesame seeds	1160	10.5
Soybean		
Curd (tofu)	128	1.9
Flour (full-fat)	199	8.4
Formula (commercial)	150	12.4
Spinach	93	3.1
Sunflower seeds	120	7.1

Source: Watt, B. K.; and Merrill, A. L. 1963. *Composition of foods. Agricultural Handbook No. 8*, U. S. Department of Agriculture, Agricultural Research Service.

sources is present predominantly as heme iron, the absorption of which is affected little or not at all by other dietary constituents. In contrast, iron from vegetable sources is present as ferrous and ferric forms in organic iron complexes. The absorption of non-heme iron is markedly depressed by phytates and vegetable fiber.

No studies of the iron status of vegetarian children are available. Because of the possibility of inadequate iron nutriture in these children, this aspect of their care deserves careful scrutiny. A daily maintenance dose of ferrous sulfate providing 10 to 15 mg of elemental iron per day may be desirable.

ZEN MACROBIOTICS

A careful inquiry into the actual dietary practices of the vegetarian family is particularly important in the case of Zen macrobiotics. People who follow Zen macrobiotics consider themselves vegetarians. In the more liberal form of the diet, 25% to 30% of total calories are provided by foods of animal origin. In its most restrictive form, only cereals, predominantly brown rice, are eaten, making it an inadequate diet for both adults and children. Adherents of Zen macrobiotics generally vary the diet depending on their state of health, time of year, and so on.

Dietary Regimens and Their Adequacy

The Zen macrobiotic regimens are said to be based on principles of diet followed by Zen Buddhist monks and brought to this country by George Ohsawa. There are ten dietary regimens, shown in Table 7-5. Diets are numbered from minus three to plus seven. Diets with negative numbers are considered by Zen macrobiotics adherents to be unhealthful for prolonged consumption. The higher the number of the diet followed, according to the proponents, the more healthful the diet. People beginning the Zen macrobiotic diet are exhorted to start with diet number seven, which is 100% cereal. Ideally, brown rice would be the cereal eaten because of the purported balance of potassium (yin) and sodium (yang) in brown rice. Brown rice is said to have a potassium to sodium ratio of 5:1; in Zen macrobiotics this is considered the ideal ratio for all diets. After consuming diet number seven for a period of days, the adherent may regress to a lower level, choosing foods so as to maintain the 5:1 yin:yang balance if possible, or discovering a new ratio that results in a better sense of health. Tables that provide the "yinness" or "yangness" of individual foods are available. Most people following Zen macrobiotic regimens probably consume diets represented by levels three to six—that is, strict vegetarian diets. A return to level seven is suggested during any illness. It is interesting that although the adult is counseled to drink liquids sparingly, some of the Zen macrobiotic literature teaches that children need less salt and more liquid.

Integral to Zen macrobiotics is the concept of natural foods. Fruits and vegetables that are artificially grown with the use of inorganic fertilizers or insecticides are avoided. Fruits and vegetables

Marginal notes:

A careful inquiry into the actual dietary practices of the vegetarian family is particularly important in the case of Zen macrobiotics.

Table 7-5

Foods are selected to balance yin and yang.

Integral to Zen macrobiotics is the concept of natural foods.

Table 7-5 Zen macrobiotic dietary regimens

Regimen number	Cereals	Vegetables	Soup	Animal products	Fruits, salads	Desserts	Drinking liquid
7	100%						sparingly
6	90%	10%					sparingly
5	80%	20%					sparingly
4	70%	20%	10%				sparingly
3	60%	30%	10%				sparingly
2	50%	30%	10%	10%			sparingly
1	40%	30%	10%	20%			sparingly
−1	30%	30%	10%	20%	10%		sparingly
−2	20%	30%	10%	25%	10%	5%	sparingly
−3	10%	30%	10%	30%	15%	5%	sparingly

Source: Abehsera, M. 1968. *Zen macrobiotic cooking.* Copyright © 1968 by Michael Abehsera. Published by arrangement with Lyle Stuart.

out of season are also avoided. Foods that are subjected to processing—including milling, canning, and, in some instances, pasteurization—are also avoided whenever possible. The preference for unprocessed foods makes it even more difficult to provide adequate amounts of protein and energy, a problem already discussed for other vegetarians.

Zen macrobiotics in its less strict form is compatible with health. Although the family may place an undue emphasis on certain types of natural or health foods, the inclusion of up to 30% of calories from animal sources provides a well-balanced diet. Individuals eating only from the higher levels will have all of the problems previously discussed for pure vegetarians; eating only from the highest level is incompatible with good health.

The highest level of Zen macrobiotics is incompatible with good health.

Nutritional Problems in Zen Macrobiotic Children

In large part, children being raised on Zen macrobiotic diets account for the increased number of nutritional problems among vegetarian children in recent years. Although breast-feeding is common, exclusive breast-feeding is not prolonged in many instances. Solid food or other "milks" may be introduced as early as 1 to 3 months of age. A word about Zen macrobiotic weaning foods is in order. Zen macrobiotic parents will often report that the child is receiving "soy milk" in addition to breast milk. Because of the distrust of processing, many of these soy milks are prepared at home by grinding soybeans and mixing them with water. The white fluid that results when the bean particles are strained out is called milk but has little nutritive value. Similar milks from almonds are also used on occasion. Another infant food is kokoh, which is apparently a mixture of whole grains and flours such as rice, wheat, and sesame. Brown rice and other vegetables, frequently raw, are also given to infants under the age of 6 months.

Both marked marasmus and kwashiorkor, in some instances severe enough to result in death, have been reported in infants fed macrobiotic diets. Severe megaloblastic anemia, hypoproteinemia, hyponatremia, and rickets have been reported. Studies of older children who are growing up in macrobiotic households have suggested a slower growth rate, as well as, in many instances, inadequate intakes of vitamin D. Many parents follow Zen macrobiotic regimens as part of a larger set of religious teachings of a sect to which they belong. Whenever a Zen macrobiotic infant or child presents with clinical nutritional problems, other children of the same religious group should be examined if possible. In many instances, it may be possible to work with the group to establish a dietary regimen that ensures that the children's requirements are met without violating the convictions of the families.

Marked marasmus and kwashiorkor, in some instances severe enough to result in death, have been reported in infants fed macrobiotic diets.

MANAGEMENT OF THE VEGETARIAN CHILD

We pointed out at the beginning of this chapter that caring for the vegetarian child requires an understanding of the parents' beliefs. Important to this understanding is knowledge of the reasons given by adults for espousing vegetarianism. Health, ethical, and metaphysical reasons lead the list, accounting for about 75% of responses. Economic, religious, and political beliefs and ecological concerns are also mentioned. For many vegetarians the desire to use diet as a means of improving health is consistent with attitudes toward other aspects of medical care. Dwyer et al (1974) found that only 26% of vegetarians would use medication prescribed by a physician. A survey of English vegans documented that only 9% approved of immunizations and only 38% would sanction a blood transfusion, compared with figures of 91% and 97%, respectively, in the general population. Data such as these indicate that a

A variety of nonnutritional practices among vegetarians may affect the child's health, well-being, and response to medical treatment as much as the food he or she eats.

variety of nonnutritional practices among vegetarians may affect the child's health, well-being, and response to medical treatment as much as the food he or she eats.

Dealing with Parental Beliefs

Of prime importance in the management of vegetarian children is the acceptance of the sincerity of the parents' beliefs. Little is to be gained by arguing that a vegetarian diet is inherently unhealthful, because, in principle, this is not correct. A more effective approach is to identify the actual dietary pattern of the family and child and to try to modify it to ensure adequate nutrition. The following is a list of principles of management to be considered:

1. Accept the parent's decision to embrace vegetarianism.
2. Encourage prolonged breast-feeding.
3. Convert infants to a lactovegetarian diet whenever possible, and suggest feeding cow milk or commercial soy-based formula.
4. Encourage use of *milled* cereals and grains whenever possible.
5. Advise vitamin supplements: B_{12} and D.
6. Advise iron supplement.
7. Maintain in traditional health-care system.

Specific Dietary Recommendations

During infancy prolonged exclusive breast-feeding is optimal. A minimum of six months without the addition of solid foods is desirable, as it is for all infants. If the infant's linear growth and weight gain are acceptable, there is no reason not to continue exclusive breast-feeding for additional months. Because lactovegetarians, in general, have fewer problems than those following stricter vegetarian regimens, breast-feeding through the end of the first year should be encouraged even after other foods have been added.

The weaned infant should be converted, if possible, to a lactovegetarian diet.

The weaned infant should be converted, if possible, to a lactovegetarian diet. In many cases parents will be content to continue cow milk in the diet. In those who follow strict vegetarianism, a *commercial* soy-based formula will provide the child with essentially the same nutrients a lactovegetarian diet would. Some parents may recoil from the suggestion of using a processed formula, preferring instead to use a homemade soy milk, as discussed previously. Because commercial soy formulas are a good source not only of readily digested protein but also of vitamins and minerals, every effort should be made to persuade the parents to accept this compromise.

The importance of cereal-legume combinations in meeting the protein requirements of vegetarians has been explained. Most vegetarians are aware of the higher protein content of unmilled and undermilled products, but most are *unaware* of the lower absorption of nitrogen from these cereals. The use of milled products such as white rice and the many forms of pasta will somewhat decrease the bulkiness of the diet and also allow for maximally efficient digestion and absorption. To help overcome the inherently low energy content of vegetarian diets, margarines and other vegetable oils should be used liberally on bread, vegetables, or salads, for example. A decreased emphasis on fruits, which are low in both energy and protein, is desirable. Finally, a vitamin and iron supplement is essential in the management of vegetarian children.

Several of the suggestions we have made for changing the diet may run counter to the beliefs of vegetarian parents. It may be helpful to point out that some modification of the usual adult diet, whether vegetarian or not, is always necessary before it will be suitable for young infants. Few parents will knowingly compromise the health of their children. A continued dialogue with the parents is the only way to manage vegetarian children successfully. If the child does poorly, further liberalization of the diet will be necessary. For the child who does well, a gradual evolution of the child's diet toward that of the parents should be possible.

> Most vegetarians are aware of the higher protein content of unmilled and undermilled products, but most are *unaware* of the lower absorption of these cereals.

> A vitamin and iron supplement is essential in the management of vegetarian children.

NATURAL FOODS, ORGANIC FOODS, AND MEGAVITAMINS

Although natural and organic foods and megavitamin therapy are not used exclusively by vegetarians, they represent an approach to diet that is more common in vegetarians than in omnivores. Consequently, it seems appropriate to comment on these dietary beliefs.

Natural Foods

A fear among some people that processing saps food of many of its nutrients has created a demand for "natural" foods. Although processing such as blanching, freezing, or fermentation (for example, in the production of yogurt), is acceptable when done at home, industrial processing of any type is considered suspect

The benefits of food processing are frequently overlooked.

by some. The benefits of food processing are frequently overlooked. A primary benefit of food processing is preservation, which may make food available both out of season and at points far removed from where it is harvested. Processing methods such as milling may improve digestibility, as is the case with the cereal grains, mentioned previously. Processing may also destroy natural toxicants, such as the trypsin inhibitor in soy or the bovine serum albumin in whole cow milk that leads to gastrointestinal bleeding in infants.

Food additives are antithetical to the natural food concept. Chemical preservation is considered unsafe.

There is no evidence that "natural" vitamins are used any differently than synthetic forms.

Some people believe that synthetic forms of vitamins are utilized less efficiently by the body than are natural forms. However, there is no scientific evidence that, for example, synthetic ascorbic acid is utilized any differently than that found in rose hips. What has come to light recently is the fact that many of the natural vitamins on the market are in fact highly fortified with synthetic forms of the vitamin. This is necessary because of the low concentrations of most vitamins in all foods. For example, the concentration of vitamin C in rose hips is approximately 2%. Natural rose hips vitamin C can achieve the 50% level at which it is marketed only by the addition of substantial amounts of synthetic ascorbic acid.

Many so-called natural products can be on the health food store shelf only with the aid of a significant amount of processing.

Many so-called natural products can be on the health food store shelf only with the aid of significant processing. Protein supplements require isolation and concentration of the vegetable protein they contain. Sesame, soy, and safflower oils must all be pressed from their seeds and then separated. Nut butters require considerable processing in their production. Protein bars and vitamin pills exist only because of the ability to process foods. What separates acceptable from unacceptable forms of food processing is not entirely clear.

Strictly from a nutritional point of view one of the major advantages to the use of processed foods is digestibility. For the vegetarian child, the increase in digestibility of some processed foods may make the difference between inadequate and adequate protein and energy intakes.

Organic Foods

Organic foods are foods that have been grown without the use of inorganic fertilizers or pesticides. Recent evidence suggests that there is some basis for concern about pesticide residues in our food supply. The potential risks of pesticides must be weighed against the increased crop yields that accompany their use. Both yield and nutrient contents of many crops are improved markedly by the use of fertilizers. Since all nitrogen must be broken down to an inorganic form before it can be fixed by plants, organic fertilizers are not better utilized than inorganic sources of the same nutrients. Controlled agricultural trials have demonstrated no differences in the nutrient contents of foods grown with organic and inorganic fertilizers.

There is no governmental regulation of the use of the term "organic." Pesticide residues in samples of food bought in organic-food stores have frequently been found to equal the levels assayed in foods purchased in supermarkets. There have also been suggestions that because of the economic pressures to maintain food yields, inorganic fertilizers are not infrequently used in the production of "organic" foods. The primary drawback to both organic and natural foods is their cost. Surveys have shown the cost of a standard market basket of foods to be from 35% to 60% more in health-food stores than in supermarkets.

> Controlled agricultural trials have demonstrated no differences in the nutrient contents of foods grown with organic and inorganic fertilizers.

> The primary drawback to both organic and natural foods is their cost.

Megavitamin Therapy

The pharmacological use of vitamins to achieve a variety of difficult-to-document effects has gained wide popularity. Yet the potential toxicity of vitamins A and D have been recognized for some time. Excessive intake of retinol (but not carotenes) produces anorexia, desquamation of the skin, bony changes, and a pseudotumor cerebri syndrome with increased intracranial pressure. Vitamin D intoxication produces hypercalcemia with metastatic calcifications. More recently, the potential toxicities of some of the other vitamins frequently used in "megadoses" have come to light.

The effects attributed to vitamin E on longevity, sexual potency, and heart disease probably limit its use primarily to adults. Ingestion of excessive amounts of vitamin E has been demonstrated experimentally to interfere with vitamin K metabolism and to cause creatinuria. Whether these effects are of clinical importance in children who may be given megadoses of vitamin E has not been studied.

Debate over the value of vitamin C in the treatment and prevention of the common cold continues; there is, however, a lack of scientific evidence that it is of value. The ingestion of more than 80 mg of vitamin C per day by most adults results in no further increase in the plasma level of ascorbic acid. Large doses have been used to acidify the urine in the treatment of urinary tract infection. Much larger doses, frequently 1000 times the physiologic dose, are recommended by some for prevention and treatment of colds. They argue that even if the ingestion of

> The potential dangers of megavitamin therapy are becoming apparent.

Prolonged ingestion of large amounts of vitamin C may increase the baseline requirement for ascorbic acid.

vitamin C in these quantities is not helpful, it is not harmful. However, studies in both humans and other animals suggest the opposite. Ascorbic acid increases the absorption of iron, a fact that is of concern probably only in the adult male. It also interferes with the absorption of vitamin B_{12}, certainly an undesirable side effect in the vegetarian. Massive doses cause infertility or abortion in animals. Human pregnancies have been terminated using ascorbic acid. Finally, the prolonged ingestion of large amounts of vitamin C may increase the baseline requirement for ascorbic acid. When intakes return to a more modest level, a conditioned deficiency of the vitamin may result.

A complete coverage of megavitamin therapy and its potential problems is beyond the scope of this chapter. The examples we have presented should serve, however, to alert the physician to the fact that even many of the water-soluble vitamins in large doses are not as innocuous as may be generally thought.

Suggested Reading

Dwyer, J. T.; Dietz, W. H.; Haas, G.; and Suskind, R. 1979. Risk of nutritional rickets among vegetarian children. *Am. J. Dis. Child.* 133:134–140.

Dwyer, J. T.; Mayer, L. D. V. H.; Dowd, K., et al. 1974. The new vegetarians: the natural high? *J. Am. Diet. Assoc.* 65:529–536.

Food faddism. 1974. *Nutrition Reviews,* Supplement to Vol. 32.

Lapatsanis, P.; Deliyanni, V.; and Doxiadas, S. 1968. Vitamin D deficiency in Greece. *J. Pediatr.* 73:195–202.

MacLean, W. C., Jr.; and Graham, G. G. 1980. Vegetarianism in children. *Am. J. Dis. Child.* 134:513–519.

MacLean, W. C., Jr.; Lopez de Romaña, G.; Klein, G. L., et al. 1979. Digestibility and utilization of the energy and protein of wheat by infants. *J. Nutr.* 109:1290–1298.

The role of processing in extending the food supply. 1977. *Dairy Council Digest.* 48:19–24.

Shull, M. W.; Reed, R. B.; Valadian, I., et al. 1977. Velocities of growth in vegetarian preschool children. *Pediatrics* 60:410–417.

Zmora, E.; Gorodischer, R.; and Bar-Ziv, J. 1979. Multiple nutritional deficiencies in infants from a strict vegetarian community. *Am. J. Dis. Child.* 133:141–144.

8 Iron Deficiency and Other Nutritional Anemias

Contents

Iron Balance **152**
  Host Factors **152**
  Iron Absorption **153**
Dietary Requirements for Iron **156**
  Requirements During the First Year **156**
  Requirements of the Older Child and Adolescent **159**
Iron Deficiency **162**
  Definition **162**
  Manifestations of Iron Deficiency **163**
  Prevalence of Iron Deficiency **167**
  Whole Cow Milk and Iron Deficiency **168**
Other Nutritional Anemias **169**
  Anemia of Protein-Energy Malnutrition **170**
  Folic Acid Deficiency **170**
  Vitamin B_{12} Deficiency **172**
  Vitamin E Deficiency **173**
  Copper Deficiency **173**

Overview

Iron deficiency is perhaps the single remaining area for justifiable concern for undernutrition in the United States. Iron deficiency is also prominent among the nutritional problems of most developing countries. This chapter *looks at the nutritional aspects of maintaining adequate iron status in children. It covers both the hematologic and nonhematologic manifestations of iron deficiency. Because the approach is primarily nutritional, no attempt is made to cover in detail the diagnosis and medical treatment of iron-deficiency anemia. The other nutritional anemias, such as those caused by folic acid deficiency or vitamin B_{12} deficiency, are far less common in pediatric practice; brief comments concerning these deficiencies are found at the end of the chapter.*

IRON BALANCE

An individual's iron balance is the net result of the interaction among the physiologic requirement for iron, dietary iron intake, and iron absorption.

An individual's iron balance is the net result of the interaction among the host's physiologic requirement for iron, dietary iron intake, and iron absorption.

Host Factors

An individual's iron requirement is determined by several factors, some of which are relatively constant for all humans and some of which vary with the individual:

Fixed loss—skin, gastrointestinal tract, nails, hair

Growth—hemoglobin, myoglobin, metalloenzymes

Menstruation

Pregnancy

Lactation

Abnormal blood loss

Although there is no physiologic mechanism for the excretion of iron from the body, a small but constant loss of iron occurs through the desquamation of cells from the skin and from the intestinal tract. Iron is also lost in the nails and hair. These fixed losses are relatively small and average about 14 μg/kg/day. Iron is also required for growth. During the first few months of life, hemoglobin concentration decreases rapidly. After this period iron must be available for the synthesis of hemoglobin so that an adequate hemoglobin concentration is maintained as plasma volume increases. Total required hemoglobin mass is a direct function of lean body mass. Iron is also required for myoglobin synthesis as muscle mass increases. Smaller amounts of iron are required for the synthesis of metalloenzymes such as the cytochromes. The requirement for iron varies considerably from individual to individual depending on the growth rate.

The onset of menstruation imposes an additional iron requirement on the adolescent girl. There is considerable variation among girls and women in the amount of iron lost during each menstrual period. When expressed as the average amount of additional iron required on a daily basis, this loss varies from approximately 0.6 to 2.0 mg of iron per day. Differences in menstrual blood loss account for most of the variability in iron requirements from girl to girl. When iron required for menstruation is added to the 1 mg of iron that must be absorbed on a day-to-day basis to cover other physiologic requirements, it is clear that iron requirements for individual girls can vary by as much as 100%, depending on menstrual flow. Pregnancy increases the need for iron even further. The amount of additional iron required during the nine months of gestation has been estimated to be between 300 and 500 mg. Some of the increased requirement is offset by the decrease in iron loss resulting from cessation of menstruation. Lactation imposes no additional net requirement for iron, since breast-feeding tends to prolong postpartum amenorrhea. The approximately 0.5 to 1.0 mg of iron required for milk secretion approximately equals the amount of iron that would be required if menstruation were resumed.

> Iron requirements for adolescent girls vary by as much as 100% because of differences in menstrual blood losses.

Abnormal blood loss in either sex affects the requirement for iron. Gastrointestinal bleeding secondary to the ingestion of whole cow milk by younger infants is thought by many to contribute significantly to the prevalence of iron-deficiency anemia. Blood loss from recurrent epistaxis, from ulcers or other intestinal diseases, or from trauma also increases the requirement for iron, though the blood loss may not result in anemia. Because each gram of hemoglobin contains approximately 3.5 mg of iron, the loss of as little as 3 mL of blood from a child with a hemoglobin concentration of 10 g/dL will carry with it 1 mg of iron.

> Each gram of hemoglobin contains approximately 3.5 mg of iron.

Iron Absorption

Iron is unique among nutrients in that absorption rather than excretion plays the critical role in determining iron balance. Most nutrients, be they macronutrients such as protein or micronutrients such as vitamin C, are consumed and absorbed in excess. The amount needed for maintenance and growth is retained in the body, and the rest is excreted, usually via the urine or bile. Because there is no effective means for the excretion of iron, iron balance is determined largely by the efficiency of iron absorption by the intestinal mucosa. Depending on the form of iron ingested, the absorption of iron (% of iron intake) from different foodstuffs may vary as much as 25 or 30 fold. Consequently, factors affecting

> Iron balance is determined largely by the efficiency of iron absorption by the intestinal mucosa.

iron absorption may be as important as or more important than actual iron intake in determining the ultimate iron status of the infant or child.

Iron is absorbed from two distinct pools, the heme iron and nonheme iron pools. *Heme iron* is iron that is complexed as part of hemoglobin or myoglobin. Whether heme is split from the hemoglobin or myoglobin molecule in the lumen of the intestine or after it is absorbed into the intestinal mucosal cell is uncertain. In either case release of iron from the heme molecule is then accomplished in the enterocyte. The absorption of heme iron is relatively efficient—up to 25% to 30% from test meals—and is virtually unaltered by other dietary constituents.

Most iron in the diet is present in inorganic forms. The absorption of this *nonheme iron* is highly variable and is subject to a variety of influences. Factors that favor absorption include:

Ferrous (Fe^{++}) form—10^{16} more soluble than Fe^{+++} at pH7

Animal protein in the diet

Ascorbic acid

Fructose

Alcohol

Factors that decrease absorption include:

Ferric (Fe^{+++}) form

Vegetable fiber in the diet

Eggs

Oxalates

Phytates

Pica—clay, coal

The ferrous (Fe^{++}) form of iron is far more readily absorbed than the ferric (Fe^{+++}) form, being approximately 10^{16} times more soluble at the neutral pH of the small intestine. Ascorbic acid is well known to improve the absorption of nonheme iron. Animal protein, in addition to being a good source of heme iron, has a beneficial effect on the absorption of nonheme iron. Fructose and alcohol also improve nonheme-iron absorption. Among the dietary constituents that reduce iron absorption are phosphorus, either as phosphate or phytate, oxalates, and vegetable fiber. Phytates are present in high concentration in many cereal grains; oxalates occur in spinach, beets, and some meats. Egg has a relatively high concentration of iron and also provides animal protein, a factor that should improve iron absorption. However, the bioavailability of

Figure 8-1

The net iron absorption from a meal as a whole will be the result of the interplay among the factors in individual foods that favor or hinder iron absorption.

iron from egg is poor, because most of the iron is complexed with a phosphoprotein in the egg yolk.

The variability of absorption of iron from a variety of foods is illustrated in Figure 8-1. When several of these foods are consumed together as a meal, the net absorption from the meal as a whole will be the result of the interplay among the factors in individual foods that favor or hinder iron absorption. It is virtually impossible to predict exactly how all these factors will balance out. Current estimates suggest an upper limit of absorption of 20% of dietary iron when more than 25% of calories in a meal are from foods of animal origin and a lower limit of no more than 10% when less than 10% of calories are from foods of animal origin. Because iron absorption may be as low as 10% of intake, the dietary requirement for iron is necessarily much higher than the physiologic requirement.

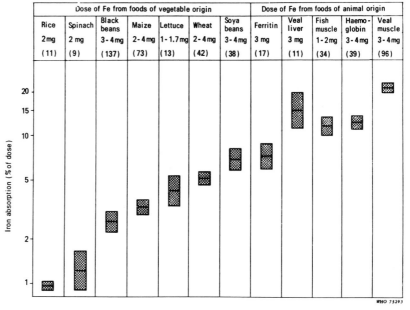

a The horizontal thick line represents the geometrical mean value; the shaded area indicates the limits of 1 standard error. Numbers in parentheses are numbers of cases. From a collaborative study of the departments of botany and medicine, University of Washington at Seattle, WA, USA, and the Department of Pathophysiology, Instituto Venezolano de Investigaciones Cientificas, Caracas, Venezuela.

Figure 8-1   Efficiency of absorption of iron from various foods. From Brown, E. G.; and Moore, C. V., editors. 1971. *Progress in hematology,* Vol. 7. New York: Grune & Stratton.

DIETARY REQUIREMENTS FOR IRON

Dietary requirements for iron are relatively higher in infants than in older children and are not as easily met without supplements.

Requirements During the First Year

Assessing iron stores and iron requirements   Placental transfer of iron from mother to fetus occurs relatively independently of maternal iron status except in extreme maternal iron depletion. The average full-term infant is born with an iron endowment of approximately 75 mg/kg, more than 75% of which is present in hemoglobin per se. Hemoglobin concentration and body weight taken together are the best means of assessing iron stores in the newborn infant.

Hemoglobin concentration and body weight taken together are the best means of assessing iron stores in the newborn infant.

When the infant leaves the relatively hypoxic environment of the uterus, the infant is able to meet its oxygen transport needs with a smaller hemoglobin mass than it needed in utero. Erythropoiesis decreases markedly and hemoglobin concentration declines slowly during the first several months. The net effect is a redistribution of iron from hemoglobin into body stores. After several months of life, when erythropoiesis becomes more rapid again, iron from body stores is gradually used. Even if there were no dietary intake of iron, the normal full-term infant could double its birth weight without becoming anemic by drawing on iron originally contained in hemoglobin and other iron stores. For example, a 3 kg infant with a blood volume of 10% and a hemoglobin concentration of 16 g/dL would have 16 g of hemoglobin per kg or 48 g of hemoglobin total. At a weight of 6 kg, blood volume would have decreased to approximately 8% of body weight. The original 48 g of hemoglobin would now be carried in a total blood volume of approximately 480 mL, giving a hemglobin concentration of 10 g/dL. As the child continued to grow, however, iron stores would be progressively depleted as iron were further used for synthesis of hemoglobin, myoglobin, and iron-containing enzymes.

Approximately 0.8 mg of iron must be absorbed daily during the second six months of life.

The difference between the total body iron desirable at 1 year of age and that present at birth has been used to estimate the net amount of iron that must be absorbed during the first year of life. These calculations suggest that approximately 0.8 mg of iron must be absorbed daily during the second six months of life, when iron stores tend to become depleted, to maintain adequate total body iron. If an average absorption from the diet of approximately 10% is assumed, a dietary intake of approximately 8 mg per day, or about 0.9 mg per day per kg average body weight, will be required during the second six months of life.

The optimal iron intake during the first year of life has been determined more directly by monitoring the hemoglobin response to different levels of dietary intake of iron. Studies of this type suggest that an iron intake of 1.0 mg/kg/day is associated with maximal hemoglobin levels. The Committee on Nutrition of the American Academy of Pediatrics (1976) recommends an intake of 1.0 mg/kg/day to a maximum of 15 mg/day based on these studies. The Committee suggests that this intake be begun by 2 months of age. Because infants born prematurely will have lower than normal iron stores at birth, the allowance for these infants has been liberalized to approximately 2 mg/kg/day, with the same 15 mg/day maximum.

Meeting iron requirements during the first year of life The iron intake of the exclusively breast-fed infant is exceedingly low. Human milk contains 0.5–1.0 mg of iron/liter initially. This concentration decreases during lactation to 0.3–0.6 mg/liter. Once nursing is established, most infants take approximately 750 mL of milk per day or about 0.2–0.5 mg of iron per day. This low intake of iron is offset to a large degree by the high bioavailability of iron in human milk. Although studies differ, most show that the absorption of iron from human milk is about 40%–60%. No one questions the adequacy of human milk as a source of iron up to the age of 4 months. This should not be surprising since an intake of virtually no iron during the first 4 months of life is still compatible with a normal hemoglobin concentration. Many pediatricians and nutritionists feel that the exclusively breast-fed infant is unlikely to become anemic or significantly iron depleted up to the age of 8 or 9 months. Others argue that a normal hemoglobin concentration in these infants is maintained only by the gradual depletion of iron stores.

It should be stressed that up to this point we have been speaking of the exclusively breast-fed infant. Although the iron in human milk is highly bioavailable, it is not heme iron; consequently, its absorption is affected by other foods in the diet. One recent study demonstrated that the addition of puréed pears to a feeding of human milk decreased the apparent absorption of iron from 24% to 6% (Oski and Landow, 1980). In one study in which increments of total body iron were estimated during four months of exclusive breast-feeding and during the subsequent two-month period when solid foods were added, the net increase in iron dropped from 20 mg/month of 0 mg/month in association with the change in feeding (Saarinen and Siimes, 1979; Figure 8–2).

The low iron intake of the exclusively breast-fed infant is offset by the higher bioavailability of iron in breast milk.

Figure 8–2

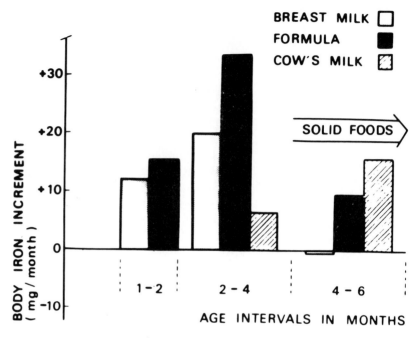

Figure 8-2 Increments of total body iron at different ages by infants being fed breast milk, modified milk formula, or cow milk. *Source:* Saarinen, U. M., and Siimes, M. A. 1979. Iron absorption from breast milk, cow's milk and iron supplemented formula: an opportunistic use of changes in total body iron determined by hemoglobin, ferritin, and body weight in 132 infants. *Pediatr. Res.* 13:143–147.

For the infant who is being exclusively breast-fed for a prolonged period of time, it is desirable to provide additional iron (1 mg/kg/day) in the form of ferrous sulfate after the age of 5 to 6 months.

Such data show that exclusive breast-feeding is desirable for good iron nutrition. As a general rule, some form of additional dietary iron should be supplied once solid foods have been introduced into the diet of the breast-fed infant. For example, iron-fortified cereals should be introduced before fruits and vegetables, which would be low in iron and which would also inhibit the absorption of iron from breast milk. For the infant who is being exclusively breast-fed for a prolonged period of time, it is desirable to provide additional iron (1 mg/kg/day) in the form of ferrous sulfate after the age of 5 to 6 months. Exclusive breast-feeding without additional iron is acceptable beyond this age only if the practitioner is willing to monitor hemoglobin concentrations on a regular basis.

For the formula-fed infant, iron-fortified formula provides the best assurance of meeting iron requirements. The iron concentration of iron-fortified formulas (12 mg/liter) assures an intake of 7–10 mg of iron per day for the average infant. If one assumes an

Exclusive formula-feeding has been shown to be associated with much more efficient iron absorption than mixed feeding has.

absorption of about 10%, actual iron absorbed from formula will be about 50% more than that absorbed from human milk. Just as exclusive breast-feeding is important to assure maximum bioavailability of iron from human milk, exclusive formula-feeding has also been shown to be associated with much more efficient iron absorption than mixed feeding has. In the study of Saarinen and Siimes (1979) the addition of solid foods to the diet resulted in a reduction of iron absorption to one-third the level previously documented with exclusive formula-feeding (see Figure 8-2). If iron-fortified infant cereal is the first food introduced, the iron in the cereal will tend to counterbalance the reduction. Dry cereals marketed in the United States contain about 14 mg of iron per ounce of dry cereal. Consequently, the consumption of ½ oz dry cereal will provide an additional 7 mg of iron. The iron preparation most commonly used in infant cereals is electrolytic iron powder, an iron of very small particle size that is easily digested and absorbed. However, phytates and other factors in cereal decrease the absorption not only of this supplemental iron but also of the iron in the formula with which the cereal is mixed. Some studies have suggested that iron absorption from cereal can be enhanced by mixing the cereal with fruit juices high in vitamin C rather than with infant formula. This is probably unnecessary as a general practice.

Whether iron fortification of infant formulas is truly required to prevent iron deficiency is debatable. One recent study showed no difference in hematologic indicators between groups of infants fed infant formulas containing 14 mg and 1.4 mg Fe per quart during the first four months of life (Picciano and Derring, 1980). Similarly, there was no difference found when infants fed iron-fortified formula for the entire first year of life were compared with infants given unfortified formula. The results of this and other studies suggest that infants who accept solid foods, particularly iron-fortified cereals, may fare well without the use of iron-fortified formula. It should be noted, however, that most of the studies that have reached these conclusions have been done in private-practice situations. These conclusions may or may not hold true for less advantages segments of the population. There is no contraindication to the use of iron-fortified formula, and consequently the recommendation of the Committee on Nutrition that iron-fortified formulas be used throughout the first year of life make good sense.

Some studies suggest that infants who accept solid foods, particularly iron-fortified cereals, may fare well without the use of iron-fortified formula.

Requirements of the Older Child and Adolescent

As growth slows during the preschool years, the requirement for iron decreases. At the same time energy intake is progressively

Table 8-1

increasing. Because iron intake is directly proportional to energy intake, it becomes progressively easier for the preschool and preadolescent child to meet his or her energy requirements from diet alone. This is well illustrated in Table 8-1, which shows the recommended dietary allowances for energy and iron intake and the calculated iron density (mg Fe/1000 kcal) of the diet required to provide the RDA of iron. Iron density is slightly overestimated in Table 8-1 because the RDA for energy represents the median intake whereas the RDA for iron represents the intake adequate to meet the needs of nearly all (~97.5%) healthy individuals. Nevertheless, the table demonstrates that it becomes progressively easier to meet iron requirements from diet alone in older children up to the onset of puberty. Although there is wide variation from family to family and from region to region, the average iron density of the typical American diet is approximately 5.5 to 6 mg/1000 kcal.

It becomes progressively easier to meet iron requirements from diet alone in older children up to the onset of puberty.

Table 8-1 Estimated iron density of the diet required to provide the RDA of iron

Age (yrs)	Energy RDA (kcal)	Fe RDA (mg)	Fe density (mg/1000 kcal)*
0.5–1	950	15	15.7
1–3	1300	15	11.5
4–6	1700	10	5.9
7–10	2400	10	4.2
Female			
11–14	2200	18	8.2
15–18	2100	18	8.6
Male			
11–14	2700	18	6.7
15–18	2800	18	6.4

Source: Based on 1980 Recommended Dietary Allowances.

*Estimates of required iron density are slightly high because the RDA for energy is the recommended median intake whereas that for iron is the amount suggested to meet the needs of nearly all (~97.5%) healthy individuals.

Table 8-2

The factors other than total energy (and consequently iron) intake that are critical in determining the adequacy of iron intake are the mix between heme and nonheme iron, the percentage of foods from animal and vegetable origin, and the effects of the various foods on the absorption of nonheme iron. FAO/WHO has taken this factor into account in its recommendations, which are shown in Table 8-2. The amount of dietary iron that must be consumed to meet the actual iron requirement of the individual varies by as much as 100%, depending on the proportion of foods from animal origin.

During the rapid growth of adolescence, the requirement for iron increases substantially for both boys and girls. At the height of the adolescent growth spurt boys may be increasing in weight at a rate of as much as 10 kg per year, girls at a rate of 9 kg per year (see Figure 6-1). Some additional iron is required for myoglobin synthesis as lean body mass increases, especially in boys. Most of the increased iron required during this period is used for the production of hemoglobin necessary to maintain an adequate hemoglobin concentration in the increasing plasma volume. In addition, there is a progressive increase in the hemoglobin concentration in the expanded plasma volume. The increase in hemoglobin concentration is greater in the male than in the female because of his

Table 8-2 Recommended daily iron intake

Group (by age and sex)	Absorbed iron required	Recommended intake according to diet		
		Animal foods below 10% of calories	Animal foods 10%–25% of calories	Animal foods above 25% of calories
Infants 5–12 months	1.0	10	7	5
Children 1–12 years	1.0	10	7	5
Boys 13–16 years	1.8	18	12	9
Girls 13–16 years	2.4	24	18	12
Menstruating women	2.8	28	19	14
Men and postmenopausal women	0.9	9	6	5

Source: Report of the FAO/WHO Expert Group on Requirements for Ascorbic Acid, Vitamin D, Folic Acid, Vitamin B_{12} and Iron. 1970. *Wld. Hlth. Org. Techn. Rep.* Ser. No. 452.

greater lean body mass. It has been estimated that during the year of peak growth approximately 350 mg of iron are required for the adolescent boy, approximately 280 mg of iron for the adolescent girl. After the slowing of growth, the iron requirement for the adolescent male decreases. The cessation of growth in girls is accompanied by the onset of menstruation; for this reason there is no decrease in the iron requirement for girls following adolescence. Because growth has stopped at this point, however, energy intake decreases, making it more difficult for the postadolescent girl to meet her iron requirements.

Children in the second half of infancy (12-24 months), because of the shift away from highly fortified infant foods, and adolescent girls are the two groups primarily at risk for dietary iron deficiency during childhood.

From the previous discussion and from Table 8-1, it is clear that children in the second half of infancy (12-24 months), because of the shift away from highly fortified infant foods, and adolescent girls are the two groups primarily at risk for dietary iron deficiency during childhood. One should not infer from the estimated iron densities that iron supplementation at these two periods is mandatory. In the United States in particular, where diets tend to be rich in heme iron and animal protein, most children are able to meet their iron requirements without further supplementation. For children in these age groups, the practitioner should obtain a brief dietary history including information about iron intake and the factors affecting iron absorption; laboratory assessment of hemoglobin concentration is also indicated.

IRON DEFICIENCY

Iron deficiency is generally acknowledged to be one of the few remaining areas of undernutrition in the United States. The lack of agreement on the prevalence and severity of iron deficiency results largely from inconsistency in the way iron deficiency is defined.

Definition

A decrease in the intake of any nutrient is followed by a predictable series of physiologic and pathologic changes. If intake is insufficient to meet the physiologic needs of the individual, the stores of the nutrient become progressively depleted. Once stores are exhausted, the serum concentration of the nutrient generally decreases. This decrease in serum concentration is followed sequentially by changes in enzyme activities, changes in organ function, and, later, obvious morbidity or mortality.

Iron deficiency has its own set of sequential changes. Some nutritionists classify the failure to meet recommended dietary allowances for iron, that is, any decreased intake, as iron deficiency. This type of "iron deficiency" is frequently used to justify government food programs. Serum ferritin can be used as a measure of iron stores and might be used as a measure of iron deficiency. Dallman et al. (1980), however, have pointed out that while the maintenance of iron reserves is desirable, it may be an unrealistic goal for the average rapidly growing infant or older child. A decreased serum-iron concentration is also used as an indicator of deficiency by some. Iron deficiency results in reduction of hemoglobin concentration, that is anemia, and also in changes in the levels of a variety of metalloenzymes—for example, cytochrome c. It is not certain whether a mild anemia (0.5–1.0 g/dL below standard) is in and of itself harmful to the individual or whether anemia of this degree correlates with functional changes in other organ systems secondary to changes in levels of iron-containing enzymes.

> While the maintenance of iron reserves is desirable it may be an unrealistic goal for the average rapidly growing infant or older child.

Manifestations of Iron Deficiency

Hematologic manifestations Because of the ease with which hematocrit and hemoglobin concentration can be measured, the hematologic manifestations of iron deficiency are those most frequently screened for. The total hemoglobin mass is affected by a variety of factors, the most important being lean body mass. Differences in lean body mass explain most of the variability in hemoglobin mass attributed to age and sex. Genetic factors and the altitude at which an individual lives also influence hemoglobin levels. Normal values for hemoglobin and hematocrit during childhood are shown in Table 8–3. There is a wide range of normal values at each age. An inference that might be incorrectly drawn from the table is that hemoglobin and hematocrit values vary around the mean with a normal Gaussian or bell-shaped distribution. If this were the case, children falling below the lower end of the normal range would represent about 2.5% of the population and would be defined statistically as anemic. However, anemia is better defined in pathophysiologic terms as a hemoglobin mass suboptimal to the oxygen transport needs of the individual. The child living at an altitude of 10,000 feet or suffering from cyanotic heart disease may be anemic with a hemoglobin of 14 g/dL, whereas a wasted child with reduced lean body mass may be normal with a hemoglobin of 9 g/dL. Figure 8–3 shows that anemic and nonanemic individuals form two distinct groups, each with its own "normal" distribution, with considerable overlap. Because this is the case, values at the lower end of the normal range of hemoglobin and hematocrit may indicate either anemic or normal status, depending on the individual.

> Table 8–3

> Anemia is better defined in pathophysiologic terms as a hemoglobin mass suboptimal to the oxygen transport needs of the individual.

> Figure 8–3
>
> Values at the lower end of the normal range of hemoglobin and hematocrit may in fact indicate either anemic or normal status, depending on the individual.

Table 8-3 Normal values of hemoglobin and hematocrit during childhood and adolescence

Age	Hemoglobin (g/dL)		Hematocrit (%)	
	Mean	Range	Mean	Range
At birth (cord blood)	16.8	13.7–20.1	55	45–65
2 weeks	16.5	13.0–20.0	50	42–66
3 months	12.0	9.5–14.5	36	31–41
6 months–6 years	12.0	10.5–14.0	37	33–42
7–12 years	13.0	11.6–16.0	38	34–40
Adolescence				
Female	14.0	12.0–16.0	42	37–47
Male	16.0	14.0–18.0	47	42–52

Source: Pearson, H. A. 1979. Diseases of the blood. *In* Vaughan, V. C., III; McKay, R. J.; and Behrman, R. E. (editors). *Nelson textbook of pediatrics,* 11th Ed. Philadelphia: W. B. Saunders Co.

The problem of using only hemoglobin or hematocrit to separate anemic from nonanemic individuals was well illustrated in a study of iron deficiency anemia in adult women (Garby et al., 1969). Using the hematologic response to iron as the criterion for iron deficiency (with the response to a placebo as a control), the investigators determined that the true prevalence of iron deficiency among otherwise healthy women in the community was approximately 17%. They then calculated the effect of choosing hematocrit levels between 35 and 41 for the definition of anemia on the *apparent* prevalence of anemia and on the number of false negative and false positive diagnoses that would be made. These data are shown in Table 8-4. It is clear that no single level of hematocrit correctly identifies those in need of iron therapy or avoids indicating treatment for a large number of those who do not need iron therapy. While the determination of hemoglobin concentration or hematocrit is a good initial screening test, other indicators (such as the MCV, serum iron or ferritin, or a blood smear) are necessary if the anemic and nonanemic populations are to be more clearly delineated. Some authorities have suggested that ultimately the question of whether a child is iron deficient can be settled only

Table 8-4

No single level of hematocrit correctly identifies those in need of iron therapy.

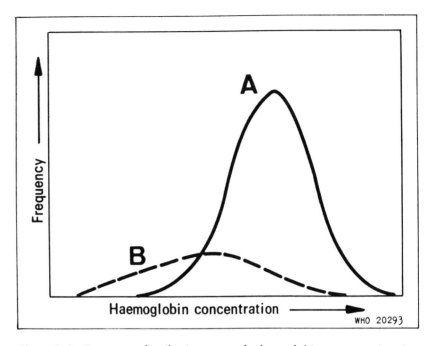

WHO 20293

Figure 8-3 Frequency distribution curves for hemoglobin concentrations in normal (A) and anemic (B) individuals. From Layrisse, M.; Roche, M.; and Baker, S. J. 1976. Nutritional anaemias. In Beaton, G. H.; and Bengoa, J. M., editors. *Nutrition in Preventive Medicine.* Geneva: World Health Organization, pp. 55–82.

by a trial of iron therapy (Dallman et al 1981). This makes good sense.

Nonhematologic manifestations A large number of signs and symptoms have been attributed to iron deficiency. Spooning of the nails (koilonychia), glossitis, angular stomatitis, and cricopharyngeal webs may accompany iron deficiency. A desire to eat ice, pagophagia, is also occasionally encountered. Some studies indicate that iron deficiency impairs host response to infection; others suggest that a reduced serum concentration of iron is protective against many kinds of infection.

Several gastrointestinal manifestations of iron deficiency have been described. Some investigators feel that iron deficiency per se can cause intestinal bleeding. It is often difficult to decide whether enteric blood loss was the cause or the result of anemia. In some studies the intestinal blood loss associated with the ingestion of whole cow milk may have been a factor causing anemia. Beeturia

Table 8-4 Effect of varying the hematocrit value as an index for the prediction of response to iron therapy among women

Hematocrit *below* which subjects are selected (%)	Proportion of potential responders that is not included (false negative) (%)	Proportion of potential nonresponders that is included (false positive) (%)	Proportion of total population that is included* (apparent prevalence) (%)
35	81	0.7	4.0
36	65	1.7	7.5
37	43	5.1	14
38	26	14	25
39	11	29	40
40	2.8	47	56
41	0	66	72

Source: Used with permission from Beaton, G. H. Epidemiology of iron deficiency. In Jacobs, A.; and Wormwood, M. (editors), *Iron in biochemistry and medicine,* copyright by Academic Press Inc. (London) Ltd.

*This may be compared to the observed "prevalence" of responders of 17.3%.

Although iron-deficiency anemia is often associated with poor growth, it is often difficult to decide whether one causes the other or whether both result independently from inadequate nutritional intake.

has been ascribed to iron deficiency and results from the apparently enhanced absorption of betanin, a red pigment in beets, in iron deficiency. Finally, several studies have indicated that some children with iron deficiency have impaired iron absorption. Such an impairment of iron absorption is the opposite of the expected response of increased iron absorption in iron deficiency. The impairment may be reversed after parenteral administration of iron.

Perhaps the most important question to resolve is whether iron deficiency impairs growth, work performance, and mental functioning. Although iron-deficiency anemia is often associated with poor growth, it is often difficult to decide whether one causes the other or whether both result from inadequate nutritional intake. Several studies have indicated that mental functioning and behavior are altered by iron deficiency, independent of hemoglobin concentration. Treatment of iron-deficient children is said to reverse behavioral abnormalities before any change in hemoglobin level is noted. The validity of these studies has been questioned because of methodologic difficulties. The findings are nevertheless intriguing and the question of the effect of iron on mental function is one that still needs resolution.

Severe anemia is known to result in decreased muscle function and work output. Experimental studies in animals that have been iron depleted but whose hemoglobin levels have been acutely adjusted upward suggest that decreased work capacity is in part due to intrinsic changes in muscle function resulting from iron deficiency. It is not clear whether significant functional changes in muscle occur at marginal levels of iron deficiency or only when more pronounced deficiency is present. A recent study by Siimes et al (1980), in which rats were fed diets containing variable amounts of iron, documented that decreases in cytochrome c levels paralleled changes in hemoglobin concentration. Diets that contained enough iron to prevent anemia also prevented reductions in cytochrome c level. Diets associated with progressively more severe iron deficiency caused parallel decrements in cytochrome c. These findings are nearly impossible to confirm in humans, at least in children, but the data suggest that degrees of iron deficiency sufficient to cause mild anemia may also result in biologically significant alterations in iron-dependent nonhematologic functions.

> It is not clear whether significant functional changes in physical and mental performance occur at marginal levels of iron deficiency or only when more pronounced deficiency is present.

Prevalence of Iron Deficiency

The prevalence of iron deficiency in childhood varies substantially with age, socioeconomic status, and race. The apparent prevalence of iron deficiency also depends on hemoglobin or hematocrit level used to differentiate between anemic and nonanemic children. The Preschool Nutrition Survey (Owen et al, 1974) found that approximately 50% of children failed to take in at least 8 mg of iron per day. When a hemoglobin concentration of 10 g/dL was used as a cut-off, 14% of 1- to 2-year-olds in the low-income group were found to be anemic. When the criterion was raised to 11 g/dL, this percentage increased to 27%. In this and other studies the apparent prevalence of iron deficiency decreased with increasing age. By 5 years of age no children in the survey had hemoglobin concentrations less than 10 g/dL; only 9% had less than 11 g/dL. The Ten State Nutrition Survey, which intentionally looked for undernutrition, found that 24% of children less than 2 years of age had hemoglobin concentrations less than 10 g/dL. Only 6% of children between the ages of 2 and 5 were below this level. A survey of 9-month-old infants in a private-practice setting showed that only 3% of the children had hemoglobin values less than 10 g/dL.

> The prevalence of anemia varies with the cut-off level of hematocrit or hemoglobin used in the individual studies.

It is difficult to know what to conclude from the data from studies of anemia. All of these studies use only a single indicator to define anemia. In addition, many of the data in Black children were interpreted prior to the recent confirmation that Black children normally have hemoglobin concentrations approximately 0.5 g/dL lower than White children, independent of socioeconomic status. In general, most studies suggest that iron deficiency is to a large degree a problem of late infancy and that, in most children, the problem corrects itself by the time the child is 4 to 5 years old. This spontaneous decline in the prevalence of iron deficiency probably reflects the greater ease of meeting iron requirements relative to energy intake with age.

Iron deficiency is to a large degree a problem of late infancy; in most children the problem corrects itself by the time the child is 4 to 5 years old.

Whole Cow Milk and Iron Deficiency

For years the stereotype of the iron-deficient infant was the relatively overweight, pale "milk baby." It was popular to ascribe anemia to the insufficient intake of iron from a diet in which cow milk provided most of the calories. In the early 1960s studies by Hoag and coworkers (1961) demonstrated that inadequate iron intake alone could not explain the degree of anemia seen in many infants. They suggested that occult blood loss, most likely from the intestinal tract, was often the cause of iron deficiency in such infants.

Subsequent studies have implicated whole cow milk in the intestinal blood loss and resultant anemia of many infants. In at least one infant studied, goat milk caused a similar problem. There is no evidence for an allergic mechanism for the blood loss. It appears rather to be a direct irritant effect of some factor in milk on the intestinal mucosa. Bovine serum albumin passed in milk may be one agent responsible for cow-milk-induced blood loss. Feeding bovine serum albumin to children who manifest this problem causes enteric blood loss that is quantitatively intermediate between that seen with whole cow milk and that seen with formula. Pasteurization of milk does not alter the response. Boiling of milk, or the processing carried out in the production of evaporated milk or of modified milk formulas, denatures the offending agent, which makes it harmless.

Bovine serum albumin passed in milk may be one agent responsible for cow-milk-induced blood loss.

The prevalence of this phenomenon is unknown. A study by Wilson et al. (1974) found that cow milk induced blood loss in 17 of 34 anemic infants studied. Despite statements to the contrary by the authors, there appeared to be a bias in the selection of infants toward those with more severe or recurrent anemia, as well as toward those who had failed to respond to usual iron

The true prevalence of milk-induced enteric blood loss in the general population is undetermined, but recent data suggest it may be lower than previously thought.

therapy. The true prevalence of whole-cow-milk-induced enteric blood loss in the general population is unknown, but it is probably far below the 50% level implied by this study. Foman et al. (1981) randomly assigned 81 normal infants to diets containing whole cow milk (39 infants) or formulas or heat-treated cow milk (42 infants) at 112 days of age and followed them to 196 days of age. Both groups had occult blood in the stools. The difference was statistically significant only to 140 days of age. Whereas 39% of the infants fed whole cow milk passed stools with occult blood (17% of stools tested), only 9% of infants fed formula or heat-treated milk passed stools with occult blood (2% of stools tested). In both feeding groups 5%–6% of stools tested had occult blood from 140 to 196 days of age. All infants received 12 mg ferrous sulfate with 50 mg ascorbic acid daily throughout the study. There were no differences measured in iron nutritional status at the end of the study.

The problem of enteric blood loss is one of the major reasons for the suggestion that unmodified cow milk be withheld from the diet of infants up to the age of 12 months. The likelihood of developing the problem is said to decrease substantially during the second six months of life. The data from Foman et al. (1981) suggest that the propensity for blood loss may decrease at an even earlier age. On the other hand, and equally important, in the study of Wilson et al. (1974), 19 of the 34 children studied were between 6 and 12 months of age, while 11 of the 34 were older than 1 year.

In summary, there is no question that cow milk or goat milk may induce gastrointestinal bleeding in some infants. Whether the data presently available can be used to justify withholding cow milk from all children until the age of 12 months or older is debatable. It should be emphasized, however, that the practitioner should look for enteric blood loss and its relationship to cow milk in the diet in all infants and children who are found to be anemic.

OTHER NUTRITIONAL ANEMIAS

The reduction of hemoglobin concentration in malnutrition may be a physiologic adaptation.

Unlike iron-deficiency anemia, which is a common condition frequently associated with a seemingly normal diet, the other nutritional anemias are rare and occur in quite characteristic clinical settings. A detailed description of the characteristic hematologic changes of each is beyond the scope of this chapter. These changes are well covered in standard pediatric textbooks. This section provides an overview of the other nutritional anemias, emphasizing the clinical conditions in which they should be suspected.

Anemia of Protein-Energy Malnutrition

Protein deficiency alone or, more commonly, a deficiency of both energy and protein, results in a mild degree of anemia even when other hematinic agents are present in the diet in adequate amounts. In clinical practice in the United States the most common form of protein-energy malnutrition is mild marasmus, a balanced starvation (see Chapter 10). Children with mild marasmus characteristically have a normochromic normocytic anemia that results from decreased production of erythrocytes. Hemoglobin concentration and hematocrit usually fall below accepted norms. Whether this should be considered anemia in the pathologic sense, however, is debatable. The reduction of total hemoglobin mass that occurs in children with this condition appears to be an adjustment appropriate to lower oxygen transport requirements associated with decreased lean body mass and decreased metabolic rate. Studies of the anemia of marasmus in animal models have shown that the capacity of the marrow to respond is normal.

Anemia encountered in malnourished patients should be attributed to deficits of protein and energy intake only when other nutritional causes of anemia can be excluded. The treatment of the anemia of protein-energy malnutrition is nonspecific. An adequate diet that results in weight gain and linear growth is accompanied by a gradual increase in hematocrit and hemoglobin concentration.

Folic Acid Deficiency

The functions of folic acid and the dietary requirement for folate were reviewed in Chapter 2. The full-term infant is born with an adequate amount of folic acid, even in the case of mild maternal folate deficiency. Deficiency of folic acid results in a megaloblastic anemia associated with hypersegmented neutrophils that is indistinguishable from vitamin B_{12} deficiency. Some of the more common causes of folic acid deficiency are summarized below:

Low dietary intake
    Evaporated-milk formula without supplementation
    Goat milk

Poor absorption
    Chronic diarrhea
    Blind-loop syndrome
    Drugs—oral contraceptives, barbiturates, diphenylhydantoin

Increased requirement
    Rapid growth or cell turnover—premature infant, hemolytic anemia
    Increased metabolic activity—hyperthyroidism, cardiac disease

Poor utilization
    Antimetabolites—methotrexate, trimethoprim
    Anticonvulsants (possibly)
    Congenital deficiencies of enzymes of folate metabolism
    Vitamin B_{12} deficiency

Inadequate dietary intake of folic acid may produce folic acid deficiency in an otherwise healthy child. Because folic acid is heat labile, its content in evaporated milk, and consequently in evaporated-milk formulas, is low. The infant who is fed an evaporated-milk formula without additional vitamins is at risk for folic acid deficiency. Goat milk is also very low in folic acid, and the use of goat milk for children with cow-milk intolerance has resulted in folic acid deficiency.

Folic acid deficiency should be considered in other clinical conditions. Chronic diarrhea and blind-loop syndromes, with their associated malabsorption, may produce folate deficiency. Certain drugs, such as barbiturates and diphenylhydantoin, interact with folic acid in the intestinal lumen, compromising absorption of the vitamin. Some conditions result in an increased requirement for folic acid. Because folic acid is integral to DNA synthesis, rapid growth or rapid cell turnover increases the need for folic acid. For example, premature infants and children with hemolytic anemias, such as sickle cell anemia, have increased folic acid requirements. Hypermetabolic states, such as hyperthyroidism and certain types of cardiac disease, also seem to generate a need for increased folic acid intake.

In some cases of folic acid deficiency, dietary intake and absorption of folate may be normal but utilization of the vitamin may be poor. Several drugs can cause this phenomenon. Methotrexate, an antineoplastic agent, is given specifically for its antifolate activity. The antibiotic trimethoprim, used with increasing frequency recently, tends to interfere with folate utilization. Anticonvulsants have been suspected of interfering with folate utilization as well. Because of the integral link of vitamin B_{12} and folic acid metabolism, vitamin B_{12} deficiency itself may result in poor recycling and poor utilization of folate.

Hematologically, folate deficiency is quite characteristic. The diagnosis is best made by ruling out vitamin B_{12} deficiency and by

Red cell concentrations of folic acid are thought to be more representative of folic acid reserves than are serum levels.

obtaining a serum and red cell folic acid level. Red cell concentrations of folic acid are thought to be more representative of folic acid reserves than are serum levels. Once folic acid deficiency is confirmed, a therapeutic dose of 500 μg per day results in rapid improvement.

Vitamin B_{12} Deficiency

In addition to producing anemia, vitamin B_{12} deficiency (see Chapter 2 for vitamin B_{12} requirements) may result in marked neurological changes. Some of the more common causes of B_{12} deficiency are:

> Low dietary intake
>> Pure vegetarian diets
>
> Poor absorption
>> Low intrinsic factor—congenital, gastric atrophy associated with endocrinopathies, gastrectomy
>> Ileal disease—for example, Crohn's, celiac disease
>> Ileal resection—for example, after necrotizing enterocolitis
>> Blind loop
>> Drugs—PAS, neomycin, oral contraceptives (possibly)
>
> Increased requirement
>> Rapid growth or cell turnover (possibly)
>> Hyperthyroidism
>
> Poor utilization
>> Malnutrition (possibly), renal or liver disease (possibly), malignancy (possibly)

Dietary vitamin B_{12} deficiency is uncommon in children except in some individuals following pure vegetarian regimes.

Dietary deficiency is uncommon in children except in some individuals following pure vegetarian regimes. Poor absorption is a more common cause of deficiency. Vitamin B_{12} is normally absorbed only after it is complexed with intrinsic factor, a protein secreted in the stomach. Congenital absence of intrinsic factor or atrophy of gastric mucosa associated with endocrinopathies may result in poor absorption. Because absorption of B_{12} occurs primarily in the ileum, diseases affecting this part of the small intestine, such as Crohn's disease, may result in deficiency. Premature infants with partial intestinal resections following necrotizing entercolitis are being encountered more and more often. Whenever ileal resection has been involved, deficiency may eventually result if the vitamin is not administered. Blind loop syndromes and certain drugs may also result in deficiency. In these cases it is uncertain whether increased requirement for or poor utilization of the vitamin is responsible for clinical vitamin B_{12} deficiency.

Vitamin B_{12} deficiency is diagnosed by the combination of appropriate hematologic findings: a normal or elevated serum or red-blood-cell folic acid level and a low serum concentration of the vitamin. After the diagnosis has been confirmed, the Shilling test, a measure of vitamin B_{12} absorption, may be indicated as a means of differentiating among the possible causes of deficiency. In most instances treatment will be by the parenteral route. Daily doses of 25–50 μg of B_{12} initially or monthly doses of ten times this amount should be adequate. Most of the conditions resulting in B_{12} deficiency are permanent, making continued treatment necessary.

Vitamin E Deficiency

The anemia of vitamin E deficiency is confined primarily to premature infants. As was pointed out in Chapter 2, vitamin E functions as an antioxidant in biological systems. The requirement for vitamin E varies directly with the content of polyunsaturated fatty acids in the diet. Sources of polyunsaturated fatty acids are generally good sources of vitamin E. Caution must be exercised with infants who are receiving prolonged parenteral alimentation, in order to assure that vitamin E intake is adequate. Because vitamin E is fat soluble, any disease resulting in steatorrhea, such as cystic fibrosis or biliary atresia, may result in poor absorption. The premature infant with poor fat absorption may not absorb vitamin E well either. Iron appears to interfere with the absorption or utilization of vitamin E. For this reason, many neonatologists manage premature infants during the first month with formula that is not iron fortified (see Chapter 12).

Because vitamin E is fat soluble, any disease resulting in steatorrhea may result in poor absorption.

Vitamin E deficiency should be suspected in premature infants with mild hemolytic anemia associated with edema of the eyelids, labia, or lower extremities. An abnormal peroxide-hemolysis test is suggestive. A serum concentration of alpha-tocopherol less than 0.5 mg/dL has been considered diagnostic. Serum tocopherol values can only be interpreted properly if total serum lipid content is known, as this affects the tocopherol level. Management of vitamin E deficiency anemia involves providing additional vitamin E (1 mg/kg/day has been suggested) and minimizing contributing factors such as increased iron in the diet.

Copper Deficiency

The full-term infant is born with adequate copper stores. Copper is excreted in bile but is efficiently reabsorbed in the intestinal tract, with very little net loss. Poor dietary intake of copper is

Poor dietary intake of copper is rarely a cause of copper deficiency.

rarely a cause of copper deficiency except in the case of prolonged parenteral alimentation with solutions inadequate in copper. Realimentation, either oral or parenteral, of the copper-depleted child without providing adequate copper will also condition deficiency. Poor absorption of copper occurs in children with chronic intractable diarrhea and also as a congenital defect in Menkes' disease. Because 90% of copper is bound to the plasma protein ceruloplasmin, any disease causing increased protein losses, such as exudative enteropathies or nephrotic syndrome, may result in an increased dietary requirement for copper. The additional quantities required are easily supplied by most diets.

Because ceruloplasmin is thought to function in part as a ferrioxidase affecting iron absorption at the intestinal level, it is not surprising that the anemia of copper deficiency resembles that of iron deficiency. Neutropenia is an earlier manifestation of copper deficiency and always precedes anemia. Copper-deficient children will have absolute neutrophil counts of less than 1500. Although a leukocytosis occurs with infection in a copper-deficient child, the response is muted. The association of neutropenia with unresponsive "iron-deficiency" anemia in the appropriate clinical setting should suggest copper deficiency. A serum copper of less than $70~\mu g/dL$ is suggestive except in young infants, whose ceruloplasmin levels are physiologically low, and in cases of severe protein deficiency. In the latter instance, the reduction in ceruloplasmin results in a low serum copper level despite adequate total body copper. Copper sulfate in a dose of approximately 0.2 mg/kg/day is indicated in the treatment of copper deficiency and results in a marked response in affected individuals.

The association of neutropenia with unresponsive "iron-deficiency" anemia in the appropriate clinical setting should suggest copper deficiency.

Suggested Reading

Committee on Nutrition, American Academy of Pediatrics. 1976. Iron supplementation for infants. *Pediatrics* 58:765–767.

Cordano, A.; Baertl, J. M.; and Graham, G. G. 1964. Copper deficiency in infancy. *Pediatrics* 34:324–336.

Dallman, P. R. 1974. Iron, vitamin E, and folate in the preterm infant. *J. Pediatr.* 85:742–752.

Dallman, P. R.; Reeves, J. D.; Driggers, D. A.; and Lo, E. Y. T. 1981. Diagnosis of iron deficiency: the limitations of laboratory tests in predicting response to iron treatment in 1-year-old infants. *J. Pediatr.* 98:376–381.

Dallman, P. R.; Siimes, M. A.; and Stekel, A. 1980. Iron deficiency in infancy and childhood. *Am. J. Clin. Nutr.* 33:86–118.

Fomon, S. J.; Ziegler, E. E.; Nelson, S. E. and Edwards, B. B. 1981. Cow milk feeding in infancy: gastrointestinal blood loss and iron nutritional status. *J. Pediatr.* 98:540-545.

Garby, L.; Irnell, L.; and Werner, I. 1969. Iron deficiency in women of fertile age in a Swedish community. III. Estimation of prevalence based on response to iron supplementation. *Acta Med. Scand.* 185: 113-117.

Hoag, M. S.; Wallerstein, R. P.; and Pollycove, M. 1961. Occult blood loss in iron deficiency anemia of infancy. *Pediatrics* 27: 199-203.

Oski, F. A. 1979. The nonhematologic manifestations of iron deficiency. *Am. J. Dis. Child.* 133:315-322.

Oski, F. A.; and Landow, S. A. 1980. Inhibition of iron absorption from human milk by baby food. *Am. J. Dis. Child.* 134:459-460.

Owen, G. M.; Kram, K. M.; Garry, P. J.; et al. 1974. A study of the nutritional status of preschool children in the United States, 1968-1970. *Pediatrics.* 53:597-646.

Picciano, M. F.; and Derring, R. H. 1980. The influence of feeding regimen on iron status during infancy. *Am. J. Clin. Nutr.* 33: 746-753.

Saarinen, U. M.; and Siimes, M. A. 1979. Iron absorption from breast milk, cow's milk and iron supplemented formula: an opportunistic use of changes in total body iron determined by hemoglobin, ferritin, and body weight in 132 infants. *Pediatr. Res.* 13:143-147.

Siimes, M. A.; Refino, C.; and Dallman, P. R. 1980. Manifestation of iron deficiency at different levels of intake. *Am. J. Clin. Nutr.* 33: 570-574.

Wilson, J. F.; Lahey, M. E.; and Heiner, D. C. 1974. Studies on iron metabolism. V. Further observations on cow's milk-induced gastrointestinal bleeding in infants with iron-deficiency anemia. *J. Pediatr.* 84:335-344.

9 Lactose Intolerance and Milk Intolerance

Contents

Lactose Intolerance 177
- Normal Lactose Digestion 177
- Physiologic Changes in Lactase Activity with Age 177
- Pathologic Changes in Lactase Activity 179
- Lactose Malabsorption 180
- Lactose Intolerance—Problems of Terminology 182
- Diagnosis of Low Intestinal Lactase and Lactose Intolerance 182
- Lactose Malabsorption and Symptomatic Intolerance 184
- Asymptomatic Lactose Malabsorption 186

Milk Protein Intolerance and Milk Allergy 188
- Problems of Identification 189
- Prevalence 190
- Clinical Pictures 190
- Diagnosis 192
- Management of Milk-Protein Intolerance or Allergy 192
- Prophylaxis of Allergy by Withholding Milk 193

Overview

No food is consumed with greater frequency or in greater quantity in infancy and early childhood than milk. Consequently, it is not surprising that when abnormal signs or symptoms appear, especially in the gastrointestinal tract, the question of milk intolerance or milk allergy is raised. Because most racial groups experience a decline in intestinal lactase levels during childhood, symptomatology associated with the ingestion of milk and resulting from lactose malabsorption is common. Reactions to the protein constituents of milk can also occur. The prevalence of these reactions and whether they are immunologically mediated are still the subjects of investigation and debate. This chapter gives an overview of the syndromes that have been ascribed to milk intolerance. However, because of its relatively greater frequency and importance, lactose intolerance is covered in greater detail.

LACTOSE INTOLERANCE

Lactose intolerance has many connotations, which range from asymptomatic malabsorption of lactose to diarrhea following ingestion of small amounts of lactose.

Normal Lactose Digestion

Lactose, a β-galactoside of glucose and galactose, is uniquely present in mammalian milk and is the principal carbohydrate in the diet of human infants. Digestion of lactose occurs at the brush border of the epithelial cells of the small intestine. Although there are two other enzymes with lactase activity, the neutral lactase of the brush border is virtually completely responsible for hydrolysis of lactose to its component monosaccharides. This hydrolysis is the rate-limiting step in the assimilation of lactose. As is the case with absorption of other carbohydrates, the absorption of lactose carries with it sodium and water. In addition, lactose absorption appears to exert a favorable effect on calcium absorption.

> Hydrolysis of lactose to its component monosaccharides by the brush border is the rate-limiting step in the assimilation of this carbohydrate.

Physiologic Changes in Lactase Activity with Age

The three principal disaccharidases—lactase, sucrase, and maltase—are all found in highest concentration in the jejunum. For reasons not understood, the fetal development of sucrase and maltase occurs quite early. These enzymes are present in significant concentrations in utero as early as 10 to 12 weeks. Lactase concentrations have been studied in only a small number of human infants, but it appears that lactase concentrations do not begin to rise until after 32 to 33 weeks of gestation (Figure 9–1). Virtually all premature infants are born with low intestinal lactase levels. Whether low enzyme concentrations should be equated with lactose intolerance and whether some other carbohydrate should be substituted for lactose in the diet of premature infants are questions that are addressed later.

> Figure 9–1
>
> Virtually all premature infants are born with low intestinal lactase levels.

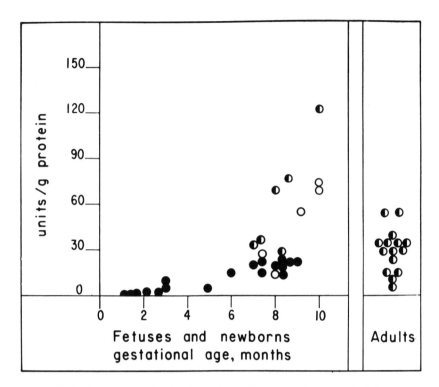

Figure 9-1 Lactase activity in the embryo, fetus, newborn, and adult. ○ indicates children less than one day of age. ● shows children older than one day of age, but before first feeding and ◑ shows individuals older than one day but after the first feeding. Reprinted from Auricchio, S.; Rubino, A.; and Mürset, G. 1965. Intestinal glycosidase activities in the human embryo, fetus and newborn. *Pediatrics* 35:944–954. Copyright American Academy of Pediatrics.

Lactase concentrations reach their highest level at term or shortly thereafter. Even at term sucrase concentration is 1½ to 2 times higher and maltase concentration is 4 to 5 times higher than that of lactase. Lactase concentrations remain high throughout infancy. In most individuals there is a gradual decline following infancy. This age-related pattern is not unique to man; it is found in most mammals past the age of weaning. Among humans, Whites, especially those of Northern European origin, deviate from the normal pattern. Lactase persists in Northern European Whites in high concentration throughout adult life.

The age-determined and racially determined loss of lactase in Blacks, Orientals, and many Whites (Figure 9–2) should not be thought of as lactase deficiency for several reasons. First, this

Figure 9-2

The age-determined and racially determined loss of lactase in Blacks, Orientals, and many Whites should not be thought of as lactase deficiency.

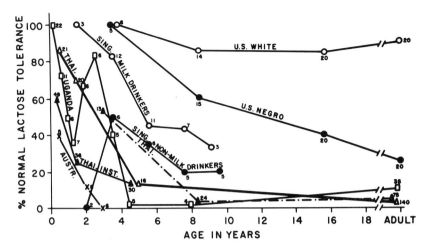

Figure 9-2 Prevalence of lactose intolerance at different ages in various racial groups. From Bayless, T. M.; and Paige, D. M. 1972. Disaccharide intolerance in feeding programs. In White, P. L.; and Selvey, N., editors. *Proceedings, Western Hemisphere Nutrition Congress III, 1971.* Mount Kisco, N. Y.: Futura Publishing Company, Inc., pp. 188–193.

pattern occurs in most humans in the absence of pathology, even if substantial quantities of milk continue to be drunk. Second, the enzyme does not disappear entirely, although its concentration may be only 10% to 20% of that seen during infancy. The practitioner should keep in mind the distinction between low intestinal lactase activity and lactase deficiency when approaching clinical lactose intolerance in the older child or adolescent in whom age-determined and racially determined loss of enzyme activity would be expected. As will be discussed in greater detail later, because some enzyme activity persists, many individuals who have abnormal lactose-tolerance tests are nevertheless able to continue to drink milk in usual quantities.

Pathologic Changes in Lactase Activity

In addition to the physiologic changes in lactase levels that occur with age, there are two pathologic forms of low lactase levels. Congenital or primary alactasia is an extremely rare condition in which the child is born without lactase activity. This absence of the enzyme is permanent.

Primary alactasia is very rare. Most lactose intolerance is secondary in nature, especially following infectious enteritis.

Far more frequent and clinically important is the loss of lactase secondary to acute infectious diarrhea or other intestinal diseases. Under normal circumstances, the enterocytes of the small intestine are produced in the crypts of the mucosa, migrating during a period of 2 to 5 days to the tips of the villi. Disaccharidase levels in the brush border of immature crypt cells are low. Maturation of disaccharidases occurs during migration. Epithelial cells at the tips of the villi have maximal enzyme concentrations. Many forms of infectious enteritis disrupt the intestinal mucosa, causing these cells to be shed into the lumen. This results in an acute and marked decrease in all disaccharidase levels. Because lactase is normally present in the lowest concentration of any of the disaccharidases, its loss is more frequently clinically apparent. During recovery cells migrate rapidly from crypts to tips, repopulating the villi with enterocytes. Rapid migration does not allow adequate time for the complete maturation of the cells. As a result, even after the villi are completely covered with enterocytes, the enzyme concentrations of these cells may be lower than normal. The time required for total recovery is uncertain and may vary with the agent responsible for the diarrhea.

Lactose Malabsorption

Factors Affecting Absorption   Up to this point we have been discussing only the normal and abnormal changes in enzyme activity that are known to occur. Carbohydrate digestion and absorption, however, depend on more than enzyme activity alone. Other factors involved are: quantity of carbohydrate ingested, enzyme concentration, total surface area of the small intestine available for absorption, and length of time the carbohydrate is in the small intestine.

Enzyme concentration per surface area may be adequate but the mucosa may be atrophic. In this case total enzyme activity (enzyme concentration × surface area) would be markedly reduced. Malnutrition often results in both a decrease in enzyme concentration and a reduction of surface area. Surface area may also be reduced following intestinal resection; there is marked mucosal hypertrophy but the total surface area frequently does not reach normal.

The amount of time that the substrate, lactose, and enzyme are in contact is also important. Any condition resulting in rapid intestinal transit will decrease the time that the substrate and enzymes have to interact.

Bolus or infrequent feeding may present the intestinal mucosa with more lactose than can be hydrolyzed during the short period of time allowed, whereas the same quantity of lactose given slowly over a longer period of time may be absorbed without difficulty.

Figure 9–3

Fermentation of unabsorbed lactose by bacteria in the colon produces many of the signs and symptoms characteristic of lactose intolerance.

Pathophysiology of lactose malabsorption   Lactose that is not hydrolyzed and absorbed in the small intestine passes into the large intestine (Figure 9–3). Here it comes in contact with the colonic microflora, and fermentation ensues. The end products of this fermentation generate many of the symptoms associated with lactose intolerance and are important in several of the tests used to make the diagnosis. Lactose is first split into its component monosaccharides; glucose and galactose are then further metabolized. Lactic acid and short-chain fatty acids (volatile fatty acids) are produced. Their presence results in the lower pH of the stools of lactose malabsorbers. The degradation of the lactose molecule into many smaller molecular forms substantially increases the osmolality of the intestinal contents, pulling water into the lumen. In addition, the acid pH tends to inhibit absorption of water by the colonic mucosa. Both the high osmolality and the low pH contribute to diarrhea. Fermentation also produces several gases, among them hydrogen and carbon dioxide. These gases explain the sometimes frothy nature of the stools seen in lactose

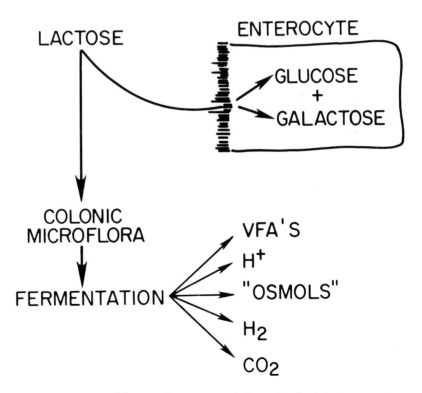

Figure 9–3   Normal lactose absorption and the pathophysiologic events in lactose malabsorption.

malabsorption. In addition, both hydrogen gas and carbon dioxide are absorbed from the colon and subsequently excreted by the lungs. The hydrogen breath test for the diagnosis of lactose intolerance makes use of this phenomenon.

Lactose Intolerance—Problems of Terminology

"Lactose intolerance" means many things to many people. The differences are of more than semantic importance.

"Lactose intolerance" is used by different people to mean different things. The lack of consistency in definition is more than a semantic problem since recommendations for diagnosis and management depend on the definition employed. Some investigators equate decreased lactase concentration in intestinal biopsy material with lactose intolerance. Decreased lactase concentration might better simply be termed low intestinal lactase. A flat or muted plasma glucose curve following the ingestion of a standard amount of lactose is the criterion used by some others. Still other investigators require associated signs and symptoms in addition to the flat glucose response. Finally, there are those who believe that the diagnosis of lactose intolerance should be a clinical diagnosis based purely on symptomatology, regardless of intestinal lactase level or plasma glucose curves. This last approach makes the most sense from a nutritional point of view.

Diagnosis of Low Intestinal Lactase and Lactose Intolerance

A variety of tests are available for the presumptive diagnosis of low intestinal lactase.

Intestinal biopsy Most direct is the assay of enzyme activity on a biopsy specimen of the jejunum. However, there is disagreement about what enzyme activity level constitutes low intestinal lactase. Determination of lactase activity is frequently used as the standard against which other tests are judged. This standard is appropriate if the final question that requires answering is whether the enzyme level is high or low. But if the question to be answered is whether milk is responsible for symptoms or whether an individual can drink milk, the use of biopsy material as a reference point is less appropriate. In addition, determination of lactase levels in infants and small children is impractical because it is difficult to obtain the mucosal specimen for assay.

Determination of lactase activity is frequently used as the standard for lactose intolerance. This may not be appropriate.

Lactose tolerance test The test most frequently relied on is the standard lactose tolerance test. In this test, lactose, 2 g/kg (maximum 50 g), is given as a 20% suspension in water after an overnight fast. Blood glucose levels are obtained prior to ingestion and 20, 40, and 60 minutes after ingestion. A rise of blood glucose of more than 25 mg/dL above baseline is considered by most to be a normal test, although some investigators use a lower figure—20 mg/dL. Determination of glucose by Dextrostix® used in conjunction with the reflectance meter designed to read them is generally sufficient for this test. Variables such as gastric emptying time, intestinal surface area, and the rate of peripheral uptake of glucose from the plasma after absorption help to explain the degree of discordance noted between the results of lactose tolerance testing and assays of intestinal lactase levels.

There is a degree of discordance between the results of lactose tolerance testing and assays of intestinal lactase levels.

During the lactose tolerance test, the practitioner should look for signs and symptoms of lactose intolerance. In older children abdominal pain is an important symptom. In younger children and infants, borborygmi should be listened for. All stools passed during the 24 hours following lactose administration should be tested for pH and reducing substance. A decrement of the stool pH to a level of 5.5 or below and a rise in reducing substance are indicative of lactose malabsorption, though not necessarily of clinical intolerance.

Standard lactose tolerance tests give unphysiologically large loads of lactose.

The standard lactose tolerance test has been fairly criticized as being unphysiologic; the dose is relatively large and the lactose is given as a pure suspension rather than as part of milk, the form in which lactose is usually consumed. Although small infants taking in 130 to 140 kcal/kg may approach an intake of 2 g lactose per kilogram at a single feeding, in general lactose intakes, even by most small infants do not approach 2 g/kg at a single feeding. In later infancy and early childhood lactose intakes relative to body weight are decreased. The 8-ounce glass of milk offered at mealtime contains 12 g of lactose. A 12 g dose of lactose has been suggested as more appropriate than the 2 g/kg test dose. Studies of the symptomatic response to 12 g of lactose either as pure suspension or as milk show that there are fewer symptoms with this dose than with the standard higher dose used in the lactose tolerance test. If the milk is ingested as part of a meal, even fewer symptoms are experienced.

Breath hydrogen lactose tolerance test The breath hydrogen lactose tolerance test is a modification of the standard lactose tolerance test. It relies on the fact that fermentation of malabsorbed lactose produces hydrogen gas, a fixed percentage (about 15%) of which is absorbed from the colon and subsequently excreted via the lungs. Because the human body produces no hydrogen gas by its intermediary metabolism, any hydrogen gas found in expired air must be the result of bacterial fermentation of unabsorbed substrate.

Breath hydrogen excretion can be used as an index of lactose malabsorption.

The breath hydrogen lactose tolerance test is performed in a manner similar to the standard lactose tolerance test. Rather than, or in addition to, blood samples for glucose determination, breath samples are obtained prior to ingestion of lactose and at 30, 60, 90, 120, and 180 minutes after the ingestion of lactose. The older child can provide an end expiratory breath sample by blowing up a bag. A small nasal cannula is used to obtain a sample from the younger child. An increase in breath hydrogen concentration of more than 10 parts per million (ppm) is considered an abnormal test. Elegant studies in adults using the nonabsorbable lactose analogue, lactulose, have demonstrated that breath hydrogen excretion by any individual is directly proportional to the amount of carbohydrate reaching the large intestine. Consequently, the magnitude of the breath hydrogen response can be used to some degree to estimate the amount of lactose being malabsorbed. The breath hydrogen lactose tolerance test is useful in diagnosing lactose malabsorption, but here again, a positive test should not be considered a positive indication of clinical lactose intolerance in the symptomatic sense or of the inability to drink milk.

Each test measures a different parameter.

The discordance between the results of various tests used to diagnose lactose intolerance is not surprising, because each test is measuring a different parameter. The practitioner should choose the test to use according to what question he or she wants answered. In the following discussion of the clinical syndromes associated with lactose intolerance, it will become clear that a clinical challenge with lactose in solution or as milk, keying on signs and symptoms, is frequently the most appropriate test to use in deciding whether milk should be continued in the diet. In those instances in which milk clearly causes symptoms, monitoring changes in blood glucose or breath hydrogen is a useful adjunct for delineating whether the intolerance is to lactose or to some other component of milk.

Lactose Malabsorption and Symptomatic Intolerance

Lactose intolerance is usually suspected in any of three clinical settings: acute diarrhea following the reintroduction of milk to a child recovering from an episode of infectious enteritis, chronic nonspecific diarrhea of childhood, and chronic abdominal pain of childhood.

Intolerance after infectious enteritis The tendency for infectious diarrhea to worsen after the reintroduction of milk has been noted for many years. The pathophysiology of this secondary type of low intestinal lactase and associated intolerance was described previously. Some practitioners change all infants recovering from acute infections to lactose-free formulas because of the possibility of lactose intolerance. While the exact incidence of secondary lactose intolerance is unknown, most infants do not seem to require lactose-free diets if milk is reintroduced gradually. We reserve lactose-free formulas for those children demonstrating signs and symptoms after milk ingestion.

Routine use of lactose-free formulas after acute diarrhea is probably not warranted.

It is not necessary to perform a standard lactose-tolerance test in this type of secondary low intestinal lactase. Some physicians carry out a modified lactose-tolerance test using the first milk feeding as the challenge. Obtaining blood for glucose determinations by finger stick before and at intervals after this first feeding may be useful in some instances, but in general the clinical response to the reintroduction of small quantities of milk provides the best guide for managing the patient. Because of the enzyme concentration, surface area, and time considerations discussed above, small amounts of lactose may be tolerated in situations where the response to a standard 2 g/kg challenge dose could lead to massive diarrhea and possibly dehydration. The smaller the infant, the less appropriate is the standard challenge because of the possible side effects if the infant is intolerant. A modified tolerance test may be more useful after milk has been successfully reintroduced; it can quantify to some degree the efficiency of lactose absorption.

Chronic nonspecific diarrhea Chronic nonspecific diarrhea of childhood is a syndrome characterized by the onset of loose stools between 7 and 20 months of age. The child is otherwise well and continues to grow adequately. One of the original reports of this syndrome by Davidson and Wasserman (1966) pointed out that the diarrhea was generally not responsive to dietary manipulations. Although lactose intolerance is frequently raised as a possible cause for chronic nonspecific diarrhea of childhood, in fact it is rarely the cause. The age of onset of the syndrome is well before the age-dependent and race-dependent decline in lactase activity should occur. Unless chronic diarrhea follows an acute episode of diarrhea, there is no reason to think that a spontaneous decline in lactase has taken place, especially in White children. Whether continued diarrhea per se can alter intestinal lactase levels is uncertain. Rarely, a trial of a milk-free diet may be indicated to gauge clinical response. A lactose tolerance test is rarely of value in management.

Lactose intolerance is rarely the cause of chronic nonspecific diarrhea.

Chronic abdominal pain Chronic abdominal pain affects 10%–15% of children between the ages 4 and 12. A number of reports have documented that lactose intolerance is responsible for the

It is uncertain how frequently lactose intolerance is responsible for chronic abdominal pain.

pain in some of these children. A recent study by Barr et al (1979), in which children were screened with a lactose tolerance test and then further studied by responses to lactose-containing and lactose-free diets suggested that the prevalence of symptomatic lactose intolerance in children with chronic abdominal pain could be as high as 28%. These studies are difficult to carry out and interpret because it is nearly impossible to "blind" both patient and observer. Because there appears to be strong psychological overlay in much of the chronic abdominal pain of childhood, a placebo effect resulting from obvious dietary manipulation cannot be ruled out.

This is well illustrated by another study (Lebenthal et al. 1981) in which 103 White children with recurrent abdominal pain were evaluated. Twenty-one (30%) of 69 children studied with lactose tolerance tests were classified as lactose malabsorbers. The same prevalence of lactose malabsorption was found in a matched control population without recurrent abdominal pain. During a diet trial of three successive six-week dietary periods—lactose-free, lactose-containing, lactose-free—48% of lactose malabsorbers and 24% of lactose absorbers reported increased pain in association with lactose consumption. However, 33% of malabsorbers and 24% of absorbers also experienced increased pain when given a lactose-free dietary supplement. After a 12-month milk elimination diet, 6 of 15 (40%) malabsorbers and 5 of 13 (38%) absorbers were pain-free. Five of 12 (42%) lactose absorbers who had not been on a milk-free diet also experienced resolution of their pain.

Lactose intolerance unquestionably explains intermittent abdominal pain in some children. For children in whom it is suspected, a lactose tolerance test may be helpful, but the response to milk-free and milk-containing diets is far more important. Ideally, it would be preferable to use a milk-free diet with the addition of capsules containing lactose and glucose separately, noting the response to each. This is seldom practicable.

Asymptomatic Lactose Malabsorption

Throughout this chapter we have repeatedly stressed the importance of using clinical response rather than the results of lactose tolerance tests in making decisions about patient management. Although this approach has always seemed appropriate, recent information about the degree to which both premature and full-term infants malabsorb lactose with no symptomatology or apparent ill effect has underscored this point. The low pH of the stool in infancy, especially of the breast-fed infant, is the result of

Table 9-1

Most full-term and premature infants malabsorb substantial amounts of lactose with no apparent ill effects.

fermentation of carbohydrate reaching the colon. Significant amounts of reducing substances (greater than 0.5%) are found in nearly half of all full-term infants fed standard formulas or human milk. Lactose, glucose, and galactose can also be found in the stool of normal infants. Some years ago Auricchio et al (1965) assayed the total lactase activity of a group of fetuses and premature infants that died shortly after birth. They then calculated the maximum amount of lactose that could be hydrolyzed by the entire small intestine every 24 hours. In Table 9-1 these calculated quantities are compared to the lactose intake that a normal infant of the same gestational age would be receiving if 120 kcal/kg/day were fed as a standard lactose-containing formula. Table 9-1 also shows the estimated percentage of ingested lactose that would be malabsorbed. The results of the study indicate that premature infants probably malabsorb large quantities of lactose.

Recent studies of breath hydrogen excretion by both full-term and premature infants show that lactose malabsorption is the rule rather than the exception. Mean breath hydrogen concentrations of 55 ± 15 ppm were evident in 10 full-term infants at 10 days of age following a formula meal containing 1.8 ± 0.2 g lactose per kg of body weight. A sequential study of premature infants fed increasing amounts of lactose also showed persistently high breath hydrogen excretions by these infants. It was estimated that as a group these infants failed to absorb up to 50%–60% of ingested lactose in the small intestine.

Table 9-1 Calculated maximal *in vitro* hydrolysis of lactose by the entire small intestine

Gestational age (lunar months)	Number studied	Lactose hydrolysis* (g/24 hr)		Mean† weight (g)	Lactose intake at 120 kcal/kg/d (g)	Estimated percent malabsorbed
		Died at <1 day of age	Died after 1 day of age			
6	1	0.3	—	875	10.8	97
7–8	6	3.8	6.4	1375	16.9	62–78
8–9	8	5.8	23.4	2100	25.8	9–22

Source: MacLean, W. C., Jr.; and Fink, B. B. 1980. Lactose malabsorption by premature infants: magnitude and clinical significance. *J. Pediatr.* 97:383–389.

*Data from Auricchio, S.; Rubino, A.; and Murset, G. 1965. Intestinal glycosidase activities in the human embryo, fetus, and newborn. *Pediatrics* 35:944–954.

†Based on intrauterine growth curve.

Despite breath hydrogen excretions that would be considered grossly abnormal in older children and adults, most premature and full-term infants do well on lactose-containing formulas. Estimated energy losses in the stools of these infants are not exceedingly high. This has suggested that the colonic microflora may have an important role in the adaptation to small intestinal lactose malabsorption. Volatile fatty acids are known to be absorbed from the large intestine of the adult and it has been hypothesized that most of the products of fermentation of lactose by colonic bacteria are also absorbed from the large intestine of the infant.

The infant, especially the premature infant, exemplifies the human organism that habitually ingests large amounts of lactose without symptoms despite apparently low intestinal lactase levels. Many of the world's population of older children and adults also have low intestinal lactase levels, yet drink milk with no ill effects. It has been recognized for some time that many individuals with low intestinal lactase can be habituated to milk ingestion; their symptoms decrease or disappear after prolonged consumption. Biopsy studies document that this is not the result of induction of the enzyme itself. The importance of the colonic microflora in the adaptation to lactose ingestion by these older individuals is uncertain at this time.

> The most important lesson to be learned from the response of normal infants to lactose loads is the importance of relying on clinical response rather than specific tolerance testing.

The most important lesson to be learned from the response of normal infants to lactose loads is the importance of relying on clinical response rather than tolerance testing. If blood sugar rises were used to determine intolerance to starch, most individuals would be judged starch intolerant because of the slow hydrolysis and absorption of these macromolecules in the intestine. Similarly, if breath hydrogen excretion, pH of less than 5.5, or the presence of reducing substance in the stool were to be used as the basis of removing lactose from the diet, almost all infants would be judged lactose intolerant. The most appropriate role for lactose tolerance testing is the differentiation of lactose intolerance from other types of intolerance in individuals experiencing symptoms after milk ingestion.

MILK-PROTEIN INTOLERANCE AND MILK ALLERGY

Milk-protein intolerance and milk allergy are not clearly understood. There seems little doubt that reactions to milk protein occur. However, there is a lack of diagnostic criteria that specifically relate intolerance to the ingestion of a food and that demonstrate an immunologic basis to the reaction that occurs.

Problems of Identification

Goldman's criteria Despite their marked shortcomings, the criteria of Goldman et al (1963) are still accepted in making the diagnosis of milk allergy. These criteria require that, on three occasions, symptoms abate when milk is eliminated and recur within 48 hours after the reintroduction of milk. While these criteria may be adequate for establishing an intolerance to milk, they in no way imply an immunologic basis for the reaction. Contaminants in the food, such as antibiotics or microorganisms, irritants such as bovine serum albumin, and lactose in the lactose-intolerant individual, would all be capable of causing reactions that would meet these criteria.

To establish a diagnosis of milk allergy the Goldman criteria should be carried one step further—that is, the reaction should be shown to be immunologically mediated. While in principle this seems like a reasonable and simple thing to do, in practice it becomes quite difficult. Milk contains at least 20 proteins that might serve to sensitize the individual. Beta-lactoglobulin, a protein not found in human milk, appears to be one of the most antigenic. During the hydrolysis of proteins that occurs in normal digestion, additional antigens may be produced.

Antibodies to milk protein The demonstration of antibodies to milk protein in plasma is of no value in substantiating milk allergy. The appearance of cow milk protein in plasma and the subsequent development of antibodies in healthy cow-milk-fed infants was demonstrated more than 40 years ago. The absorption of these whole proteins has been shown to be due to incompletely developed intestinal secretory IgA. The extent of antibody formation depends in large part on the age at which cow milk protein is introduced. Antibodies to milk protein are common in childhood but are almost never seen in the adult, who develops an immunologic tolerance.

Skin testing and RAST Skin testing with milk protein has also been used to try to substantiate milk allergy. Standardization of preparations and dosages is lacking. As a rule, a negative skin test with appropriate antigen rules out allergy to cow milk. However, a positive skin test may be seen in many atopic individuals and is unhelpful; there is a high frequency of positive tests coupled with asymptomatic responses after ingesting cow milk. It was hoped that the development of the radioallergosorbent test (RAST) would provide a more precise way of diagnosing food allergy. Here again, the correlation between a positive test and clinical problems has been found to be low. These difficulties in diagnosis caused

While the usual criteria used for diagnosis *may* be adequate for establishing an intolerance to milk, they in no way imply an immunologic basis for the reaction.

Antibodies to milk protein are common in childhood.

As a rule a negative skin test with appropriate antigen rules out allergy to cow milk.

Davidson (1969) to state, "Some of us regularly sift through the host of confusing papers which appear in the field of gastrointestinal allergy in the fond hope that we may substantiate our suspicion that the entity must exist." In the discussion that follows we will concentrate on intolerance to milk proteins, pointing out those areas in which an immunologic mechanism may be operative.

Prevalence

The prevalence of milk "allergy" has been estimated to be as low as 0.1% and as high as 7.5%. In one study (Gerrard et al. 1973) that used criteria similar to Goldman et al. but with only two challenges required, 7.5% of infants were felt to have milk allergy as manifested by diarrhea, vomiting, eczema, rhinorrhea, bronchiolitis, or asthma. Similar studies designed to answer the same question have yielded much lower figures. It seems likely that the differences in results of various studies relates more to the design and criteria of the studies themselves than to actual differences in prevalence from one experimental population to another.

Clinical Pictures

A number of clinical conditions have been attributed to milk allergy. Systemic anaphylaxis has occurred on rare occasions following the ingestion of milk, and no one doubts the allergic basis of this response. Atopy is frequently related to the ingestion of a variety of foods and, as will be discussed, the use of a milk-free diet for the prevention of atopic disease in infants at risk has been studied on several occasions.

Four discrete gastrointestinal syndromes have been attributed to milk allergy.

There are four principal gastrointestinal syndromes ascribed to intolerance to cow milk protein.

Acute colitis   Acute colitis following the ingestion of cow-milk protein in milk or in commercial formula has been seen in a number of infants. This may occur in infants as young as several days of age. Blood and mucus are passed in the stools. Elimination of milk from the diet results in prompt reversal of symptomatology.

Malabsorption associated with intolerance   A syndrome of malabsorption associated with cow-milk intolerance has been studied extensively by Kuitunen and coworkers (1975). Diarrhea and failure to thrive were the presenting problems. Blood and mucus were not prominent. Characteristic were the early age of onset—average age 9 weeks—and the prompt response to withdrawal of milk.

Symptoms of intolerance disappeared in most children by 1 year of age. It should be stressed that the syndrome must be relatively uncommon since an average of only six cases per year were seen in a relatively large children's hospital by a group known to be interested in the problem.

Blood-losing and protein-losing enteropathy An enteropathy characterized by protein and blood loss rather than by malabsorption has also been described in association with the ingestion of cow milk. The presence of large numbers of eosinophils on biopsy material has heightened the suspicion that this syndrome is mediated on an allergic basis. (The apparently unrelated phenomenon of enteric blood loss following the ingestion of whole cow milk that has not been heat treated was discussed in Chapter 8.)

Heiner's syndrome In 1967 a syndrome of poor growth, gastrointestinal symptoms, iron deficiency anemia, and pulmonary hemosiderosis in association with precipitins to cow milk protein was described. This has come to be known as Heiner's syndrome. Clinically the problem presented between 13 days and 6 months of age. Growth below the 10th percentile was characteristic. Recurrent pulmonary disease with changing signs on x-ray was also seen. Three-quarters of the patients had an eosinophilia of more than 10%. When precipitins to cow milk were studied, all patients reacted to at least five different fractions. Although Heiner's syndrome is generally thought of as a manifestation of intolerance to cow-milk protein, it should be noted that of seven infants carefully studied, three developed symptoms while being exclusively breast-fed. Sensitivity to cow-milk protein in infants being nursed by mothers drinking cow milk has been documented. Unfortunately, the dietary history of the nursing mothers in the study whose infants developed Heiner's syndrome is unknown.

All the syndromes described present at a rather young age with dramatic symptoms. All improve strikingly when milk is withdrawn from the diet.

There are several things that all of the previously described syndromes have in common: All present at a rather young age with dramatic symptoms. All improve strikingly when milk is withdrawn from the diet. Finally, judging from the size of the series of patients reported, none seems to be exceedingly common.

Tension-fatigue syndrome For the sake of completeness, the tension-fatigue syndrome should be mentioned. Those who believe in it suggest that a variety of symptoms—from clumsiness, photophobia, sluggishness, and pallor, to tiredness, increased sweating, and enuresis—are all the result of allergy to foods, milk among them. We are unaware of any credible scientific evidence supporting the validity of this syndrome. Although withholding milk from the diet in such cases can conceivably have a placebo effect, it unnecessarily deprives the child of an excellent food and distracts the physician from approaching the actual cause of the problem.

Diagnosis

One must document that milk causes the reaction and exclude other possible causes of the reaction.

May (1975) has listed three general principles on which the diagnosis of milk allergy or any other food allergy should be based. First, it must be documented that milk results in an adverse reaction. Second, other possible causes of the reaction must be excluded. Finally, an immunologic mechanism for the reaction must be demonstrated. This last step is exceedingly difficult under the best of circumstances and for practical purposes is probably not necessary; once the cause of the reaction has been identified as milk, the management of either milk intolerance or milk allergy involves a milk-free diet.

Because milk is drunk so frequently, almost any sign or symptom is preceded by recent ingestion of milk.

The diagnosis of milk allergy should be approached with a healthy skepticism. Because of the frequency with which milk is drunk, a temporal relationship usually exists between the ingestion of milk and almost any sign or symptom. Add to this the general awareness by parents of the concept of milk allergy, and it is not surprising that many parents arrive in the office wondering whether milk is the cause of their child's problems. A detailed history should be taken at this point.

It is very important to make the challenge a blind one whenever possible.

If milk intolerance in any form seems likely, milk should be withdrawn from the diet for a period of several weeks. If symptoms subside, a challenge with milk should be carried out; the practitioner should look for the previously reported signs and symptoms. It is very important to make the challenge a blind one whenever possible. Many parents become so convinced that their child is allergic to milk, that the psychologic overlay of placing a glass of milk on the table in front of the child may in and of itself help to produce signs and symptoms. In addition, parents may unconsciously take note of changes in behavior or other symptoms during the period of milk challenge that had been present and ignored during the milk-free period. Because milk and lactose can be obtained in powdered forms, both can easily be given in capsules in a blind fashion. May (1975), whose experience with food allergy is extensive, states that only a small minority of suspected reactions will be proven to be due to the food in question when verification by blind challenge is required.

Management of Milk-Protein Intolerance or Allergy

Management of milk-protein intolerance revolves around a cow-milk-free diet. In the past goat milk was frequently used as a substitute for cow milk. That this should have produced beneficial results in as many children as it did is of interest, because there is considerable cross reactivity of the proteins in goat milk and cow milk.

Soy-based formulas are currently the mainstay in the treatment of cow-milk intolerance. Soy protein has acquired an unwarranted reputation for being hypoallergenic. Yet the proteins of the soybean appear to be every bit as antigenic as those of cow milk, although there is apparently little cross reactivity. Sensitivity to soy protein is well documented and occasionally may manifest in a child who has previously been diagnosed as sensitive to cow milk. It is tempting to speculate that if soy-protein formula were introduced at as early an age and with the same frequency as cow-milk formula, the prevalence of sensitivity to soy protein would be greater than that currently observed. Hydrolyzed protein and amino acid mixtures are more expensive than soy-based formula, but they may be the only remedy for true protein intolerance.

Soy protein has acquired an unwarranted reputation for being hypoallergenic.

Prophylaxis of Allergy by Withholding Milk

Nearly 30 years ago Johnstone and Glaser (1953) published the results of a study in which cow milk was withheld from the diets of 91 infants from birth to between 6 and 9 months of age. A soybean formula was used instead. The authors were not completely successful in withholding cow milk—more than 25% of their study group received cow milk in the first 3 months of life. The prevalence of allergy in the test group was compared with that found in the case histories of 65 older siblings and in a review of cases of 175 additional children previously seen in the authors' allergy practice. Only 15% of the test group manifested major allergic problems during the 2- to 5-year period of follow-up. This compared with 64% of the sibling controls and 52% of the other controls. The authors concluded that a milk-free diet was beneficial in preventing the development of allergy in infants at risk. A subsequent editorial (Lowell and Schiller, 1954) pointed out the fact that half of the children developing major allergy in all three groups had been diagnosed as allergic to milk.

More recent studies (Brown et al, 1969) of the same problem have reached opposite conclusions about development of allergy (Table 9-2). A milk-free diet was suggested for 183 infants; 85 families agreed, but 98 rejected the idea. An additional 196 children were followed as a control group. The prevalence of allergy subsequently found in all three groups was similar regardless of dietary management. Saarinen et al (1979), however, demonstrated that the prevalence of atopic disease was significantly

Table 9-2

Table 9-2 A prospective study of milk-free diet in the prophylaxis of allergy

	Number in group	Percent with subsequent allergy
Offered	183	9.8
Accepted	85	10.6
Rejected	98	9.2
Control	196	13.3

Source: Brown, E. B.; Josephson, B. M.; Leveine, H. S.; and Rosen, M. 1969. A prospective study of allergy in a pediatric population. The role of heredity in the incidence of allergies and experience with milk-free diet in the newborn. *Am. J. Dis. Child.* 117:693. Copyright 1969, American Medical Association.

lower in a group of infants who were predominantly breast-fed and received no cow milk for the first 6 months than in infants introduced to whole cow milk earlier in life. This effect was limited to infants with a family history of allergy. The authors speculated that a protective effect of breast-feeding through secretory IgA could have prevented absorption of potentially antigenic proteins. There are data available to confirm such an effect in young animals other than humans.

There is no question that withholding cow milk from the diet of an infant will delay, if not prevent, the manifestations of cow-milk intolerance. It would seem prudent to recommend a cow-milk-free diet for the newborn younger sibling of a child previously demonstrated to have cow-milk intolerance. The best means of accomplishing this is by prolonged breast-feeding. Whether cow milk should be withheld from the diet of the nursing mother in such a case is unsettled. Should the nursing infant begin to develop signs or symptoms, especially gastrointestinal bleeding, a history of maternal ingestion of cow milk should be investigated as a possible contributing factor.

> It would seem prudent to recommend a cow-milk-free diet for the newborn younger sibling of a child previously demonstrated to have cow milk intolerance. The best means of accomplishing this is by prolonged breast-feeding.

Suggested Reading

Auricchio, S.; Rubino, A.; and Mürset, G. 1965. Intestinal glycosidase activities in the human embryo, fetus, and newborn. *Pediatrics* 35:944–954.

Barr, R. G.; Levine, M. D.; and Watkins, J. B. 1979. Recurrent abdominal pain of childhood due to lactose intolerance: a prospective study. *New Eng. J. Med.* 300:1449–1452.

Davidson, M. 1969. *In* Gellis, S. B. (editor), *Yearbook of pediatrics.* Chicago: Year Book Medical Publishers, p. 95.

Davidson, M.; and Wasserman, R. 1966. The irritable colon of childhood (chronic nonspecific diarrhea syndrome). *J. Pediatr.* 69:1027–1038.

Eastman, E. J.; and Walker, W. A. 1979. Adverse effects of milk formula ingestion on the gastrointestinal tract: an update. *Gastroenterology* 76:365–375.

Gerrard, J. W.; MacKenzie, J. W. A.; Galuboff, N., et al. 1973. Cow's milk allergy: prevalence and manifestations in an unselected series of newborns. *Acta Paediat. Scand.*, Suppl. 234:1–21.

Goldman, A. S.; Anderson, D. W., Jr.; Sellars, W. A., et al. 1963. Milk allergy. I. Oral challenge with milk and isolated milk proteins in allergic children. *Pediatrics* 32:425–443.

Heiner, D. C.; Sears, J. W.; and Kniker, W. T. 1967. Multiple precipitins to cow's milk in chronic respiratory disease. *Am. J. Dis. Child.* 103:40–56.

Johnson, J. D.; Kretchmer, N.; and Simoons, F. J. 1974. Lactose malabsorption: its biology and history. *In* Schulman, I. (editor), *Advances in pediatrics.* Chicago: Year Book Medical Publishers, Vol. 21, pp. 197–237.

Johnstone, D. E.; and Glaser, J. 1953. Use of soybean milk as an aid in the prophylaxis of allergic disease in children. *J. Allergy* 24:434–436.

Kuitunen, P.; Visakorpi, J. K.; Savilhati, E.; and Pelkonen, P. 1975. Malabsorption syndrome with cow's milk intolerance. Clinical findings and course in 54 cases. *Arch. Dis. Child.* 50:351–356.

Lebenthal, E.; Rossi, T. M.; Nord, K. S.; and Branski, D. 1981. Recurrent abdominal pain and lactose absorption in children. *Pediatrics* 67:828–832.

Lowell, F. C.; and Schiller, I. W. 1954. It is so—it ain't so (editorial). *J. Allergy* 25:57–59.

MacLean, W. C., Jr.; and Fink, B. B. 1980. Lactose malabsorption by premature infants: magnitude and clinical significance. *J. Pediatr.* 97:383–388.

May, C. D. 1975. Food allergy: a commentary. *Pediatr. Clinics of N. Am.* 22:217–220.

Saarinen, U. M.; Backman, A.; Kajosaari, M.; and Siimes, M. A. 1979. Prolonged breastfeeding as prophylaxis for atopic disease. *Lancet* 2:163–166.

Solomons, N. W.; Viteri, F. E.; and Rosenberg, I. H. 1978. Development of an interval sampling hydrogen (H_2) breath test for carbohydrate malabsorption in children: evidence for a circadian pattern of breath H_2 concentration. *Pediatr. Res.* 12:816–823.

10 Protein-Energy Malnutrition (PEM)

Contents

Marasmus   198
    Etiology   198
    Signs and Symptoms   200
    Laboratory Findings   201
    Management   201
Kwashiorkor   201
    Etiology   202
    Signs and Symptoms   203
    Laboratory Findings   204
    Management   204
    Marasmic Kwashiorkor   205
Classification and Diagnosis of PEM   205
    Gomez Classification   206
    Waterlow's Classification   207
    McLaren Score   207
Changes in Gastrointestinal Function in PEM   209
Effect of PEM on Ultimate Stature   209
    Infancy   209
    Older Childhood   210
Effect of PEM on Subsequent Mental Development   210
    Animal Studies   210

Human Studies **211**

Anorexia Nervosa **213**

Clinical Presentation **214**

Social and Psychologic Antecedents **214**

Management **215**

Long-term Prognosis **216**

Overview

Protein-energy malnutrition (PEM) is a significant problem for many infants, especially those with chronic disease. The child with failure to thrive is most often exhibiting a mild form of marasmus. Depending on the diet that has been fed and the infections the child has had, cystic fibrosis may present as either marasmus or kwashiorkor or as an intermediate syndrome. Both marasmus and kwashiorkor have characteristic physical and biochemical changes and an underlying pathophysiology on which the primary disease process is superimposed. This chapter concentrates on PEM, which is basically generalized undernutrition. Except for iron deficiency (Chapter 8), specific nutrient deficiencies, such as beriberi (thiamine deficiency) and scurvy (vitamin C deficiency) are uncommon in the United States. In the sections that follow, marasmus and kwashiorkor will be described in their pure, more severe forms. Although it is convenient to approach this description of protein-energy malnutrition by examining these two distinct diseases, the practitioner should recognize that many children in the United States present mixed forms of less severity.

MARASMUS

Etiology

Marasmus may be thought of as balanced starvation.

Conceptually, marasmus may be thought of as balanced starvation. In many cases it is a form of protein-calorie malnutrition in which the diet is particularly low in calories. Marasmus will result when a relatively well-balanced diet is consumed or absorbed in amounts that are inadequate to meet the host's requirements. Because nutrients are being consumed in proper proportion to one another, signs and symptoms of single-nutrient deficiencies are uncommon. In other clinical situations an unbalanced diet may be consumed in inadequate amounts, but the cessation of growth that accompanies inadequate energy intake prevents single-nutrient deficiencies from being expressed.

Table 10-1

The clinical situations in which marasmus is encountered are numerous. Some of the more common ones have been classified in Table 10-1. Many cases of failure to thrive, or mild infantile marasmus, are the result of child neglect or deliberate abuse. The common presentation is a child who is not growing adequately at home despite a history of good intake. Rapid weight gain ensues with

Table 10-1 Common causes of marasmus

Inadequate Intake

Abuse or neglect

Errors in formula preparation—overdilution

Psychosocial dwarfism

Congestive heart failure

Anorexia of chronic renal disease, chronic infection

Elimination diets—suspected food allergy, chronic nonspecific diarrhea

Vegetarian or natural foods—bulkiness, low energy density

Chronic vomiting—chalasia, achalasia, rumination, pyloric stenosis

Anorexia nervosa

Inadequate Absorption

Postintestinal resection

Decreased surface area—chronic diarrhea, celiac disease, Crohn's disease

Pancreatic disease—cystic fibrosis, Schwachman-Diamond syndrome

Chronic liver disease

Poor digestibility of foods—pure vegetarian, some natural foods

Increased Requirements

Hypermetabolic states—for example, hyperthyroidism

Increased "work," as with chronic lung disease, cardiac failure, and spasticity, or with competitive athletics

nothing more than proper feeding in the hospital. Poor growth in slightly older children has frequently been attributed to psychosocial factors. Although the early literature suggested that psychosocial dwarfs consumed large quantities of foods that were poorly utilized, the weight of current evidence points to neglect and inadequate intake as the cause of this syndrome. Inadequate intake of a balanced diet may also be seen in infants with congestive heart failure, whose poor ability to suck and difficulties with fluid overload often restrict intake; in children with anorexia due to chronic renal disease or chronic infection; or, in older girls, in anorexia nervosa, which is discussed at the end of this chapter.

A variety of diseases may result in malabsorption of a degree severe enough to alter nutritional status—for example, chronic diarrhea, celiac disease, or Crohn's disease; the loss of absorptive surface resulting from intestinal resection can also result in severe malabsorption. Inadequate pancreatic enzyme activity, most commonly in cystic fibrosis, or poor secretion of bile acids in chronic obstructive liver disease may also result in malabsorption. Parents who follow pure vegetarianism or who rely heavily on "natural" and undermilled foods may feed their children a diet that is relatively indigestible even with normal gastrointestinal function. Less commonly, marasmus may result when food intake is normal but nutrient requirements are uncommonly high. Several conditions that fall into this category are also listed in Table 10–1.

Signs and Symptoms

The physical appearance of the infant or child with marasmus depends on the degree of inadequacy of the diet. Marginal decreases in intake in infancy first result in a slowing in the rate of weight gain. Linear growth may continue at a normal rate or may be decreased slightly. These signs are typical of the mildly marasmic infant or "failure-to-thrive" case seen most commonly in outpatient practice. A more marked inadequacy of intake leads to a complete cessation of linear growth and weight gain. Weight loss may follow. This more severe form of marasmus is characteristic of chronically ill infants—for example, those with cystic fibrosis or chronic intractable diarrhea. Older children with marginal intakes over prolonged periods of time often grow more slowly than their peers but do not show any great disparity between weight and height; these children are the so-called hypocaloric dwarfs. More marked or acute decreases in intake in older children may result in the cessation of linear growth and in weight loss. The differentiation between the former case, stunting, and the latter, wasting, is further discussed later in this chapter.

> The marasmic child may be wasted, stunted, or both.

The infant who is marasmic is frequently irritable, somewhat listless, and withdrawn. Anthropometric measurements are all well below standard. The infant may appear only slightly thin or may be frankly wasted. There is a loss of subcutaneous fat as well as muscle mass. In the most severe form of marasmus the child appears to be "skin and bones." The eyes may lack luster and be somewhat sunken and the skin may tent, giving the examiner the false impression that the child is mildly dehydrated. A striking feature of the physical examination, other than the obvious wasting, is the absence of skin rashes, edema, or other signs of single-nutrient deficiency.

> A striking feature of the physical examination is the absence of skin rashes, edema, or other signs of single-nutrient deficiency.

Laboratory Findings

Most of the laboratory
findings in marasmus are
not specific.

Most of the laboratory findings in marasmus are not specific. A mild degree of "anemia" is frequently found. Hematocrits in the range of 29 to 30 with hemoglobins of 9.5 to 10 g/dL are frequently encountered. As discussed in Chapter 8, these values probably reflect an adjustment of the total red-cell mass appropriate for changes in lean body mass and metabolic rate, rather than actual anemia. In mild forms of marasmus, serum electrolytes are normal. In more severe forms there is a tendency to slight hyponatremia ($Na = 130-135$ meq/L). Infants with severe marasmus retain sodium, and therefore total body sodium is actually increased. Total body water increases even more, however, and the result is hyponatremia. Plasma glucose concentration may be low (50–50 mg/dL); the severely marasmic infant may develop hypoglycemia if a source of calories is not provided frequently. Finally, serum total protein and albumin concentrations are normal. Other serum proteins, such as prealbumin and transferrin, are also normal. In the child who has had frequent exposures to infectious agents, serum globulin concentrations may actually be elevated.

Management

The marasmic infant is metabolically well adapted to chronic undernutrition. Basal metabolic rate and oxygen consumption are markedly decreased. While such adaptations permit survival despite grossly inadequate intakes, they also make treatment difficult because of their resistance to reversal. Deadaptation occurs slowly and only after provision of a steady supply of nutrients.

The initial management of infants with marasmus must address questions of infection and hydration. Following this, oral feedings are cautiously reintroduced, beginning with intakes as low as 25 kcal/kg/day and increasing progressively (frequently to 175 kcal/kg/day) until weight gain and linear growth ensue. Attempts at rapid rehabilitation may induce diarrhea, further compromising nutritional status. The choice of diet and the details of nutritional management of marasmus are covered in Chapter 11.

KWASHIORKOR

At the other end of the spectrum of protein-energy malnutrition is kwashiorkor. Kwashiorkor is far less commonly seen than marasmus in the United States and in many cases is iatrogenic. Simplistically, kwashiorkor results when protein in the diet is inadequate relative to the intake of energy and other nutrients.

Etiology

The disparity between protein and energy intakes creates a situation in which the fuel necessary to run synthetic metabolic processes is present but the amino acid building blocks are not. In this situation proteins stored in muscle, serum albumin, and other sites are catabolized to provide amino acids for synthesis of proteins of a more critical nature.

The genesis of kwashiorkor is complex. In many environments, for example, the diet leading to kwashiorkor is not different from that resulting in marasmus. In otherwise healthy children, a progressive decrease in protein intake without a concommitant decrease in energy intake may result in slow growth because of inefficient use of dietary energy rather than in kwashiorkor. Infection frequently plays a role in producing kwashiorkor. Both bacterial and viral infections may induce a state of negative nitrogen balance. An acute episode of infection in the child whose protein intake is marginal in either quantity or quality may tip the balance from positive to negative. Measles is one of the most commonly recognized antecedents of kwashiorkor in many developing countries.

Some of the more common conditions associated with kwashiorkor in pediatric practice in the United States are listed in Table 10–2. Protein intake is rarely inadequate in American children in a free-living situation. Inappropriate parenteral or enteral therapy, however, may result in a wide disparity between energy and protein intakes in hospitalized children. The prolonged use of intravenous glucose, especially 10%–20% glucose, in an effort to provide more calories, without attention to providing amino acids sets up a classic situation in which kwashiorkor may occur. Commercial infant formulas are frequently altered by the addition of nonprotein energy in the form of polymers of glucose or medium chain triglycerides in an effort to "push calories." The result is that the percentage of calories supplied by protein in the formula may be reduced to well below the 8% that is desirable. In inappropriate parenteral or formula feeding, the stress of the primary condition or an episode of hospital-acquired infection is all that is needed to complete the development of kwashiorkor.

Inadequate absorption of nitrogen can produce kwashiorkor. Although cystic fibrosis is frequently associated with a generalized malabsorption and marasmus, a number of infants have presented with hypoalbuminemia and edema. Common to these infants has

Infection is often as important as low protein intake in the genesis of kwashiorkor.

Table 10–2

Table 10-2 Common causes of kwashiorkor

Inadequate intake

Prolonged intravenous glucose without amino acids

Excessive addition of fat or carbohydrate to infant formulas

Inadequate absorption

Cystic fibrosis—especially with human milk and soy formulas

Celiac disease

Inadequate utilization

Infection—measles, bacterial sepsis

Inborn errors of amino acid metabolism

Increased requirements

Protein-losing states: enteropathy, lymphangiectasia, nephrosis

Possibly burns

been a history of consumption of a diet of low protein content (human milk) or lower protein quality (soy formula). Older infants with celiac disease may present with the clinical picture of kwashiorkor. Inadequate utilization of protein because of infection has already been discussed. Finally, several clinical conditions may increase dietary requirements for nitrogen because of persistent protein loss.

Signs and Symptoms

Kwashiorkor is often superimposed on marasmus.

The child with kwashiorkor is frequently listless and irritable. Although kwashiorkor is often superimposed on marasmus, in its pure form kwashiorkor may be associated with normal height and weight for age. Because of the adequacy of energy in the diet, subcutaneous tissue may be well preserved. Initial appearances can be deceiving if there is edema. The child admitted with mild edema and apparently little loss of subcutaneous tissue may appear far more marasmic than anticipated when edema fluid has been completely mobilized several days or weeks later.

In kwashiorkor, one looks for hair changes, "flaky paint rash," hepatomegaly, and edema.

Several physical findings on examination are quite characteristic of kwashiorkor. The hair is silky, sparse, and straighter than normal. There is a change in the pigmentation of hair: black hair turns auburn or red. In addition, the hair can easily be plucked from the scalp. Microscopic examination of the hair root shows a characteristic disorganization of the root cells. Depigmentation of the skin occurs frequently. Quite characteristic is the so-called "flaky paint rash." This rash resembles dry desquamating skin but when peeled off leaves open raw areas. The distribution of the rash is not distinctive. It may occur on all extremities and on the trunk as well. Enlargement of the liver secondary to fatty infiltration is a hallmark. Livers palpable 2 to 5 cm below the right costal margin are not uncommon. In children whose serum albumin concentration has fallen to less than 2 g/dL, pitting edema is almost invariably present.

Laboratory Findings

Hematocrit and hemoglobin concentrations are depressed to a degree similar to that seen in marasmus. This may result either from protein deficiency per se or from changes in oxygen transport requirements. Serum electrolytes are usually abnormal. The serum sodium concentration is frequently decreased below 135 meq/L, often to a level of 130 meq/L or less. This should not be interpreted as sodium depletion. Total body sodium is markedly increased, as is total body water. Serum chloride concentration is at the low end of the normal range or lower. The serum potassium concentration is often quite low (<3 meq/L); this low serum potassium level represents a potentially life-threatening derangement. Total body potassium depletion has been documented in kwashiorkor. It is thought to result from an intracellular accumulation of sodium and a corresponding loss of potassium.

Derangements of serum sodium and potassium are common in kwashiorkor.

Many of the commonly measured serum proteins are low in kwashiorkor. Serum albumin, prealbumin, and transferrin are all decreased to some degree. There appears to be a hierarchy with which serum proteins are preserved. For example, normal concentrations of serum globulins, important in host defense against infections are maintained. For most clinical purposes, the measurement of serum albumin concentration is sufficient both for defining the severity of kwashiorkor and for assessing the clinical response to treatment. A number of other serum proteins with shorter half-lives have been shown to be more sensitive indicators but their superiority as indicators in the day-to-day diagnosis and management of most patients has not been clearly demonstrated.

Management

The child with kwashiorkor is far less well adapted to his inadequate dietary intake than the child with marasmus, which makes the child with kwashiorkor both more precarious and, in some respects,

Paramount in initial management of children with kwashiorkor is the recognition that these children are waterlogged and potassium depleted.

Providing generous amounts of potassium not only effects an increase in the serum potassium concentration but also results in the excretion of sodium.

easier to treat. Paramount in initial management of children with kwashiorkor is the recognition that these children are waterlogged and potassium depleted. It is extremely important *not* to give solutions containing high concentrations of sodium in an effort to improve the serum sodium concentration. Conversely, quantities of potassium above those normally provided for maintenance are required. Potassium intakes should be increased from 3 meq/kg/day to at least 5 meq/kg/day during the first week. Providing generous amounts of potassium not only effects an increase in the serum potassium concentration but also results in the excretion of sodium. Serum sodium concentration increases slowly over a period of days. Mobilization of edema fluid may take several weeks and usually occurs before the serum albumin concentration reaches a level of 2 g/dL, indicating the role of electrolyte imbalance in the genesis of edema in these infants.

As with marasmus, the treatment of severe infection can be lifesaving in kwashiorkor. Once the child is considered stable, cautious reintroduction of oral feeding is begun. Detailed management of this phase of treatment is covered in Chapter 11.

Marasmic Kwashiorkor

Pure kwashiorkor is exceedingly uncommon in the United States. In most instances, signs of protein depletion are superimposed on the clinical picture of marasmus. The development of kwashiorkor may be a gradual process heralded by a gradually enlarging liver and slowly falling serum albumin concentration in a chronically under-nourished hospitalized child. Alternatively, a child with marasmus secondary to short gut or chronic intractable diarrhea may suffer an acute episode of infection, rapidly manifesting signs of kwashiorkor. The fluid and electrolyte management outlined briefly for kwashiorkor is appropriate for marasmic kwashiorkor. Once acute derangements have been corrected, the practitioner is left with a marasmic child, whose treatment will generally be prolonged and somewhat difficult.

CLASSIFICATION AND DIAGNOSIS OF PEM

A variety of different classification systems for malnutrition exist. None is without its strong points and shortcomings. Many systems of classification have been designed with field studies in mind and thus may be more useful in assessing the prevalence of a specific type of malnutrition in a population than in making a diagnosis in a specific child. Classifications designed for field studies rely on laboratory determinations as little as possible.

There are three classifications of potential value for the primary-care practitioner. Two of these are used to assess the degree of undernutrition and to decide whether the child is stunted or wasted. The third provides a useful set of criteria for differentiating among marasmus, marasmic kwashiorkor, and kwashiorkor.

Gomez Classification

Table 10-3

The oldest and simplest approach to classifying undernourished children is that of Gomez et al (1956) shown in Table 10–3. This classification is based on the 50th percentile of weight-for-age using the Boston growth standard. The National Center for Health Statistics (NCHS) standard can be used equally well. In this classi-

Classification is based on weight and height for age and on weight-for-height.

fication the child's weight as a percentage of the appropriate 50th percentile weight-for-age is calculated and classified as normal or as first-degree, second-degree, or third-degree malnutrition, according to the value. Gomez derived this classification based on mortality rates of malnourished children. In general, children with second-degree and third-degree malnutrition begin to manifest important functional changes in organ systems such as the gastrointestinal tract or in those systems involved in host defense. Treatment is most difficult and mortality highest in children with third-degree malnutrition. Children classified as normal or as first-degree rarely show functional changes of significance in organ systems. The Gomez classification has two major drawbacks. First, because the 50th percentile is used as the reference point

Table 10–3 The Gomez classification of malnutrition

Percent of weight-for-age*	Classification
91–100	Normal
76–90	First degree
61–75	Second degree
≤60	Third degree

Source: Gomez, F.; Galvan, R. R.; Frenk, S.; et al. 1956. Mortality in second and third degree of malnutrition. *J. Trop. Ped.* 2:77.

*Based on the 50th percentile of the Boston growth standard.

children in the upper range of first-degree malnutrition will in fact fall between the 3rd and 25th percentiles of the Boston or NCHS growth curves and may well be normal. Second, the classification fails to distinguish between the acutely malnourished or wasted child and the more chronically malnourished stunted child.

Waterlow's Classification

Table 10-4

A system that takes both height-for-age and weight-for-height into account and that overcomes the difficulties of the Gomez classification has been developed by Waterlow (1976) (Table 10-4). Height-for-age, a measure of stunting, is classified as normal or as mildly, moderately or severely retarded. Intervals of 5% are used because they represent about two standard deviations of the distribution of height-for-age around the median. Weight-for-height, a measure of wasting, is graded in decrements of 10%, about one standard deviation. Combining these two measures, the child can be classified as stunted, wasted, or both. Wasting requires acute nutritional intervention. Stunting necessitates a more long-term approach to nutritional management. Stunting with wasting is the most severe form of marasmus and requires both acute and chronic care.

Wasting requires acute nutritional intervention. Stunting necessitates a more long-term approach to nutritional management.

McLaren Score

Neither of the first two classifications distinguishes marasmus from kwashiorkor. The diagnosis of kwashiorkor relies on the findings of

Table 10–4 Waterlow's classification of protein-energy malnutrition

Index	Degree of wasting or stunting*			
	Normal	Mild	Moderate	Severe
Stunting (low height-for-age)	>95%	90–95%	85–90%	<85%
Wasting (low weight-for-height)	>90%	80–90%	70–80%	<70%

Source: Waterlow, J. C. 1976. Classification and definition of protein-energy malnutrition. *In* Beaton, G. H.; and Bengoa, J. M. (editors), *Nutrition in preventive medicine*. Geneva: WHO, pp. 530–555.

*Percent of height-for-age and weight-for-height based on the 50th percentile of the Boston growth standard.

Table 10-5

The McLaren score is useful in making the diagnosis of kwashiorkor.

liver enlargement, low serum albumin concentration, edema, and characteristic skin and hair changes. The McLaren score (Table 10–5) assigns points for each of these findings and may be a useful approach to the assessment of sicker, hospitalized children whose nutritional status is poor.

The system is not foolproof, however. Severe kwashiorkor superimposed on a marasmic child will be classified as pure kwashiorkor rather than marasmic kwashiokor if this system is used. In practice, either the Gomez or Waterlow classification provides a useful guide in assessing the degree of undernutrition. The McLaren score will prove most useful in making the diagnosis of kwashiorkor in the hospital setting.

Table 10–5 The McLaren score for the classification of severe malnutrition

Physical or laboratory finding	Points	Classification	
Edema	3	Marasmus	0–3 points
Dermatosis	2	Marasmic kwashiorkor	4–8 points
Edema + dermatosis	6	Kwashiorkor	9–15 points
Hair changes	1		
Hepatomegaly	1		
Serum albumin concentration (g/dL)			
>3.5	0		
3.0–3.4	1		
2.5–2.9	2		
2.0–2.4	3		
1.5–1.9	4		
1.0–1.4	5		
0.5–0.9	6		

Source: McLaren, D. S.; Pellett, P. L.; and Read, W. C. 1967. A simple scoring system for classifying the severe forms of protein-calorie malnutrition in early childhood. *Lancet* i:533.

CHANGES IN GASTROINTESTINAL FUNCTION IN PEM

Although there are differences in the changes in gastrointestinal function seen in marasmus and kwashiorkor, there are several common features. Morphologically, in PEM there is a variable degree of mucosal atrophy in the small intestine. Disaccharidase levels are decreased, particularly in the case of lactase. Concentrations of pancreatic proteases, lipase, and amylase are also reduced. The functional significance of these alterations is minor in many instances, because these enzymes are normally secreted in excess. Bile acid concentrations are also decreased, and it has been demonstrated that malnourished children have difficulty in achieving the critical micellar concentration required to solubilize lipids in the intestinal lumen (see Chapter 11).

Generalized malabsorption accompanies PEM and helps to perpetuate poor nutritional status.

The net result of the changes in gastrointestinal function is generalized malabsorption. Digestion and absorption of protein is less affected than digestion and absorption of fat and carbohydrate. Malabsorption tends to perpetuate malnutrition. A vicious cycle is set up in which poor absorption further compromises nutritional status, which in turn leads to further derangement in digestion and absorption. A nutritional approach to interrupting this cycle is discussed fully in Chapter 11.

EFFECT OF PEM ON ULTIMATE STATURE

Infancy

The degree to which catch-up growth is possible after severe malnutrition in infancy or early childhood has been the subject of much study. It was frequently stated that growth that failed to occur during critical periods was lost, never to be regained. Recent evidence contradicts this idea. Growth retardation on a nutritional basis is associated with a parallel retardation of bone age. Both head circumference and bone age will generally be appropriate for actual height, which suggests that the capacity exists for growth not yet achieved.

Both head circumference and bone age will generally be appropriate for actual height, which suggests that the capacity exists for growth not yet achieved.

Long-term follow-up studies of infants severely malnourished in infancy have demonstrated that complete catch-up growth is possible. Even children who were little above birth weight at 6 to 9 months of age have achieved heights and weights within the normal range. The extent of catch-up depends on the adequacy of the diet and freedom from further nutritional insults or severe infections during subsequent years. Whether full genetic potential for height is attainable by these children is a question that cannot be answered.

Older Childhood

It is more difficult to be certain of the effect on ultimate stature of a period of nutritional inadequacy in older childhood. Mild insults probably cause no problems. It is uncommon to see an American child past the age of 3 or 4 years with markedly impaired nutritional status on the basis of inadequate food intake alone. In the older child chronic diseases such as renal failure or Crohn's disease often underlie growth failure. Decreased food intake secondary to anorexia may be partly responsible. To what extent the disease processes themselves influence growth velocity is uncertain. What is clear, however, is that there is a limited number of years left for catch-up growth when growth retardation occurs in late childhood or early adolescence. This limitation is especially critical in girls, whose epiphyses close following menarche. Boys may grow until their early 20s and thus theoretically have a better chance of catching up once the underlying disease process is brought under control and nutrition is improved.

> There is a limited number of years left for catch-up growth when growth retardation occurs in late childhood or early adolescence.

EFFECT OF PEM ON SUBSEQUENT MENTAL DEVELOPMENT

Whether a period of severe malnutrition in infancy results in a permanent deficit in mental ability is a far more critical question to answer than whether there is a relationship between malnutrition and subsequent size. Whereas the loss of a few centimeters of ultimate stature is of minor importance, any reduction in subsequent learning abilities and mental development is considered a definite handicap. Ten years ago the prevailing point of view was that malnutrition during critical periods of brain growth resulted in irreversible reductions in brain cell number and mental function. More recent studies have called this point of view into question. While clearly no one suggests that malnutrition is desirable or beneficial, studies in both lower animals and humans have suggested that the mental deficits associated with malnutrition may not be as devastating as previously thought.

> Mental deficits associated with malnutrition may not be as devastating as previously thought.

Animal Studies

Because of the ease with which studies of rats are carried out, the malnourished rat has been used most frequently to study the relationship of malnutrition and mental development. Malnutrition of rats during early infancy produces a number of changes. Overall brain size is decreased. Cell number, reflected by total DNA, is also reduced, especially in the cerebellum. Both the protein and lipid contents are also low. Functionally, the animals are listless and learn poorly. Many of the biochemical and functional changes appear to be permanent even if adequate nutrition is provided subsequently.

It is difficult to apply findings in rats to humans because of the differences in the timing of brain development.

It is difficult to apply these findings to humans for several reasons. The most important is the marked difference in the timing of development of the brain in rats and humans. For example, there is normally a large increase in neuronal cell number in the rat early in extrauterine life, a phase of development that occurs in the human during the second trimester *in utero*. The rat brain at birth is developmentally similar to that of the 17–week human fetus. Malnutrition of the rat in early infancy primarily affects processes that normally occur *in utero* in the human at a time in development when the fetus is relatively well protected from the effects of maternal malnutrition.

Many studies in animals have been criticized because the severity of malnutrition produced experimentally is far worse than that generally seen in humans. More importantly, animal studies have rarely tried to control for environmental effects on mental development. The technique often used to malnourish infant rats—that is, expanding the number of pups in the litter—leads not only to malnutrition but also to psychological deprivation. Maternal deprivation alone may produce changes in the degree of arborization of dendrites in well-nourished but maternally deprived rats (see Greenough 1975). Findings such as these emphasize the importance of controlling for effects of environment in interpreting human studies and also indicate a direct link between environmental deprivation and physical and biochemical changes in the brain.

Human Studies

Not surprisingly, there are few studies of the biochemical changes in the human brain following severe malnutrition. Early studies by Winick and his coworkers (see Winick 1971) confirmed that many of the deficits previously demonstrated in the rat were also present in the human. When total DNA, protein content, lipid content, and lipid:DNA ratio (a crude measure of myelinization) were determined in a group of nine infants who had died from malnutrition, all of the values obtained were low in comparison to those of nonmalnourished children of the same age. The meaning of these findings is not clear. It is unreasonable to expect brain growth during

It is unreasonable to expect brain growth during malnutrition to parallel that seen in normal children of the same age.

malnutrition to parallel that seen in normal children of the same age when growth of the rest of the body is markedly retarded. When each child's values for DNA, protein, lipid, and so on were plotted against height, most values fell within the normal range, the exceptions being those of several infants in whom there was some question of intrauterine growth retardation. A further problem with autopsy studies is that they do not address either the potential for recovery or the functional changes associated with biochemical alterations.

Virtually all early studies of the subsequent mental development of previously malnourished children were carried out in underdeveloped countries where there was a high prevalence of infantile malnutrition. These studies indicate that a child malnourished in infancy will function at a suboptimal level later in life. However, a cause-and-effect relationship between malnutrition and suboptimal functioning cannot be assumed. Studies done in poor environments have rarely been controlled for factors such as parental IQ, the degree of physical recovery of the infant, the extent to which chronic undernutrition is present, and, most importantly, aspects of the environment itself, such as mental stimulation. Children who have become malnourished in underdeveloped countries seldom return to an optimal environment in which adequate food and mental stimulation are provided. Rather, they return to the same environment that was initially responsible for their malnutrition. It is completely plausible that the malnutrition in infancy and the subsequently poor mental development are separate effects resulting from a common cause. It is doubtful that studies carried out in suboptimal environments can ever settle this question.

Studies of mental development after malnutrition in underdeveloped countries cannot be expected to separate environment from nutritional effects.

Several studies carried out in the United States surmount these difficulties. The study groups comprised children who suffered a finite period of severe malnutrition resulting from treatable illnesses and who were afterward returned to good home environments with adequate nutrition. Klein and coworkers (1975) used pyloric stenosis as a model of malnutrition. Most infants were below expected weight for age at the time of admission, and all recovered rapidly following surgery. Subsequent mental development was compared to a sibling control group and a matched control group that had not required hospitalization. A weight deficit of as little as 10% (based on the 50th percentile) was found to be associated with measurable deficits in some functions. Children with deficits of 21%–42% were most severely affected.

Whether infants with pyloric stenosis are an appropriate model for malnutrition is questionable. Much of the weight deficit manifested by these children was most certainly the result of dehydration. Serum electrolyte values were not reported. Dehydration and electrolyte imbalance of the severity frequently seen in pyloric stenosis are known to affect the brain directly and could have been responsible for the observed differences. Anesthesia and surgery of an infant in suboptimal condition could also have contributed to the deficits observed.

Several other studies have used cystic fibrosis and other forms of malabsorption in infancy as their model. Lloyd-Still and his coworkers (1974) followed up a group of 41 infants who had been malnourished in infancy, 34 as a result of having cystic fibrosis. Using the criteria of Gomez, 58% of the infants were classified as showing third-degree malnutrition. Appropriate dietary management had resulted in good physical recovery in all instances. When recovered children under the age of 5 were tested and compared with sibling controls, their scores on standardized tests, which rely to a large degree on physical development, were found to be inferior. Children over the age of 5 showed no difference from sibling controls when Wechsler intelligence tests were administered. These data were interpreted as showing that deficits of mental functioning resulting from malnutrition were reversible but that this reversal required a number of years of good nutrition and mental stimulation. Ellis and Hill (1975) have reported similarly good results in studies of children slightly less malnourished as the result of cystic fibrosis. Finally, Winich and coworkers (1975) have reported normal IQ values in a group of Korean children chronically undernourished during early childhood but subsequently adopted into higher socioeconomic circumstances in the United States.

Many children who have been severely malnourished and returned to good home environments have achieved intelligence in the normal range. Whether a deficit that is unmeasurable remains and why some children do not appear to recover fully are questions that remain unanswered. Nevertheless, when parents ask about the future mental potential of a child malnourished as a result of a correctable disease process, the practitioner has good reason to be optimistic.

> Studies on the effects of nutrition and environment support the contention that a finite period of malnutrition is not necessarily associated with subsequent poor mental development.

ANOREXIA NERVOSA

Anorexia nervosa is a psychologic disorder affecting primarily teenage girls. Although severe malnutrition, almost always in the form of marasmus, is the feature that precipitates diagnosis and treatment, the emotional disability that eventually results in self-enforced weight loss is present for years before nutritional status is affected. Similarly, the reestablishment of adequate food intake and appropriate body weight, which is relatively easily achieved on an inpatient if not on an outpatient basis, often does little to correct the cause of the disorder, and relapse is common in severe cases if prolonged psychiatric therapy is not pursued.

Clinical Presentation

Ninety percent of patients with anorexia nervosa are girls. Weight loss begins sometime after the age of 10, generally shortly after the pubertal growth spurt. This weight loss is voluntary. In retrospect, many patients can pinpoint a comment or event that convinced them they were too fat and that led to the institution of rigid weight control. Anorexia in the true sense of the word is absent; many girls experience constant hunger—bulimia—and go on eating binges when they lose control over their appetite. Bulimia may be followed by self-induced vomiting. Purgative abuse in an effort to control weight is also occasionally encountered in anorexia. Other anorexic patients display an undue concern for food by spending excessive amounts of time preparing food for others while refusing to eat themselves. There is a complete denial of any problem, emotional or nutritional, as weight loss becomes progressive. Secondary sexual characteristics are gradually lost and menstruation ceases or fails to begin. Although some experts suggest that at least 25% of body weight must have been lost for the diagnosis of anorexia nervosa to be secure, it seems inappropriate to allow weight loss to continue to this point once the characteristic pattern of anorexia nervosa is obvious.

> There is a complete denial of any problem, emotional or nutritional.

Physical examination reveals signs and symptoms characteristic for marasmus, with moderate to severe degree of emaciation. Hypothermia and bradycardia may be present. Lanugo hair is common. The hematocrit may be low, as may be the peripheral white blood cell count. Serum electrolytes, total protein, and albumin concentrations are generally in the normal range. A variety of endocrinologic changes have been noted. These and the defects in intestinal absorption that are often found are probably nonspecific alterations related to the marasmic state. Low plasma retinol and carotene levels have been noted, but overt clinical vitamin A deficiency does not appear to be a problem.

Social and Psychologic Antecedents

Children with anorexia nervosa tend to come from families of higher social class, but this is not uniformly the case. Parents of children with anorexia nervosa are generally college educated.

Family turmoil is common despite an exterior appearance of well-being. The patients themselves are generally described as bright, perfectionist, high achieving. Mean IQ has not been found to be above average, and many children may have invested long hours to attain the high degree of achievement expected of them by their parents.

Detailed descriptions of the psychopathology of this disorder are available elsewhere (see Bruch, 1973). Briefly, these children have a pervasive sense of inadequacy and ineffectiveness. There has generally been a strong dependence on parents, especially for decision making, with a lack of autonomy. Body image is very distorted; most anorexics consistently overrate the size of their body in relation to others. Anxiety and depression are frequent, especially in response to loss of control—that is, weight gain or excessive eating. Malnutrition and hunger superimpose their own behavioral changes on this premorbid personality.

These children have a pervasive sense of inadequacy and ineffectiveness.

Management

Treatment of anorexia nervosa should not be undertaken by the primary-care practitioner alone. Although nutritional status may be so poor as to require immediate hospital intervention, successful treatment will require months to years. Outpatient management is frequently tried. In mild cases this may be successful. In many instances office visits may serve primarily to convince all concerned that a problem exists and to gain acquiescence for hospital admission.

The hospital approach to management generally involves nutritional therapy in association with behavioral modification techniques, psychotherapy, and occasionally the use of medication in the form of antidepressants or drugs that promote weight gain. The efficacy of drug therapy in general is unproven.

Depending on the hospital, patients are admitted to a children's psychiatric ward or to the appropriate general ward. Both approaches have their pluses and minuses and both seem to work. Patients with anorexia nervosa generally require 5000 calories or more per day to sustain steady weight gain. There are reports of the use of total parenteral nutrition to reverse deteriorating nutritional status. Most patients are treated enterally, eating four meals a day. The diet should be well balanced and should take into account known likes and dislikes of the patient. High-protein diets, food supplements, and so on are not required. Initially the patient is confined to her room and the acquisition of ward privileges, such as time in the game room, use of telephone, and receipt of mail, is contingent on food intake initially and on weight gain subsequently. The exact

Management generally involves nutritional therapy in association with behavioral modification techniques and psychotherapy.

approach used varies from unit to unit (one such routine is described in detail in the study by Schmidt and Duncan, 1974). All seem to agree on the necessity of good primary-care nursing and a nonpunitive approach to the patient.

Regular psychotherapy is begun during hospitalization. This treatment may involve the parents as well as the child. During sessions with the child, criteria for discharge are frequently negotiated. Hospitalization for 10–12 weeks or more is common. Long-term psychiatric treatment is usually required following discharge, especially in more severe cases.

Long-term Prognosis

Up to 15% of patients may relapse following discharge and require rehospitalization. In some reports death has occurred in up to 10% of patients, either from acute metabolic complications of starvation or by suicide. With competent treatment these figures should not be so high, especially in the pediatric age group. Early onset of the disease is one factor associated with good prognosis. Factors that may augur poorly include late onset, a history of self-induced vomiting and laxative abuse, and severe depression.

Suggested Reading

Bruch, H. 1973. *Eating disorders.* New York: Basic Books.

DeMaeyer, E. M. 1976. Protein energy malnutrition. In Beaton, G. H.; and Bengoa, J. M. (editors), *Nutrition in preventive medicine.* Geneva: WHO, pp. 23-54.

Ellis, C. E. and Hill, D. E. 1975. Growth, intelligence and school performance in children with cystic fibrosis who have had an episode of malnutrition during infancy. *J. Pediatr.* 87:565–568.

Graham, G. G.; and Adrianzen, T. B. 1971. Growth, inheritance and environment. *Pediatr. Res.* 5:691–697.

Greenough, W. T. 1975. Experimental modification of the developing brain. *American Scientist* 63:37–46.

Klein, P. S.; Forbes, G. B.; and Nader, P. R. 1975. Effects of starvation in infancy (pyloric stenosis) on subsequent learning abilities. *J. Pediatr.* 87:8–15.

Latham, M. C. 1974. Protein calorie malnutrition in children and its relation to psychological development and behavior. *Physiol. Rev.* 54:541–565.

Lloyd-Still, J. D.; Hurwitz, I.; Wolff, P. H.; and Schwachman, H. 1974. Intellectual development after severe malnutrition in infancy. *Pediatrics* 54:306–311.

McLaren, D. S.; Pellett, P. L.; and Read, W. C. 1967. A simple scoring system for classifying the severe forms of protein-calorie malnutrition in early childhood. *Lancet* i:533–535.

Schmidt, M. P. W.; and Duncan, B. A. B. 1974. Modifying eating behavior in anorexia nervosa. *Am. J. Nurs.* 74:1646–1648.

Vigersky, R. A. (editor). 1977. *Anorexia nervosa.* New York: Raven Press.

Waterlow, J. C. 1976. Classification and definition of protein-energy malnutrition. In Beaton, G. H.; and Bengoa, J. M. (editors), *Nutrition in preventive medicine.* Geneva: WHO, pp. 530–555.

Winick, M. 1971. Cellular growth during early malnutrition. *Pediatrics* 47:969–978.

Winick, M.; Meyer, K. K.; and Harris, R. C. 1975. Malnutrition and environmental enrichment by early adoption. *Science* 190:1173–1175.

11 Nutritional Management of Malabsorption and Malnutrition

Contents

Normal Mechanisms of Digestion and Absorption 219
- Protein 219
- Fat 220
- Carbohydrate 223

Malabsorption and Malnutrition in Infancy 223
- Formulas Available for Management 224
- Products Available for the Modification of Formulas 225
- Specific Clinical Conditions 230

Malabsorption and Malnutrition in the Older Child 238
- Crohn's Disease 238
- Ulcerative Colitis 239

Overview

Malabsorption is a common complication of many diseases in infancy and childhood. A number of acute and chronic intestinal diseases directly impair absorption to variable degrees. Equally important and often unrecognized is the relationship between poor nutritional status and malabsorption. Many diseases may result in moderate to severe malnutrition by mechanisms other than malabsorption (see Tables 10-1 and 10-2), and the accompanying intestinal changes may in turn lead to malabsorption, which further impairs nutritional status, setting up a vicious cycle. This chapter covers the pathophysiology of malabsorption, grouping clinical conditions according to the mechanisms by which they produce malabsorption. First, important features of the normal physiology of digestion and absorption are discussed. The nutritional rationale of specialized formulas used in the treatment of malabsorption is discussed next. Finally, the management of a number of common clinical conditions representative of different pathophysiologic problems is treated.

NORMAL MECHANISMS OF DIGESTION AND ABSORPTION

To understand the pathophysiology of digestion and absorption as it occurs in infants and children, one must first understand how these processes normally occur in healthy individuals. The sections immediately following—on digestion and absorption of protein, fat, and carbohydrate—provide a basis for understanding the departures from these norms caused by disease.

Protein

Figure 11-1

The end result of pancreatic digestion is a mixture of predominantly oligopeptides and amino acids.

The hydrolysis of protein to polypeptides is initiated by acid and pepsin in the stomach. This hydrolysis is completed in the small intestine by pancreatic enzymes. There are several pancreatic proteases, each with specificity for particular types of peptide linkages. The result of the intraluminal phase of protein digestion is a mixture of oligopeptides, predominantly, and, to a much lesser extent, free amino acids (Figure 11-1). The mucosal phase of protein digestion and absorption occurs at two sites. Peptidases capable of hydrolyzing oligopeptides with chain lengths of up to five to six amino acids are located in the brush border. Di- and tripeptides are hydrolyzed at the brush border as they are absorbed. Peptides with chain lengths of more than two or three peptides are partially hydrolyzed, the resulting dipeptides or tripeptides being transported into the cytoplasm of the enterocyte, where other peptidases complete the hydrolysis to free amino acids. Amino acids then enter the portal vein and are transported to liver and muscle.

Several aspects of digestion and absorption deserve special attention as we provide background for nutritional management of malabsorption. First, because pancreatic proteases are normally secreted in great excess, a marked reduction in their concentration must occur before a clinically apparent effect is noted. Reductions of this magnitude are rarely seen except in diseases specifically affecting the pancreas, such as cystic fibrosis. Even in severe protein-energy malnutrition, any pancreatic deficiency that does exist is usually rapidly corrected during the first 3 to 5 days of

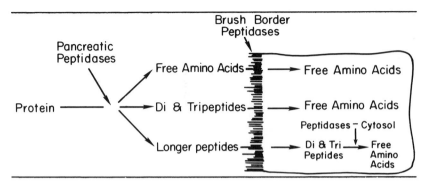

Figure 11-1 Digestion and absorption of protein in the small intestine.

Most of the nitrogen absorbed from the intestinal lumen enters the enterocyte in the form of peptides, not free amino acids.

treatment. Next, most of the nitrogen absorbed from the intestinal lumen enters the enterocyte in the form of peptides, not free amino acids. Experimental studies have shown clearly that nitrogen absorption from mixtures of peptides occurs more rapidly than from mixtures of free amino acids. Findings such as these raise questions about the usefulness of therapeutic formulas that provide nitrogen predominantly in the form of free amino acids, especially for conditions in which there is no reason to doubt the adequacy of pancreatic function. Finally, unlike malabsorption of fat and carbohydrate, malabsorption of protein does not cause significant diarrhea. Equally important, some degree of nitrogen malabsorption is tolerable because normally only a percentage of nitrogen absorbed is actually retained, the rest being excreted in the urine. Reduced nitrogen absorption, especially early in treatment, can be offset by increased retention. Because of their role as energy sources, there is no corresponding means by which malabsorption of fat or carbohydrate can be offset.

Some degree of nitrogen malabsorption is tolerable because only a percentage of nitrogen absorbed is actually retained.

Fat

The process by which triglycerides, which constitute most of dietary fat, are digested and absorbed is complex. Little digestion occurs in the stomach. As fat moves from the stomach into the duodenum, it comes in contact with pancreatic lipase and bile acids. The interaction of long-chain triglycerides with pancreatic lipase results in a mixture of free fatty acids and 2-monoglycerides. Neither is highly water soluble. Because digestion is taking place in the aqueous environment of the intestinal lumen, a further step is required to solubilize these products so that they can move freely to the surface of the enterocyte. This is accomplished by bile acids (Figure 11-2).

Figure 11-2

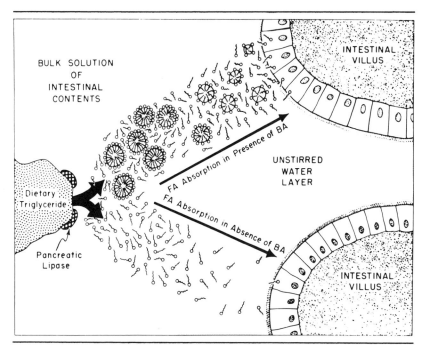

Figure 11-2 Intestinal phase of fat absorption showing the effect of the presence or absence of bile acid micelles. From Westergaard, H.; and Dietschy, J. M. 1974. Normal mechanisms of fat absorption and derangements induced by various gastrointestinal diseases. *Med. Clin. of N. Amer.* 58:1413–27.

Bile acids are large molecules with a polar (hydrophilic) and a nonpolar (hydrophobic) end. When secreted above a certain concentration, bile acids spontaneously group together to form a micelle. This concentration, about 2 mM, is known as the critical micellar concentration. The micelle is an aggregation of bile acids with all the hydrophilic parts turned toward the exterior, the hydrophobic parts forming a central core. Free fatty acids and 2-monoglycerides move into the core, thereby forming the mixed micelle. Once solubilized by this physiologic detergent (the micelle), these products are ferried across the unstirred water layer, which lies just above the mucosa, where they come in contact with and are absorbed by the enterocyte. Resynthesis to triglyceride and attachment to a lipoprotein occurs in the enterocyte. The resulting chylomicron is then transferred into the lymphatic system.

The process of fat digestion described thus far pertains to long-chain triglycerides. The absorption of medium-chain triglycerides (MCT) differs in two important respects. First, absorption of

Bile acids act as physiologic detergents in the aqueous environment of the small intestine.

The free fatty acids derived from the hydrolysis of MCT are far more water soluble than the corresponding molecules derived from long-chain triglycerides.

MCT without prior hydrolysis *may* occur to a limited extent. Second, because of their shorter chain length, the free fatty acids derived from the hydrolysis of MCT are far more water soluble than the corresponding molecules derived from long-chain triglycerides. This increased solubility allows them to cross the unstirred water layer in the absence of micelles. MCT are most useful in treatment of conditions in which there is an inability to secrete bile acids in quantities sufficient to reach the critical micellar concentration. This deficiency of bile acids occurs in such diverse conditions as marasmus and chronic obstructive liver disease.

Table 11-1

Fat absorption improves considerably during the first three months of life (Table 11-1). Further improvement occurs up to about the age of 3 years. Beyond the age of 3 years excretion of more than 10% of ingested fat, or 5 g/day in absolute terms, is abnormal. Fomon et al. (1970) have suggested that fat losses of more than 2 g/kg should be considered nutritionally significant. Although fat losses of a lesser magnitude may be indicative of gastrointestinal dysfunction, one should be reluctant to attribute growth failure to marginal fat absorption by itself.

In addition to causing significant energy losses, steatorrhea may result in diarrhea.

In addition to causing significant energy losses, steatorrhea may result in diarrhea. This diarrhea is clearly not the result of an osmotic phenomenon, because the malabsorbed lipids are insoluble in water. Rather, long-chain fatty acids entering the colon are hydroxylated by bacteria. These hydroxy-fatty-acids cause a net secretion of water into the colon, the end result being increased

Table 11-1 Normal values for fecal fat and fecal weight during the first 3 months of life in infants consuming a standard infant formula

Age (days)	Number	Fat intake (g/kg/d)	Stool fat		Stool weight (g/d)
			(g/d)	(% of intake)	
8–13	32	6.7 ± 1.1	3.8 ± 2.1	18.1 ± 11.2	63 ± 31
31–36	15	8.3 ± 0.7	4.4 ± 2.9	15.4 ± 12.4	86 ± 33
61–66	16	8.5 ± 1.2	4.8 ± 1.8	12.1 ± 5.3	102 ± 45
91–96	21	7.9 ± 1.1	3.9 ± 2.5	10.7 ± 7.6	96 ± 49

Source: MacLean, W. C., Jr.; Klein, G. L.; Lopez de Romaña, R.; et al. 1978. Transient steatorrhea following episodes of mild diarrhea in early infancy. *J. Pediatr.* 92:562–565.

stool output. This is the same mechanism by which castor oil produces its effect.

Carbohydrate

The digestion of complex carbohydrates begins in the mouth. Salivary amylase begins the hydrolysis of starch, changing the viscosity of food and making swallowing easier. The acid pH of the stomach ends hydrolysis abruptly. In the small intestine pancreatic amylase completes the intraluminal hydrolysis of amylose and amylopectin to short-chain polymers of glucose (Figure 11-3). Further digestion and absorption of these carbohydrates, as well as of the disaccharides maltose, sucrose, and lactose, takes place at the brush border of the enterocyte.

Because pancreatic amylase is secreted in excess, the intraluminal phase of carbohydrate digestion is rarely impaired except in diseases affecting the pancreas per se. Pathologic conditions affecting the intestinal mucosa may result in marked diminutions of the disaccharidases. The pathophysiology of the diarrhea produced by disaccharide malabsorption was discussed in Chapter 9.

MALABSORPTION AND MALNUTRITION IN INFANCY

An increasing number of specialized dietary products are being marketed for the management of malabsorption in infants, children, and adults. All of these products have been designed to overcome deficiencies of digestion and absorption at specific points in the process.

Margin notes:

Figure 11-3

The intraluminal phase of carbohydrate digestion is rarely impaired except in diseases affecting the pancreas per se.

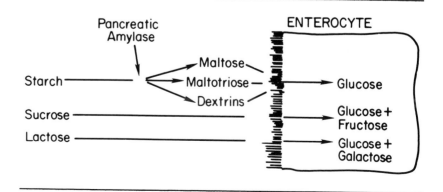

Figure 11-3 Digestion and absorption of carbohydrate in the small intestine.

Formulas Available for Management

Although the wide array of formulas available for management of malabsorption and malnutrition appears confusing at first, only a limited number of modifications of the sources of protein, fat, and carbohydrate are possible. All formulas fall into certain general groups, with minor variations from product to product within a group. The modifications made are most easily understood using the standard infant formula as a point of reference.

Therapeutic formulas usually have a different source of protein or hydrolyzed cow-milk protein.

Modification of protein source The protein of the standard infant formula is whole protein derived from cow milk. Therapeutic formulas alter this protein in one of three ways. First, another source of protein may be used. Soy protein is most commonly substituted for cow-milk protein. This substitution is often used in the treatment of cow-milk hypersensitivity (see Table 4–3 and Chapter 9). A second possible modification is the use of hydrolyzed protein (mixtures of peptides) rather than whole protein. Most formulas that provide nitrogen in this way are based on cow milk. The principal use for formulas containing hydrolyzed protein is the treatment of pancreatic insufficiency. Hydrolyzed protein is also less antigenic than whole protein and may be useful in the management of cow-milk-protein intolerance. Third, free amino acids may be used as the source of nitrogen. Some formulas that contain hydrolyzed protein also have a significant percentage of nitrogen in the form of free amino acids. At least one formula on the market provides all nitrogen as single free amino acids. Because nitrogen from peptides is absorbed more quickly than that from amino acids, there seems to be little physiologic basis for this modification, especially since increased osmolality results when free amino acids are substituted for hydrolyzed or whole protein.

Modification of fat source The source of fat in standard infant formulas is usually one or a mixture of several vegetable oils. All therapeutic formulas provide long-chain fats from these same efficiently absorbed vegetable oils. In addition, many formulas substitute medium-chain triglycerides (MCT) for a part of the long-chain triglycerides. The proportion of fat provided by MCT in those formulas that contain it varies from 18% to 88%. The substitution of MCT is made because it is more readily absorbed in the absence of bile acids than are long-chain triglycerides.

Modification of carbohydrate source All therapeutic formulas are lactose free. Carbohydrate is provided principally by polymers of glucose (corn syrup solids, maltodextrins), sucrose, and small amounts of starch. The exact proportions differ somewhat from formula to formula. Several formulas are sucrose-free and consequently may be of value in treating sucrose intolerance.

Tables 11-2, 11-3, and 11-4 show the proximate compositions of a number of commonly used therapeutic formulas. These formulas have been grouped according to protein source. Formulas containing whole protein should be considered the mainstays of treatment except where severe pancreatic insufficiency is expected. Either cow-milk protein or a mixture of milk protein and soy protein is the preferable source of whole protein because of the higher quality of the protein. The four formulas listed all provide a generous 13%–14% of calories as protein. There is a wide range in the percentage of fat provided by MCT. Two formulas contain sucrose and two are sucrose free.

The formulas that contain hydrolyzed protein shown in Table 11-3 are indicated for the treatment of pancreatic insufficiency or protein intolerance. Because a hydrolysate is used, the osmolality of these formulas tends to be slightly higher than that of other therapeutic formulas. The same variety of fat and carbohydrate sources available in formulas with whole protein is seen here. Table 11-4 shows the proximate composition of a single formula based on free amino acids. This formula has two major disadvantages. One is the high osmolality; the other is the unnecessarily low fat content. It is questionable whether a diet this low in fat can meet essential fatty acid requirements.

There appears to be considerable variation in the mineral and vitamin contents of the formulas shown. When prepared as directed and consumed in quantities sufficient to meet energy requirements, all provide adequate amounts of these essential nutrients.

Whenever possible, a proprietary formula such as those discussed here should be used. The practitioner is well advised to become familiar with one or two formulas containing whole protein and a formula containing hydrolyzed protein. In general, success of management depends more on how specific formulas are used than on what formula is chosen.

Products Available for the Modification of Formulas

Several products available for the modification of existing formulas are listed in Table 11-5. Casec® is a commercial brand of calcium caseinate that can be used to add protein to the diet. Because all of the currently marketed therapeutic formulas provide more than 8% of total calories as protein, the use of such a product is rarely

---

Margin notes:

Table 11-2

Formulas containing whole protein should be considered the mainstays of treatment except where severe pancreatic insufficiency is expected.

Table 11-3

Hydrolyzed protein is indicated for the treatment of pancreatic insufficiency or protein intolerance.

Table 11-4

Whenever possible, a proprietary formula should be used.

Table 11-5

Table 11-2 Proximate composition of several formulas with whole protein useful in the management of malabsorption

Nutrient	Formula			
	Portagen (Mead Johnson Nutritional Div.) (0.67 kcal/mL)	Ensure (Ross Laboratories) (1.06 kcal/mL)	Ensure Osmolite (Ross Laboratories) (1.06 kcal/mL)	Isocal (Mead Johnson Nutritional Div.) (1.06 kcal/mL)
kcal distribution (%)				
Protein	14	14	14	13
Fat	40	31.5	31	37
Carbohydrate	46	54.5	55	50
Source				
Protein	Casein	Casein, soy protein isolate (SPI)	Casein, SPI	Casein, SPI
Fat	Medium-chain tri-glycerides (MCT) 88%, corn oil 12%	Corn oil	MCT 50%, corn oil & soy oil 50%	Soy oil 80%, MCT 20%
Carbohydrate	Corn syrup solids (CSS) 73%, sucrose 25%, other 2%	CSS, sucrose	Hydrolyzed corn syrup	CSS
Sodium (meq/L)	14	37	26	23
Potassium (meq/L)	22	40	26	34
Chloride (meq/L)	16	40	25	30
Calcium (mg/L)	630	530	530	630
Phosphorus (mg/L)	470	530	530	530
Calcium:phosphorus	13:1	1:1	1:1	1.2:1
Magnesium (mg/L)	137	210	211	211
Copper (mg/L)	1.1	1.1	1.1	1.1
Iodine (μg/L)	48	79	79	80
Iron (mg/L)	12.7	9.5	9.5	10
Zinc (mg/L)	6.3	15.9	15.9	10.6
Vitamin A (IU/L)	5232	2650	2650	2640
Vitamin D (IU/L)	523	212	212	210
Vitamin E (IU/L)	21	32	32	40
Vitamin C (mg/L)	54	160	160	158
Vitamin B_1 (mg/L)	1.0	1.6	1.6	2.1
Vitamin B_2 (mg/L)	1.3	1.8	1.8	2.0
Niacin (Eq/L)	13.6	21.1	21.1	26
Vitamin B_6 (mg/L)	1.4	2.1	2.1	3.0
Vitamin B_{12} (μg/L)	4.0	6.3	6.3	8.0
Folate (μg/L)	107	211	211	211
Renal solute load (milliosmoles/L)	146	266	225	225
Osmolality (milli-osmoles/kg H_2O)	158	450	300	300

Table 11-3 Proximate composition of several formulas with hydrolyzed protein useful in the management of malabsorption

	Formula		
Nutrient	Pregestimil (Mead Johnson Nutritional Div.) (0.67 kcal/mL)	Nutramigen (Mead Johnson Nutritional Div.) (0.67 kcal/mL)	Vital (Ross Laboratories) (1.0 kcal/mL)
kcal distribution (%)			
Protein	11	13	16.7
Fat	35	35	9.3
Carbohydrate	54	52	74
Source			
Protein	Casein hydrolysate (CH) + cystine, tyrosine, tryptophan	CH	Soy, meat, whey hydrolysate, free amino acids
Fat	Corn oil 60%, MCT 40%	Corn oil	Sunflower oil
Carbohydrate	Corn syrup solids (CSS) 85%, modified tapioca starch (MTS) 15%	Sucrose 72%, MTS 28%	Maltodextrin 73%, sucrose 17%, hydrolyzed corn syrup 10%
Sodium (meq/L)	14	14	17
Potassium (meq/L)	18	17	30
Chloride (meq/L)	16	13	19
Calcium (mg/L)	630	630	667
Phosphorus (mg/L)	420	470	667
Calcium:phosphorus	1.5:1	1.3:1	1:1
Magnesium (mg/L)	74	74	267
Copper (mg/L)	0.6	0.6	1.3
Iodine (μg/L)	48	48	100
Iron (mg/L)	12.7	12.7	12.0
Zinc (mg/L)	4.2	4.2	10
Vitamin A (IU/L)	2090	1675	3333
Vitamin D (IU/L)	419	419	267
Vitamin E (IU/L)	15.4	10.7	20
Vitamin C (mg/L)	53.6	53.6	60
Vitamin B_1 (mg/L)	0.5	0.5	1.0
Vitamin B_2 (mg/L)	0.6	0.6	1.1
Niacin (Eq/L)	8.4	8.4	13.3
Vitamin B_6 (mg/L)	0.4	0.4	1.3
Vitamin B_{12} (μg/L)	2.0	2.0	4.0
Folate (μg/L)	107	107	267
Renal solute load (milliosmoles/L)	122	131	233
Osmolality (milliosmoles/kg) H_2O	348	479	420

Table 11-4 Proximate composition of a specialized formula in which all nitrogen is provided by free amino acids

Nutrient	Vivonex (Norwich-Eaton Pharmaceuticals) (1.0 kcal/mL)
kcal distribution (%)	
Protein	8.2
Fat	1.3
Carbohydrate	90.5
Source	
Protein	Crystalline amino acids
Fat	Safflower oil
Carbohydrate	Glucose oligosaccharides
Sodium (meq/L)	20.4
Potassium (meq/L)	30
Chloride (meq/L)	20.4
Calcium (mg/L)	550
Phosphorus (mg/L)	550
Calcium:phosphorus	1:1
Magnesium (mg/L)	222
Copper (mg/L)	1.1
Iodine (μg/L)	83
Iron (mg/L)	10
Zinc (mg/L)	8.3
Vitamin A (IU/L)	2778
Vitamin D (IU/L)	222
Vitamin E (IU/L)	16.7
Vitamin C (mg/L)	33
Vitamin B_1 (mg/L)	0.8
Vitamin B_2 (mg/L)	0.9
Niacin (Eq/L)	11.1
Vitamin B_6 (mg/L)	1.1
Vitamin B_{12} (μg/L)	3.3
Folate (μg/L)	220
Renal solute load (milliosmoles/L)	158
Osmolality (milliosmoles/L)	550

Table 11–5 Products commonly used to modify formulas

Nutrient	Casec* (Mead Johnson Nutritional Div.) (3.7 kcal/g)	MCT (Mead Johnson Nutritional Div.) (8.3 kcal/g; 7.7 kcal/mL)	Polycose liquid† (Ross Laboratories) (2.0 kcal/mL)
kcal distribution (%)			
Protein	94		
Fat	6	100	
Carbohydrate			100
Source			
Protein	Calcium caseinate		
Fat	Butter fat		
Carbohydrate	—		Glucose polymers
Sodium (meq)	6.5		2.7
Potassium (meq)			<1.0
Chloride (meq)			3.0
Calcium (mg)	1600		<40
Phosphorus (mg)			<30

*One packed level tablespoon = 4.7 g.

†Also available in powder: 94 g carbohydrate per 100 g.

necessary except in extremely complex therapeutic situations. Medium-chain triglycerides are also marketed in pure form. They may be added to formulas containing little or no medium-chain triglycerides but should never be used to supplement formulas in which most of the fat is already provided as MCT—for example, Portagen—because of the danger of decreasing essential-fatty-acid intake to an unacceptable level. Polycose is a commercially marketed carbohydrate in the form of glucose polymers. It is used principally to add calories to the diet.

If additional energy is to be added in the form of medium-chain triglycerides or glucose polymers, care should be taken not to reduce the percentage of calories provided by protein to a level below 8%.

Certain guidelines should be followed in using these products to modify existing formulas. Whenever possible, commercial formulas should be used unaltered. If additional energy is to be added in the form of medium-chain triglycerides or glucose polymers, care should be taken not to reduce the percentage of calories provided by protein to a level below 8%. Besides decreasing the ratio of protein to energy, the addition of large quantities of medium-chain triglycerides or glucose polymers to commercial formulas also reduces the nutrient density of all minerals and vitamins in the formula. The intakes of these nutrients may become inadequate as a result. There is no place for the addition of either MCT or glucose polymers to human milk, as is occasionally done in some premature nurseries.

Specific Clinical Conditions

All-inclusive coverage of the many clinical conditions associated with malabsorption in infancy is beyond the scope of this text. Seven conditions have been chosen because of the frequency with which they occur in clinical practice and because each represents a different type of clinical problem in malabsorption.

Antibiotic-induced diarrhea The use of antibiotics to treat infections such as otitis media or urinary tract infections is frequently associated with watery diarrhea several days into treatment. The causative mechanism for the diarrhea is not always clear, although alterations of the gut flora presumably play a role in many instances. In early infancy, for example, when the colonic microflora appears to play a role in the conservation of malabsorbed carbohydrate (see Chapter 9), antibiotics could change the flora and disrupt this normal mechanism for salvaging carbohydrate passing into the colon. In some instances antibiotic use is associated with overgrowth of bacteria not normally part of the flora or with the growth of fungi. Pseudomembranous colitis caused by the toxin of *Clostridium difficile* has followed the use of clindamycin and other antibiotics used more frequently in the pediatric age group, such as ampicillin and chloramphenicol.

In most instances antibiotic-induced diarrhea clears spontaneously when antibiotic treatment is stopped. No special dietary treatment is required, although some practitioners temporarily remove lactose from the diet of the young infant. Although some antibiotics can be shown experimentally to interfere with the absorption of specific nutrients, this is not of practical concern in children receiving chronic suppressive antibiotic therapy as long as it is not associated with diarrhea. Any interference with absorption is far outweighed by the positive results of the suppression or eradication of chronic infection, which can be expected to result in improved nutritional status.

Acute infectious diarrhea   Acute diarrhea is the most frequently encountered form of malabsorption in pediatric practice. Most cases resolve spontaneously. In early infancy, however, prolonged malabsorption of a minor degree may follow an acute episode of diarrhea. Inappropriate management at this point may perpetuate diarrhea and malabsorption, which can result in chronic intractable diarrhea with marasmus.

In early infancy prolonged malabsorption of a minor degree may follow an acute episode of diarrhea.

Acute infectious diarrhea of a mild nature requires little more than a slight reduction in food intake for several days. Although milk has traditionally been removed from the diet entirely, several studies (see, for example, Rees and Brook 1979) have presented data that question whether this removal indeed leads to more rapid improvement. This is an important question to resolve, especially as it relates to the breast-fed infant, because one is always reluctant to interrupt breast-feeding, especially during the early weeks.

More serious diarrhea, especially that which seems to be exacerbated by the ingestion of food, should be treated initially with an oral glucose-electrolyte solution. The two commercially marketed oral rehydration solutions commonly used in pediatrics are listed in Table 11–6. Also included in this table is the composition of the oral rehydration solution endorsed by the World Health Organization. The latter solution was originally developed for the treatment of cholera, in which stool electrolyte losses tend to be higher than in most other infectious diarrheas; it is now suggested for use in all types of diarrhea. The commercial solutions currently marketed provide sodium, potassium, and chloride in lower concentrations, which are sufficient to meet maintenance requirements but not truly sufficient for restoration of deficits. Use of a solution of higher sodium content is preferable when deficits are large. Finberg (1980) and others, however, have questioned the desirability of a solution containing 90 meq of sodium per liter for routine use in pediatrics because of the dangers of hypernatremia and circulatory overload. A solution of intermediate sodium concentration may be preferable for generalized uses in pediatrics.

Table 11-6

For diarrhea not associated with severe dehydration, one of the commercial glucose-electrolyte solutions should be used for 24 to 36 hours. An intake of 150 mL/kg is sufficient to meet fluid requirements, unless a marked degree of fever is present. *Ad libitum*

Table 11-6 Oral rehydration solutions

	Solution		
Nutrient	Pedialyte (Ross Laboratories)	Lytren (Mead Johnson Nutritional Div.)	Oral rehydration solution (WHO)
kcal/L	200	300	80
Carbohydrate source	Glucose	Corn syrup solids	Glucose
Sodium (meq/L)	30	30	90
Potassium (meq/L)	20	25	20
Chloride (meq/L)	30	25	80
Calcium (meq/L)	4	4	—
Magnesium (meq/L)	4	4	—
Citrate (bicarbonate-ORS)	28	36	30
Sulfate	—	4	—
Phosphate	—	5	—
Osmolality (milliosmoles/kg H_2O)	380	290	331

intakes much above this amount should be avoided, as they may occasionally perpetuate diarrhea due to carbohydrate intolerance. Therapy with oral glucose-electrolyte solutions is usually associated with marked reduction in stool output. Starvation stools—small green mucous stools that are often passed after each feeding— should not be mistaken for continuing diarrhea and are not reason to delay the reintroduction of food.

Formula may be reintroduced over a period of 3 to 4 days. This is frequently done by reintroducing "half strength" formula and then returning to "full strength" formula, both fed *ad libitum.* This approach to the problem is inappropriate, because it gives little control over the total dietary intake of the infant. An infant who was previously consuming 100 kcal/kg/day will be restarted at an intake of 50 kcal/kg/day; an infant previously consuming 150 kcal/kg/day will be restarted as 75 kcal/kg/day. Although the final prescription may be presented to the parents in "half strength"–

Starvation stools can be mistaken for continuing diarrhea.

The diet should be reintroduced gradually with attention to volume and actual calorie intakes.

"full strength" terminology, a more precise recommendation of actual intake should be made by the physician. This involves determination of volume, and concentration of the formula. An initial intake of 30–50 kcal/kg/day is reasonable, depending on the age and size of the child and the duration of the diarrhea. Once tolerance at this level has been demonstrated, caloric intake can be increased in one or two steps by successively concentrating the formula.

Some practitioners routinely remove all lactose from the diet for several weeks after an acute episode of diarrhea. This usually involves a change to a soy-based lactose-free formula. However, if formula is reintroduced in a graded fashion with attention to intake, it should not be necessary to treat all acute diarrheas with lactose-free formulas. If diarrhea recurs after the reintroduction of a lactose-containing formula, a switch to a lactose-free diet is appropriate. This change in diet does not guarantee success; cautious refeeding with the lactose-free formula in graded increments of intake should be prescribed.

Balance studies carried out with healthy infants recovering from seemingly innocuous episodes of diarrhea have demonstrated that it may take several weeks for stool weights to return completely to normal. Although this may reflect a mild degree of carbohydrate intolerance, impaired fat absorption is also common. It has been speculated that this impairment results from the depletion of the bile-acid pools during diarrhea, which results in an inability to secrete bile acids above the critical micellar concentration. In most instances, the degree of fat malabsorption is mild, and no specific dietary alteration is indicated. However, if loose stools and poor weight gain persist, use of a formula with medium-chain triglycerides should be instituted.

Chronic diarrhea and malnutrition Protein-energy malnutrition, especially marasmus, is the end point of many disease processes (see Table 10–1). Chronic diarrhea is both the most frequent antecedent and a frequent result of PEM. From a management point of view, PEM represents a comprehensive decrease in gastrointestinal function. Initially there is some decrease in the output of pancreatic enzymes, but in most cases this is not severe enough by itself to require special formula. Bile acids are secreted in decreased concentration, reducing fat absorption. The intestinal mucosa may show mild to severe atrophy, but in general there is a loss of overall surface area. Disaccharidase levels are depressed. Cellular peptidases are reasonably well preserved. The management of this clinical problem can serve as a model for the management of most other forms of malabsorption in infancy.

PEM represents a comprehensive decrease in gastrointestinal function.

Faced with intestinal dysfunction of the severity we have outlined, many institutions reflexively initiate total parenteral alimentation. While it is frequently desirable to provide amino acids, an energy source, and micronutrients by vein in the *severely* malnourished infant, there are compelling reasons why oral alimentation should generally be begun as early as possible, even in these children. Healthy animals who are totally parenterally fed experience a marked decrease in intestinal weight. Similarly, intestinal bypass surgery for obesity results in atrophy of the bypassed segment, despite the generally "excellent" nutritional status of the host. Regeneration of the intestinal mucosa depends on the presence of nutrients and intestinal secretions in the lumen of the intestinal tract. "Gut rest" usually generates gut atrophy and is inappropriate except in diseases with severe inflammation of the mucosa, such as Crohn's disease. Although total parenteral alimentation may lead to weight gain and overall improvement in nutritional status, a parallel improvement in intestinal function is not to be expected from this therapy. Children in whom parenteral alimentation is begun should be started on oral feedings as early as possible to induce intestinal regeneration.

Regeneration of the intestinal mucosa depends on the presence of nutrients and intestinal secretions in the lumen of the intestinal tract.

Exclusively oral feeding, which is appropriate for most infants with PEM, can be carried out in the following way. During the initial 24 hours an oral glucose-electrolyte solution establishes the ability to maintain water and electrolyte balance. Following this, a lactose-free formula with whole protein and a high proportion of the fat as medium-chain triglycerides can be begun. An appropriate intake for the first day is 25 kcal/kg. These 25 kcal/kg can be diluted in 125 to 150 mL/kg and fed in divided feedings every 3 to 4 hours. Alternatively, 25 kcal/kg can be fed as formula of normal concentration (0.67 kcal/mL or 20 kcal/oz). This will provide 37.5 mL/kg/day. Remaining fluid requirements can be met by an oral glucose-electrolyte solution or by the intravenous route.

Most infants can be managed entirely by oral feeding.

Once an intake of 25 kcal/kg/day has been tolerated for a period of 1 to 2 days, the diet may be advanced to 50 kcal/kg/day. The most important consideration in advancing the diet is stool output and character. Stool outputs of between 100 and 150 g/day are considered acceptable. Although obtaining daily stool weights is desirable, this is frequently not possible. If stools are gradually becoming more formed, the diet should continue to be advanced. If dilute formula has been used, the total volume of intake is held constant and the formula is progressively concentrated. If formula of normal concentration has been used, the volume is increased with a concomitant decrease in oral glucose-electrolyte or intravenous fluids. The diet should be advanced in this way no more often than every 1 to 2 days in increments of 25 kcal/kg/day.

An increase in intake may lead to increased stool output. Many practitioners interpret this to mean that the child cannot tolerate the formula in a qualitative sense, and the response is a change to another formula. However, more often than not, increased stool output is indicative of a quantitative intolerance—that is, too much is being fed. Intake should be reduced to the level previously tolerated for several more days and then should be advanced again.

Dietary intolerances are rarely absolute. Rather they result from the amount being fed.

Many infants require intakes as high as 150 to 175 kcal/kg/day before weight gain ensues. As long as the diet can be advanced every 2 to 3 days without causing excessive stool output, progress should be considered satisfactory. An unrealistic expectation of weight gain too early in treatment and a fear of later mental retardation leads many practitioners to advance the diet too rapidly, which results in the recurrence of diarrhea.

The seemingly high energy requirements of undernourished infants has three causes. For one thing weight is usually used to calculate nutrient requirements on the assumption that it is a good proxy for lean body mass. But weight is not a good indicator of lean body mass in malnourished infants. Whereas a normal infant may have 20% to 25% of its body weight as fat, the recovering malnourished infant may have only 5%. Consequently, kilogram for kilogram the malnourished infant is more metabolically active and requires greater quantities of nutrients. Second, because of malabsorption, calculated oral intake may considerably exceed the amount actually absorbed. Finally, malnourished children have been found to be inefficient in their energy utilization, requiring more calories for production of each gram of weight eventually gained. An estimation of the energy intake that will be required can be made as follows. The ideal weight for the child's length is multiplied by a slightly liberalized calorie intake of 120 kcal/kg/day. This estimate of total calorie intake is then divided by the child's actual weight to yield the estimated desirable intake in kcal/kg/day.

Malnourished children have very high energy requirements.

Short gut Pathophysiologically the child with a short gut presents problems similar to those of the child with chronic malnutrition. Concentrations of pancreatic enzymes and bile acids may be normal. However, there is a marked reduction of overall intestinal surface area because of resection. A degree of undernutrition during the period surrounding surgery may have resulted in some atrophy of the remaining segment. A lactose-free formula with whole protein, preferably milk protein, and some medium-chain triglycerides is

In short gut there is a marked reduction of overall intestinal surface area because of resection.

desirable. Initial maintenance with at least partial parenteral alimentation is usually required. Early introduction of enteral alimentation in graded amounts, often by continuous drip, is essential if compensatory hypertrophy of the intestinal mucosa is to occur. An approach similar to that used for chronic malnutrition is appropriate here.

Clinical course and ease of management of short gut depend to a large degree on the length of small intestine remaining following resection and on whether the ileocecal valve is intact. In one series of children, following intestinal resection no child with a small-intestinal length of less than 40 cm and without an ileocecal valve survived. In contrast, half the children with ileocecal valves and a small-intestinal length of 15–38 cm survived. And nearly all children with an ileocecal valve and more than 40 cm of small intestine had a good outcome (Wilmore, 1972). Because the proximal small intestine tends normally to be more hyperplastic than the distal part, resection of the lower part of the small intestine may result in fewer initial problems in absorption of macronutrients. Resection of the terminal ileum, however, results in an impairment of the absorption of both bile acids and vitamin B_{12}. Bile-acid malabsorption may cause diarrhea and secondary fat malabsorption. Parenteral vitamin B_{12} will eventually be required.

Cystic fibrosis Cystic fibrosis is the most common form of pancreatic insufficiency in childhood. Intestinal mucosal function is usually good, although lactose intolerance has been reported in older children. Pancreatic insufficiency necessitates the use of a formula containing hydrolyzed protein. Disaccharides and short-chain polymers of glucose, which are well absorbed in the absence of pancreatic amylase, are also indicated. Medium-chain triglycerides have been recommended because of their ability to be absorbed in the absence of pancreatic lipase, although a recent study has questioned the degree to which this occurs. Because of the difficulty of giving enzyme replacement in infancy, a formula such as Pregestimil, with hydrolyzed protein, is useful. Some malabsorption will persist, and intakes of 150 kcal/kg/day or more are frequently required to induce adequate rates of weight gain. Fat-soluble vitamins in water-miscible form should be used for supplementation.

Both breast milk and soy formulas should be avoided for infants with cystic fibrosis. Both have been associated with the development of hypoproteinemia and edema. The amount of protein in human milk and the quality of protein in soy formulas appear to be inadequate for the child with impaired nitrogen absorption.

Both breast milk and soy formulas should be avoided for infants with cystic fibrosis. Both have been associated with hypoproteinemia and edema.

Because of the expense of diets such as Pregestimil, the older child with cystic fibrosis is usually managed on a more conventional diet with pancreatic enzyme replacement. Low-fat diets are also frequently used for management of older children with cystic fibrosis. In our judgment fat restriction is indicated only if steatorrhea becomes a problem for the child. Providing adequate dietary energy in a low-fat diet is difficult at best. While liberalizing fat intake will undoubtedly result in an increase in fecal fat excretion, with appropriate enzyme therapy it should also result in a net increase in fat absorption.

Cholestatic liver disease   The child with cholestatic liver disease—for example, neonatal hepatitis or biliary atresia—has a selective defect of fat absorption because of an inadequate concentration of bile acids in the lumen of the small intestine. Protein and carbohydrate are digested and absorbed normally, and no specific alteration in their dietary sources is required. A diet in which a high proportion of fat is provided by medium-chain triglycerides will effectively overcome fat malabsorption in these children. In addition, some long-chain fats must be provided to cover essential-fatty-acid requirements. Intakes of the fat-soluble vitamins should also be increased and should be given in water-soluble or water-miscible form.

Congestive heart failure   The infant with congenital heart disease and congestive heart failure presents several problems of nutritional management. Because these children tire easily, they are often unable to take adequate amounts of formula spontaneously. Also, fluid restriction imposed for the management of congestive failure limits the volume in which nutrients can be delivered. The increased cardiac output and increased work of breathing involved in congestive heart failure increase the child's energy requirements. Marginal intakes often result in mild to moderate marasmus.

Digestion and absorption of protein, fat, and carbohydrate is normal or nearly so. For the initially well-nourished infant no special formula is required. For the child with marginal malnutrition a lactose-free diet may be preferable. To assure adequate intakes for the infant who tires with sucking, feedings may need to be given by a nasogastric tube, either as a bolus or by continuous infusion. Intakes of formula at standard concentrations (0.67 kcal/mL) should be increased until the child's fluid limit is reached. If weight gain has not resulted at this point, further nutrient intakes can be achieved by progressively concentrating the formula. In some instances, concentrations as high as 1.5 kcal/mL or more

> The increased cardiac output and increased work of breathing involved in congestive heart failure increase the child's energy requirements.

may be required to meet protein and calorie requirements without exceeding fluid tolerance. The high caloric requirement necessitates the use of a formula with low renal solute load. The serum sodium and urea nitrogen concentrations must be monitored carefully for signs of dehydration. Occasionally the formula must be modified by the addition of vegetable oil and glucose polymers to reduce renal solute load and sodium intake while keeping calorie content high. The practitioner should consult a trained nutritionist for help in carrying out dietary modifications of this kind.

MALABSORPTION AND MALNUTRITION IN THE OLDER CHILD

The nutritional management of malabsorption in older children differs from that in infants in several respects. Nutrient requirements relative to size are decreased in the older child, lessening the impact on nutritional status of mild to moderate degrees of malabsorption. There is less reliance in treatment on the use of specialized formulas, although there is no reason why they cannot be used. In many instances the treatment of malabsorption in older children is the treatment of the disease process itself rather than of the resulting malabsorption. A good example of this is the management of celiac disease. Celiac disease is associated with altered amino acid absorption, protein-losing enteropathy, significant steatorrhea, and, not infrequently, some degree of disaccharide intolerance. Although a therapeutic formula may be of value in initial treatment, the most critical aspect of dietary management is the complete removal of gluten from the diet. The introduction of a gluten-free diet based on table foods (see Appendix A) results in rapid repair of the intestine with subsequent clearing of malabsorption.

Crohn's Disease

Growth failure is a common presentation in Crohn's disease. A significant percentage of children with Crohn's disease have some degree of steatorrhea, especially if involvement of the terminal ileum impairs the absorption and recirculation of bile acids. Bacterial overgrowth in dilated areas proximal to strictures may also result in malabsorption. Total parenteral alimentation has been used successfully in children with severe Crohn's disease, which may be one of the few conditions in which there is an indication for putting the gut at rest. Alternatively, low-residue diets have been advocated in

Total parenteral alimentation has been used successfully in children with severe Crohn's disease, which may be one of the few conditions in which there is an indication for putting the gut at rest.

an effort not to distend the intestine with excessive contents. Whether the low-residue (also called elemental) diets offer any real advantage over the other therapeutic formulas, most of which are associated with very low stool output, has not been demonstrated.

Although malabsorption and growth failure in Crohn's disease are frequently encountered in the same child, they are not always causally related. The definition of malabsorption may be important as a clue to diagnosis, but the malabsorption may not be nutritionally significant. Several studies have demonstrated that most children with Crohn's disease are anoretic and that, in many cases, their decreased intake is a more than adequate explanation for poor growth. An important objective of the management of children with Crohn's disease is to increase food intake, which can best be done by increasing the number of feedings. In some instances it may be necessary to use prescribed volumes of standard formula diets to ensure the intake of 50% to 75% of the RDA; the rest of the RDA can be provided by table foods.

Ulcerative Colitis

Because there is no involvement of the small intestine in ulcerative colitis, malabsorption is generally not a problem in this disease. About 40% of individuals with ulcerative colitis have decreased intestinal lactase activity. Many of these can still tolerate milk in normal amounts. Protein and blood losses in the large intestine increase protein and energy requirements. Dietary management includes providing a palatable diet to overcome anorexia, while respecting documented food intolerances.

Suggested Reading

Finberg, L. 1980. The role of oral electrolyte-glucose solutions in hydration for children—international and domestic aspects. *J. Pediatr.* 96:51–54.

Fleisher, D. S.; DiGeorge, A. M.; Barness, L. A.; and Cornfield, D. 1964. Hypoproteinemia and edema in infants with cystic fibrosis of the pancreas. *J. Pediatr.* 64:341–348.

Fomon, S. J.; Thomas, L. N.; Filer, L. J., Jr.; et al. 1970. Excretion of fat by normal full-term infants fed various milks and formulas. *Am. J. Clin. Nutr.* 23:1299–1313.

Greene, H. L.; McCabe, D. R.; and Merenstein, G. B. 1975. Protracted diarrhea and malnutrition in infancy: changes in intestinal morphology and disaccharidase activities during treatment with total intravenous nutrition or oral elemental diets. *J. Pediatr.* 87:695–704.

Kelts, D. G.; Grand, R. J.; Shen, G., et al. 1979. Nutritional basis of growth failure in children and adolescents with Crohn's disease. *Gastroenterology* 76:720–727.

MacLean, W. C., Jr.; Lopez de Romaña, G.; Massa, E.; and Graham, G. G. 1980. Nutritional management of chronic diarrhea and malnutrition: primary reliance on oral feeding. *J. Pediatr.* 97: 316–323.

Rees, L.; and Brook, C. G. D. 1979. Gradual reintroduction of full-strength milk after acute gastroenteritis in children. *Lancet* ii:770–771.

Viteri, F. E.; and Schneider, R. E. 1974. Gastrointestinal alterations in protein calorie malnutrition. *Med. Clin. N. Amer.* 58: 1487–1505.

Williamson, R. C. N. 1978. Intestinal adaptation. 1. Structural, functional and cytokinetic changes; and 2. Mechanisms of control. *New Eng. J. Med.* 298:1393–1402; 1444–1450.

Wilmore, D. W. 1972. Factors correlating with successful outcome following extensive intestinal resection in newborn infants. *J. Pediatr.* 80:88–95.

12 Feeding the Premature Infant

Contents

Gastrointestinal Function of the Premature Infant   242

     Protein   242

     Fat   242

     Carbohydrate   243

     Minerals and Vitamins   243

Nutrient Requirements of the Premature Infant   244

     Energy   245

     Protein   245

     Fat and Carbohydrate   246

     Minerals and Vitamins   246

Feeding the Premature Infant   247

     Human Milk and the Premature   247

     Specialized Formulas for Low-Birth-Weight Infants   249

     Introduction of Oral Feeding   251

     Complications Associated with Feeding   252

Overview

The last 10 weeks of normal fetal life comprise a period of rapid growth. Between the 30th and 40th weeks, length increases nearly 25% and weight more than doubles. An estimated two-thirds of all skeletal mineral accretion occurs during this time. The infant born prematurely must rely on its intestinal tract rather than on the placental circulation to meet the high nutrient requirements of this period. Because gastrointestinal function is incompletely developed, the nutritional management of premature infants can be difficult. This chapter addresses the nutritional management of the healthy premature infant weighing between 1500 and 2000 g. Infants in this weight and gestational age range who do not have other complications may fall within the purview of the primary care practitioner. The nutrient requirements of this group and the ability of human milk and special and routine formulas to meet these requirements are covered. Some of the complications associated with feeding are discussed.

GASTROINTESTINAL FUNCTION OF THE PREMATURE INFANT

The normal mechanisms of digestion and absorption were discussed in Chapter 11. They form a basis for this brief overview of the development of gastrointestinal function. Many digestive enzymes begin to develop as early as 11 weeks *in utero.* Activities of most begin to increase rapidly somewhere between the 24th and 28th week of gestation. From this time until term there is a continual development of digestive and absorptive function. Digestive development is incompletely studied in humans, but animal evidence suggests that development accelerates again during the first postnatal week in the term infant. Whether a similar acceleration occurs postnatally in the premature infant is unknown. The deficiencies of digestive function seen in premature infants are much less pronounced for infants born closer to term than those born earlier in gestation.

Protein

The inefficiency of protein digestion by the premature infant is not of major significance.

The pancreatic phase of protein digestion develops rapidly after 28 weeks of gestation. Cellular peptidases in the brush border of the small intestine can be demonstrated as early as 11 weeks, rising slowly thereafter. Although there may be some inefficiency in digestion and absorption of protein by the 30-week premature infant, this appears to be of little or no nutritional significance, and no modification of the source of protein is required for these infants.

Fat

Malabsorption of fat is well documented in the premature infant. Pancreatic lipase levels are inadequate to hydrolyze dietary triglycerides completely. The synthesis, secretion, and reabsorption of bile acids are also poorly developed. Bile-acid pool size in premature infants is well below that of term or older infants. An inability to reach a critical micellar concentration of bile acids in the intestinal lumen is to a large degree responsible for the malabsorption of long-chain triglycerides. Medium-chain triglycerides are water soluble after hydrolysis in the absence of micelles and consequently are well absorbed by premature infants.

Carbohydrate

Pancreatic amylase, required for the hydrolysis of complex carbohydrates, is present in adequate quantities by the 28th week of gestation. Thus, although complex carbohydrates are not normally part of the infant's diet, the capacity to digest them in reasonable quantities is present. Two of the disaccharidases, sucrase and maltase, develop early in gestation and are thought to reach normal concentrations by 28 to 30 weeks of gestation. Lactase concentrations, on the other hand, remain low during much of gestation, increasing toward the levels seen at term only during the last month. This fact suggests that the premature infant should be relatively lactose intolerant. Lactose malabsorption by the premature infant is discussed extensively in Chapter 9.

Minerals and Vitamins

Most of the major minerals are very well absorbed. The absorption of calcium parallels fat absorption and varies with the source of fat in the diet. Studies in full-term infants have suggested that about 40%–60% of calcium intake is absorbed. Absorption is presumably somewhat less in the premature infant.

Trace mineral balance in the premature infant is just beginning to be studied. Limited data are available to date. Iron is well absorbed, as evidenced by the increase in the hematocrit of the premature infant in response to iron therapy. In contrast, copper and zinc appear to be poorly absorbed. When fed the quantities usually contained in human milk or formula, the infant may have a negative zinc and copper balance for a period of 4 to 8 weeks. This could be because of increased excretion during this time. Whether this negative balance can be reversed by feeding increased quantities has yet to be determined.

Indirect evidence suggests that premature infants absorb water-soluble vitamins adequately. The absorption of vitamin B_{12} in the terminal ileum has not been studied specifically in the premature infant, but vitamin B_{12} deficiency is generally not a problem. Absorption of the fat-soluble vitamins parallels fat absorption and consequently may be somewhat compromised.

NUTRIENT REQUIREMENTS OF THE PREMATURE INFANT

Determination of the nutrient requirements of the premature infant has been a difficult task and is far from complete. Because human milk has supported adequate growth in term infants for generations, its composition has been used as a reference for estimating the nutrient requirements of the term infant. A similar approach to the estimation of the requirements of the premature infant is inappropriate because its growth rate and intestinal function are markedly different.

Human milk cannot be used as a reference for determining nutrient requirements of the premature infant.

Ziegler et al. (1976) have introduced the concept of the reference fetus. Using data on body composition of infants born at different gestational ages, it is possible to calculate the percentage of weight gained as protein, fat, water, minerals, and so on during different weeks of gestation. Once the composition of the weight gained is known, the theoretical cost of the growth (kcal/g) can also be calculated. From these two values the calorie intake and nutrient densities (the amount of any nutrient per 100 kcal) required to support normal growth can be estimated. In using this approach to determine nutrient requirements, one assumes that the growth of the "extrauterine fetus" should parallel the intrauterine growth curve. The first several weeks after premature birth are marked by weight loss as the infant adapts to the extrauterine environment and gradually achieves adequate oral intake. Whether it is desirable for weight gain to parallel the intrauterine growth curve subsequently has not been determined. Because intestinal function in the premature infant may limit the rate of accretion of many minerals, it can be argued that a slower rate of weight gain should result in more normal body composition. This point has not been settled.

Whether it is desirable for weight gain to parallel the intrauterine growth curve has not been determined.

In addition to the theoretical calculations of nutrient requirements, a number of growth and balance studies have been carried out in an effort to define the requirement for certain nutrients, most notably protein and several of the major minerals. These studies have often yielded conflicting results and there remain wide gaps in our knowledge.

Energy

The energy requirement of the premature infant is highly variable. Thermoregulation is unstable in the small premature infant. The importance of maintaining the infant in a thermal neutral temperature range to reduce energy consumption is well known. Activity varies from infant to infant. The work of breathing is significant activity for the infant with mild respiratory distress. The efficiency of digestion and absorption is also quite variable. Finally, with increasing gestational age, the percentage of weight gained as fat rises. Because of the higher energy stored in this kind of tissue, the energy cost of weight gain increases progressively during the last 8 to 10 weeks of gestation.

Both theoretical calculations and experience suggest that an intake of between 110 and 140 kcal/kg/day is required to support an adequate rate of weight gain. If the intrauterine growth curve is to be used as a standard, a rate of weight gain of approximately 17 g/kg/day would be desirable between weights of 1600 and 2200 g. It may take several weeks before intakes sufficient to support this rate of weight gain can be achieved.

Protein

The Committee on Nutrition of the American Academy of Pediatrics concluded that the protein requirement of the premature infant lay somewhere between 2.5 and 5 g/kg/day. Clearly it is important to define these requirements with more precision.

After reviewing the studies available to them in 1977, the Committee on Nutrition of the American Academy of Pediatrics concluded that the protein requirement of the premature infant lay somewhere between 2.5 and 5 g/kg/day. Clearly it is important to define these requirements with greater precision. Inadequate protein intakes slow growth. High protein intakes are not without their complications; elevated ammonia and serum urea nitrogen and an increased incidence of late metabolic acidosis have all been associated with elevated protein intakes. In addition, there is concern that the relatively increased plasma amino acid levels attendant to high protein intake may have an adverse effect on the developing brain.

Several clinical studies have suggested that protein intakes in excess of those supplied by human milk result in more rapid rates of weight gain. Fomon *et al.* (1977) have estimated that the premature infant requires approximately 2.54 g protein/100 kcal or 10.2% of energy as high-quality protein, well above the 6% protein-calories of mature human milk.

The premature infant may have more stringent requirements for protein quality than the term infant.

Soy-based formulas are not appropriate for premature infants.

The premature infant may also have more stringent requirements for protein quality than the term infant. The ability to convert methionine to cystine and tyrosine to phenylalanine is reduced in the premature. In addition, the synthesis of taurine, a β-amino compound derived from cystine, is impaired. Based on these considerations, some investigators have suggested that for the premature infant, the whey:casein ratio (60:40) of human milk with its higher taurine content is preferable to the 18:82 ratio found in many standard infant formulas. Soy protein is less than ideal for the premature infant because of its lower percentage of total amino acids as essential amino acids.

Both theoretical calculations and experimental data to date support the concept of a higher protein requirement for the premature infant. As a general rule, a formula providing 9%–11% of calories as high-quality protein is desirable. The question of the adequacy of the protein content of human milk for feeding the premature infant is discussed later in this chapter.

Fat and Carbohydrate

Essential-fatty-acid requirements are approximately 3% of total calories or 300 mg of linoleic acid per 100 kcal. Most commonly used vegetable oils average approximately 40% of fatty acids as linoleic acid. If an allowance is made for some degree of fat malabsorption, 10% of total dietary calories from long-chain fats would assure adequate essential-fatty-acid intakes. There are no formulas commercially marketed at present in which long-chain fats provide less than this amount.

There are no essential carbohydrates other than vitamin C. Despite the low intestinal lactase concentration in premature infants, some lactose in the diet may be desirable to promote calcium absorption. The amount of lactose required to maximize calcium absorption has not been determined. Lactose malabsorbed in the small intestine and entering the colon may be one factor that favors the development of a fecal flora with a predominance of lactobacilli rather than coliforms.

Minerals and Vitamins

Because of the rapid accretion of minerals during the last 8 to 10 weeks of gestation, the requirements for many minerals are increased. Sodium requirements appear to be elevated in the very small premature but not in the infant weighing more than 1.5 kg. Both theoretical calculations and experimental data support the conclusion that calcium and phosphorus requirements are higher in premature than in term infants. Calcium is required primarily for mineralization of the skeleton; phosphorus is a major intracellular cation for all tissues. Hemoglobin mass and iron stores are low in the premature, resulting in an increased requirement for iron later in infancy. Because of the interaction of iron with vitamin E, however, iron supplementation is not recommended for the first several months. Whether it is necessary to withhold iron is questionable. Bell and Filer (1981) recently reviewed the studies on which the recommendation to withhold iron is based and concluded that significant hemolysis occurred only in infants receiving diets with both low vitamin E:PUFA ratios and additional iron. Iron is not required during the first several months of life and consequently some neonatologists prefer to wait to introduce it. When iron is started, a dose of 2 mg elemental iron per kg of body weight per day is appropriate. The requirements for the other trace minerals have not been established with any certainty.

Withholding iron from the premature infant because of concerns for vitamin E may not be warranted.

Vitamin requirements of the low-birth-weight infant weighing more than 1.5 kg are similar to those of the full-term infant, with two possible exceptions. Vitamin D requirements may be elevated above the usual RDA of 400 IU per day, although we feel 400 IU per day is adequate. Some nurseries provide 600 to 800 IU per day routinely, a practice that is not unreasonable. There is also a suggestion that the folic acid requirement may be increased in the preterm infant, but routine supplementation is not advocated.

FEEDING THE PREMATURE INFANT

Human milk was used extensively for feeding premature infants until 1940. At that time clinical studies suggested that rates of weight gain improved with higher protein intakes. Although standard and specialized formulas are still commonly used, the last decade has seen the reintroduction of human milk in many nurseries.

Human Milk and the Premature

Human milk has been reintroduced largely because of the suggestion that it may protect to some degree against necrotizing enterocolitis. The humoral and cellular components in human milk that are important in host defense were discussed in Chapter 3.

The nitrogen content of milk is highest early in lactation and declines during the first month.

Whether the nutrient content of human milk is adequate to meet the requirements of the premature infant is still debated. The closer the infant is to term, the less important this concern is. As discussed previously, the protein requirement of the premature infant appears to be higher than that of the term infant. Mature human milk provides approximately 6% of calories as protein, substantially lower than the 10% estimated as desirable for the small premature infant by Fomon et al. (1977). Recent studies have suggested that the nitrogen content of milk from mothers delivering prematurely may be higher and consequently better suited to the needs of the premature infant. In one study (Atkinson et al., 1978) the nitrogen content of milk during the first three days of lactation from mothers who delivered prematurely was 350 mg N/dL. The corresponding value for a group of mothers delivering at term was 302 mg N/dL. While other studies tend to confirm these findings, nitrogen content has varied greatly from study to study, and the differences between the milks of mothers delivering at term and those delivering prematurely have not been so great nor have they been statistically significant in all studies.

There is considerable variation from woman to woman in energy and protein contents of human milk.

The energy density of preterm milk is also increased because of its increased fat content. Anderson et al. (1981) recently reported that the energy density of milk from mothers delivering at 26–33 weeks gestation rose from 59 kcal/dL in the first week to 71 kcal/dL during the second, third, and fourth weeks of lactation. As with nitrogen content, there was wide variation from mother to mother. In Anderson's study the protein content of milk from mothers of premature infants was also higher than that of the milk produced at similar stages of lactation by mothers delivering at term. Protein-calories expressed as a percentage of total calories fell to below 10% in the third week and to 8% during the fourth week. Clearly the apparent advantage derived from feeding an infant its own mother's milk is likely to be lost if pooled milk is used. Although many infants, especially larger prematures, have done well on human milk, growth rates are usually somewhat slower than those achievable with formulas of higher protein content.

Calcium and phosphorus contents of breast milk may be inadequate for very small premature infants.

The adequacy for premature infants of calcium and phosphorus in human milk has also been questioned. Using the reference fetus approach, Fomon et al. (1977) have calculated that human milk contains only one-third the amount of calcium required for the very small premature. Experimental studies support this conclusion. The phosphate content of human milk may also prove inadequate for some preterm infants. Hypophosphatemic rickets of nutritional origin has been seen in a number of very small premature infants fed human milk. Sodium intake from human milk may also be inadequate, although we are not aware of documented problems in prematures fed human milk.

It must be reemphasized that the closer to term the infant is born, the more likely human milk is to be adequate. Many of the presumptions of inadequacy of human milk are based on the assumption that growth that parallels the intrauterine growth rate is desirable. As discussed earlier, this may not be the case. Many premature infants have been nourished adequately on human milk. Whenever human milk is used, every attempt should be made to use milk from the infant's mother rather than pooled milk. This will help to assure maximum nutrient concentrations relative to the infant's requirements. In addition, a multivitamin preparation should be used. In particular, vitamin D should be supplied to provide at least 400 IU per day. To assure adequate phosphorus intake, 25–30 mg/kg/day of elemental phosphorus should be supplied.

Additional carbohydrate and fat must *never* be added to human milk.

If volume considerations limit intake, a rate of weight gain below the intrauterine growth curve should be expected and is completely acceptable. Additional carbohydrate and fat must *never* be added to human milk in an effort to increase the energy density and improve weight gain. These additions only serve to reduce the density (amount per 100 kcal) of protein, vitamins, and minerals, thereby accentuating any marginal inadequacies of the milk.

Specialized Formulas for Low-Birth-Weight Infants

Table 12-1

All three major formula manufacturers in the United States market formulas specifically for the premature infant (Table 12-1). Several modifications from the standard formula have been made. The protein content has been increased from 9% to 10%–12% of total calories. The whey:casein ratio has been altered to 60:40 in Enfamil Premature and Similac Special Care but not in Similac Low Birthweight. Preemie SMA has a 60:40 whey:casein ratio, as does the full-term formula from which it is derived. The Similac and Enfamil products provide approximately 40%–50% of fat as medium-chain triglycerides in an effort to improve fat absorption; Preemie SMA contains only 10% of fat as medium-chain triglycerides. The content of lactose has been reduced to 40%–50% of total carbohydrate in all formulas, the rest being provided as glucose polymers of different chain lengths. There have been no major

Table 12–1 Proximate composition of formulas for premature infants

	Formula			
Nutrient	Enfamil Premature (Mead Johnson Nutritional Div.) (0.8 kcal/mL)	Similac LBW (Ross Laboratories) (0.8 kcal/mL)	Similac Special Care (Ross Laboratories) (0.8 kcal/mL*)	Preemie SMA (Wyeth Laboratories) (0.8 kcal/mL)
kcal distribution (%)				
Protein	12	11	11	10
Fat	44	47	47	42
Carbohydrate	44	42	42	48
Source				
Protein	Whey:casein 60:40	Whey:casein 18:82	Whey:casein 60:40	Whey:casein 60:40
Fat	Corn oil 40%; Medium-chain triglycerides (MCT) 40%; coconut oil (Coco) 20%	MCT 50%; coconut oil 30%; soybean oil 20%	MCT 50%; corn oil 30% Coco 20%	oleo, coconut, oleic (safflower), soy 90%; MCT 10%
Carbohydrate	Corn syrup solids (CSS) 60%; lactose 40%	CSS 50%; lactose 50%	CSS 50%; lactose 50%	Maltodextrins 50%; lactose 50%
Sodium (meq/L)	13.7	16.2	15.2	13.9
Potassium (meq/L)	22.9	30.8	25.6	19.2
Chloride (meq/L)	19.3	24.8	18.3	14.9
Calcium (mg/L)	950	729	1440	750
Phosphorus (mg/L)	480	559	720	400
Calcium:phosphorus	2:1	1.3:1	2:1	1.9:1
Magnesium (mg/L)	84	80	100	70.0
Copper (mg/L)	0.7	0.8	2.0	0.7
Iodine (μg/L)	64	120	150	83
Iron (mg/L)	1.5	3.0	3.0	3.0
Zinc (mg/L)	8.0	8.0	12.0	5.0
Vitamin A (IU/L)	2533	3000	5500	3200
Vitamin D (IU/L)	507	480	1200	510
Vitamin E (IU/L)	15.8	18.0	30	15
Vitamin C (mg/L)	69	100	300	70
Vitamin B_1 (mg/L)	0.6	1.0	2.0	0.8
Vitamin B_2 (mg/L)	0.7	1.2	5.0	1.3
Niacin (Eq/L)	10.1	8.4	24.0	6.3
Vitamin B_6 (mg/L)	0.5	0.5	2.0	0.5
Vitamin B_{12} (μg/L)	2.5	1.6	4.5	2.0
Folate (μg/L)	240	100	300	100
Renal solute load (milliosmoles/L)**	152	154	125	128
Osmolality (milliosmoles/kg H_2O)	300	300	300	268

*Similac Special Care is also marketed in a concentration of 0.67 kcal/mL; vitamin and mineral concentrations are approximately 16% lower and parallel the reductions in energy and protein.
**Estimated by the method of Ziegler & Foman (1971). Because premature infants who are growing rapidly retain considerable amounts of solute, actual renal solute loads are overestimated by this method (see Ziegler & Ryu, 1976).

changes in the sodium or potassium content. The calcium density has been substantially increased, but to different degrees, in all four formulas. Phosphorus has been increased in Similac Special Care. Because of the interaction of iron with vitamin E, the formulas are not iron-fortified. There are minor modifications in the vitamin contents of Enfamil Premature, Similac Low Birthweight, and Preemie SMA in comparison with the corresponding formula for full-term infants. Special Care has substantially higher amounts of most minerals and vitamins.

Many neonatologists and nutritionists continue to use standard infant formulas at a concentration of 20 or 24 kcal/oz (0.67–0.8 kcal/mL) with satisfactory results, especially for larger premature infants.

These specialized formulas may be useful in managing the small premature infant. However, many neonatologists and nutritionists continue to use standard infant formulas at a concentration of 20 or 24 kcal/oz (0.67–0.8 kcal/mL) with satisfactory results, especially for larger premature infants.

Introduction of Oral Feeding

Most premature infants in the 1500–1600 g range will require intravenous fluids for the first 24 hours of life, until they are stable and free of respiratory distress. Infants weighing closer to 2000 g may be able to be managed with oral fluids alone from birth.

Oral feeding should be begun slowly.

When oral feedings are begun, an initial feeding of about ½ oz of sterile water may be given. In some nurseries a second feeding with sterile water is given. In others the next feeding is with breast milk or formula. It is best to abide by the nursery routine in these matters. Once the infant has tolerated one or two sterile water feedings, milk feeding may be begun. A standard 0.67 kcal/mL (20 kcal/oz) formula may be used. There is often no need to use "half-strength" formula, as discussed earlier (Chapter 11), formula intakes should always be prescribed with attention to volume and calorie intake per kilogram, allowing "strength" or concentration to be determined on this basis. It is generally recommended that formulas of 0.8 kcal/mL (24 kcal/oz) not be used until feeding is well established. This suggestion seems to be prompted by problems of gastric retention rather than by difficulties with small intestinal intolerance.

Weight gain may not begin for 7 to 10 days.

Most smaller infants should be fed every 2 or 3 hours. One-half ounce fed every 3 hours will provide between 60 and 80 mL/kg during the first day for the infant weighing 1.5 to 2.0 kg. Intakes can be increased on a daily basis as tolerated. The healthy infant in this weight range can often reach intakes of 100 kcal/kg/day by the end of the first week. Full intake and the initiation of weight gain will occur some time during the second week.

Most infants weighing close to 2.0 kg will be able to be nipple-fed from the outset. Smaller infants may require gavage feeding initially. Continuous nasogastric or nasojejunal infusions should be reserved for sick infants or very small prematures, who should be cared for by a neonatologist.

Complications Associated with Feeding

Necrotizing enterocolitis Although less common in the infant weighing more than 1500 g, necrotizing enterocolitis is thought by most investigators to be related in some way to feeding practices. The disease has developed in infants who have not yet been fed, but this is distinctly unusual. Commonly, 1 to 3 days after the initiation of feeding the infant develops abdominal distention and begins to have diarrhea, usually with occult or gross blood. A flat plate of the abdomen may show pneumatosis of the intestinal wall, air in the biliary tract, or, if perforation has occurred, free air in the abdomen. The factors that appear to predispose to necrotizing enterocolitis are mucosal injury and the presence of bacteria with a suitable metabolic substrate. Necrotizing enterocolitis may be a single disease or a common final pathway for a number of intestinal insults. It appears, however, that in many instances overaggressive oral alimentation may be at least in part responsible. Infants who have suffered peripartum asphyxia or who are possibly septic should be fed with great caution. One group of neonatologists attributes the virtual disappearance of necrotizing enterocolitis from their nursery during the past 5 years to extreme caution in the rate at which oral feedings are introduced and advanced in preterm infants (Brown and Sweet, 1978).

Necrotizing enterocolitis may relate in some way to overaggressive feeding.

Lactobezoars In the last few years, several nurseries have reported the development of lactobezoars in premature infants. Many but not all of these infants were being fed formulas specifically modified for the premature infant. Abdominal distention is the most common symptom; other symptoms include gastric retention and diarrhea. In most instances the mass can be demonstrated on a plain film of the abdomen. The treatment advocated consists of withholding formula for a period of 24 to 36 hours and then reinitiating feeding with a different formula. Most lactobezoars have occurred in infants consuming formulas with a whey:casein ratio of 18:82. Lactobezoars have not been reported in infants being fed human milk or for formulas with whey:casein ratios of 60:40. It may be that the higher curd tension of formulas containing a higher proportion of casein may be partly responsible for the development of lactobezoars in infants consuming these formulas.

Suggested Reading

Anderson, G. A.; Atkinson, S. A.; and Bryan, M. H. 1981. Energy and macronutrient content of human milk during early lactation from mothers giving birth prematurely and at term. *Am. J. Clin. Nutr.* 34:258–265.

Atkinson, S. A.; Bryan, M. H.; and Anderson, G. H. 1978. Human milk: difference in nitrogen concentration in milk from mothers of term and premature infants. *J. Pediatr.* 93:67–69.

Bell, E. F.; and Filer, L. J., Jr. 1981. The role of vitamin E in the nutrition of the premature infant. *Am. J. Clin. Nutr.* 34:414–422.

Brown, E. G.; and Sweet, A. Y. 1978. Preventing necrotizing enterocolitis in neonates. *JAMA* 240:2452–2454.

Committee on Nutrition. 1977. Nutritional needs of low-birth-weight infants. *Pediatrics* 60:519–530.

Fomon, S. J.; Ziegler, E. E.; and Vazquez, H. D. 1977. Human milk and the small premature infant. *Am. J. Dis. Child.* 131:463–367.

Goldman, H. I.; Goldman, J. S.; Kaufman, I., et al. 1974. Late effects of early dietary protein intake on low birth weight infants. *J. Pediatr.* 85:764–769.

Heird, W. C. 1977. Feeding the premature infant. Human milk or an artificial formula? *Am. J. Dis. Child.* 131:468–469.

Raiha, N. C. R.; Heinonen, K.; Rassin, D. K.; Gaull, G. E. 1976. Milk protein quantity and quality in low birth weight infants. I. Metabolic responses and effects on growth. *Pediatrics* 57:659–674.

Ziegler, E. E.; O'Donnell, A. M.; Nelson, S. E., et al. 1976. Body composition of the reference fetus. *Growth* 40:329–341.

Ziegler, E. E.; and Ryu, J. E. 1976. Renal solute load and diet in growing premature infants. *J. Pediatr.* 89:609–611.

13 Obesity

Contents

Definition of Obesity **255**
    Normal Changes of Fatness with Age **255**
    Criteria **255**
Energy Balance **257**
Origins of Obesity **259**
    Genetics **259**
    Exercise **259**
    Cultural Attitudes **260**
Morbidity Associated with Obesity **261**
The Relationship of Childhood Obesity to Adult Obesity **262**
Management of Obesity **263**

Overview

Defining obesity is difficult because of our inability to relate specific degrees of overfatness to morbidity in childhood or later in life. The development of obesity is related to energy balance. Current views suggest that there may be substantial variation among individuals in their abilities to dissipate excess energy as heat and, thereby, avoid obesity. Cultural attitudes toward body image also play a role in development of obesity. Although the progression of obesity in childhood to obesity in later life is not as clear cut as once thought, it is prudent to try to maintain body weight in a reasonable range. Once established, obesity is extremely resistant to treatment.

DEFINITION OF OBESITY

Obesity is best defined as an excessive proportion of body weight as fat. The extension of this conceptual definition to a working definition using height and weight or some measure of fatness is not an easy task. Although the skinfold caliper has provided a simple and reliable indirect way of measuring fatness, deciding how much fat is too much can be difficult; one must take into account the normal changes in body fatness that take place during infancy, childhood, and adolescence. Food intake, exercise, and innate efficiency of energy utilization all affect energy balance. Cultural attitudes toward body weight play a large role in the origins and treatment of obesity.

Deciding how much fat is too much can be difficult.

Normal Changes of Fatness with Age

Man is normally one of the fattest of all mammals. During the last trimester of gestation body fat increases from 5% to 16% of body weight. Fat continues to accumulate during the first 6 months of life; at the end of this period it accounts for 26% of body weight. Body fat decreases slowly during the preschool years, representing about 14%-15% of weight at age 5, and then increases again slowly in both boys and girls until puberty (Figure 13-1). During puberty there is a decrease in fatness in boys, a marked increase in girls. At age 16 fat represents only 11% of body weight in the average boy, but 24% in the average girl.

Figure 13-1

Criteria

Weight for age Body fat can be measured by several techniques. More precise measures such as total body water determination, ^{40}K counting, and underwater weighing (densitometry) are useful research tools and have been used to validate less cumbersome indirect measures. Until recently most definitions of obesity have relied on body weight. In instances in which body weight alone is used, individuals whose weight is greater than the 90th or 97th percentile are frequently classified as obese.

Weight for height It is preferable to relate weight to height, taking into account the fact that heavier individuals may simply be bigger. Obesity is then usually defined as 20% (occasionally 10%) over ideal weight for height. The height and weight relationship has been further refined by use of the ponderal index in which height in inches is divided by the cube root of weight in pounds. A value of less than 12 is considered to indicate obesity.

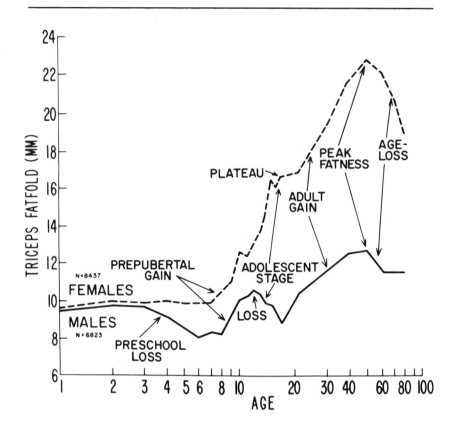

Figure 13-1 Trends in fatness throughout the life cycle as reflected in triceps fatfold measurements. From Garn, S. M.; and Clark, D. C. 1976. Trends in fatness and the origins of obesity. *Pediatrics* 57:443-456. Copyright American Academy of Pediatrics.

Skinfold measurement   Although the use of some relationship between weight and height is an improvement over the use of weight alone, all the definitions of overweight still implicitly equate overweight with overfat. The measurement of skinfold or fatfold thicknesses overcomes this difficulty and provides an easy way of estimating total body fat. There is a high degree of correlation ($r > 0.8$) between skinfold thickness and total body fat as determined by densitometry. Skinfold measurement technique was described in Chapter 1. Reference standards were also provided in Table 1-1.

Even though a simple means of estimating total body fat with some precision is available, we are still left not knowing how to define obesity. Ideally obesity should be defined in health terms rather than in statistical terms. The knowledge that a certain level of body fatness at a given age carried with it an increased risk of morbidity in childhood or later in life would provide a rational basis for deciding when an individual is too fat. Limited morbidity and mortality data by weight are available for adults; they suggest that longevity may be influenced unfavorably when body weight is more than 20% above ideal weight. We are unaware of similar data for children. In the absence of a biologic basis for the definition of obesity, the upper limit of acceptable triceps skinfold is often arbitrarily taken as the median plus one standard deviation. This automatically classifies 16% of the population as obese. By setting the cutoff at this level the practitioner can identify children who are becoming obese at an earlier stage, when management may be somewhat easier. Use of a two-standard-deviation cutoff would decrease the apparent prevalence of obesity to 3%. Diagnosis of the markedly overfat infant or child who falls into this 3% should require neither scale nor caliper.

Ideally obesity should be defined in health terms rather than statistical terms.

ENERGY BALANCE

Energy balance is the relationship of energy intake to energy output. When energy intake exceeds energy output, the excess is stored as fat. The energy requirement for an individual is determined by several factors: basal metabolic rate, postprandial heat production (so-called specific dynamic action), level of activity, and in the case of the child, growth. Energy requirements are estimated on the assumption that individuals of the same size and sex, in the same environment, whose level of activity is similar will have similar energy requirements. This approach makes activity a key variable in the difference in energy requirements among individuals and implies an exquisite sensitivity of appetite control over intake if body weight is to be maintained. Studies of food intake by adults demonstrate no correlation between day-to-day food consumption and day-to-day activity. Observations of children's eating patterns suggest that the same is true for them. With activity level constant there is great variation in an individual's daily food intake, although when intake is analyzed on a weekly basis there is less variability. There are also variations in intake among similar-sized individuals with similar activity levels. A study of army recruits undergoing basic training (Edholm, 1955) showed marked differences in food consumption by similar-sized individuals, all of whom were

When energy intake exceeds energy output, the excess is stored as fat.

Daily food intake does not correlate well with day-to-day activity.

maintaining steady weight. Although there is less information available concerning children, the range of food intake that supports adequate growth at a particular age is quite wide. Energy intakes by children age 3 have been found to vary by as much as 50%.

Under normal circumstances all nutrients are consumed in excess of need. Balance is maintained either by excretion of unused quantities (e.g. nitrogen, sodium, and calcium) or less often, by limiting absorption (e.g. iron). Balance of most nutrients does not depend on appetite to regulate intake with great precision. Fortunately, this appears to hold true for energy intake and energy balance as well. Maintenance of suitable body weight would be nearly impossible if intake regulated by appetite were the key controlling variable. For example, a daily intake of 20 kcal in excess of the individual's daily requirement over 1 year would create a positive balance of 7300 kcal, the equivalent of slightly more than 1 kg of fat. This excess calorie intake is the equivalent of 1 oz of formula a day for an infant and less than one cookie or one-quarter of an apple per day for an older child. Energy appears to be similar to other nutrients in that there is a wide range of energy intakes that will maintain weight or support growth in a given individual. Energy consumed somewhat in excess of requirement is "excreted," or more properly, dissipated as heat, although there is clearly an upper limit to the amount of energy that can be dissipated as heat. Additionally, certain types of diets, patterns of eating, and physiologic states appear to alter the degree to which this thermogenesis occurs.

To a point, excess energy can be dissipated as heat.

Most of the energy in food is necessarily converted to heat. No more than 33%–34% of the energy in protein or 38%–40% of that in fat and carbohydrate can be converted to high-energy phosphate bonds useful in running metabolic processes. It is unlikely that these theoretical maxima are ever reached. It also appears that there is considerable variation in the efficiency of energy conversion from individual to individual and within an individual at different times. Miller and Mumford (1967) fed adult volunteers diets providing 1300 kcal/day above their habitual intakes for a period of 8 weeks. High-protein and low-protein diets were studied. The anticipated weight gain from excess energy intake was nearly 6 kg. Weight gain during consumption of the high protein diet was 60% of that expected. During the period of low protein intake the average weight gain was less than 1 kg. Changes in activity, digestibility, and body composition were all ruled out as possible explanations. Oxygen consumption studies demonstrated that increased energy loss was accomplished by heat production and dissipation, especially immediately postprandially. The factors that alter the efficiency with which energy is utilized in the adult, much less in the growing child, are just beginning to be understood. Intraindividual and interindividual variations should prove extremely important in the future in understanding obesity.

ORIGINS OF OBESITY

Genetics

The idea that an individual's genetic makeup is in part responsible for the propensity to develop obesity is an attractive theory that is supported by several lines of evidence. Genetically obese strains of rats and mice have been discovered. In at least one instance, the ob/ob mouse, obesity is transmitted as a recessive characteristic. In the human there is greater concordance of weight between identical twins than between fraternal twins. There is no question that a child whose parents are obese is more likely to be obese than the child raised by thin parents, but environment may be the critical factor in the equation. Completely uninvestigated to date is the possibility that differences in intermediary metabolism and hence in the efficiency of energy utilization are genetically determined and transmissible. Although in the future we may find that genetic makeup explains why energy requirements vary so considerably among individuals or why some individuals have a smaller capacity to excrete excess energy ingested, excess food intake or decreased activity will still remain the critical environmental variable causing the genetic predisposition to be expressed as obesity.

Genetic factors may explain the variability in energy requirements, but food intake and exercise will still remain the critical factors causing obesity.

Exercise

Although lack of exercise may contribute to obesity, many children and adults who have relatively sedentary existences nevertheless maintain optimal body weight without conscious efforts to restrict food intake. Children who are obese have been found to be less active than their lean counterparts. However, reduced activity should not necessarily be equated with decreased energy utilization. Because of their increased weight, obese children may expend more energy than lean children in carrying out the same activity. Whether inactivity is a cause or the result of obesity in most cases has not been established. Although the importance of exercise in weight control should not be disregarded,

Table 13-1

when the calories expended as the result of exercise are compared with those in portions of common foods, one can clearly see how easily uncontrolled food intake can undo even the most strenuous exercise program. For example, an hour of slow running by the obese 13-year-old (Table 13–1) would catabolize approximately 250 kcal, the energy content of 2½ oz of hamburger. Carrying out the same activity, his lean brother would utilize approximately 100 kcal, the energy content of a glass of orange juice. Even given the inefficiency of converting food energy to useful energy, one can see that increasing energy expenditure by exercise without attention to the energy intake side of the equation can be a losing proposition.

Cultural Attitudes

In his review of the causes of obesity Weil (1977) concluded: "The forces derivative from social status, attitudes, and customs are probably the dominant ones in the establishment of obesity. Social factors, to the extent that they are effective, must operate through individuals; two of the most significant are the mother and the physician." The degree of fatness in children correlates closely with socioeconomic status. The Ten-State Nutrition Survey demonstrated that on the average children of higher-income families tended to be

Table 13–1 Laboratory values for energy expenditures by obese and nonobese brothers in different activities

	Energy Expenditure (kcal/min)					
	Standing		Walking		Slow running	
Age	Obese	Nonobese	Obese	Nonobese	Obese	Nonobese
4 & 5 yr	0.5	0.7	1.2	1.2	1.7	1.3
6 & 5 yr	1.2	1.1	3.1	2.1	3.7	2.6
11 & 10 yr	1.1	0.7	2.7	1.4	3.1	2.0
13 & 12 yr	1.4	0.8	3.6	1.8	4.1	1.7

Source: Modified from Waxman, M.; and Stunkard, A. J. 1980. Caloric intake and expenditure of obese boys. *J. Pediatr.* 96:187–191.

fatter than those of lower-income families. Attitudes toward food consumption and toward weight vary considerably among different racial and cultural groups. Families working their way up the socioeconomic ladder may subconsciously regard increased weight in themselves and their children as signs of increasing affluence.

Physicians, grandparents and friends alike have for generations inculcated new mothers with the idea that the chubby baby was a happy, healthy baby. A thin baby has rarely received the same adulation. The current unfounded fear of some parents and physicians that even mild degrees of malnutrition may lead to mental dysfunction may also contribute to overfeeding, especially in infancy. Finally, the use of food as the predominant means of soothing the unhappy infant or as a reward for the older child may induce overconsumption. The availability in this country of relatively inexpensive convenience foods makes overconsumption especially easy.

The practitioner must be sensitive to his or her own social and cultural values as well as to those of the child and his family. Most parents will not have the same degree of concern as the practitioner does about mild to moderate degrees of obesity. What may represent a state of overnutrition for one may simply be a sign of good health for the other. The reasons parents overfeed their children are complex and highly variable, and the practitioner can make little progress in the prevention of obesity within individual families unless he or she makes some attempt to understand these reasons.

> The reasons parents overfeed their children are complex and highly variable.

MORBIDITY ASSOCIATED WITH OBESITY

Medical concern for obesity in childhood is justifiable only if obese children are subject to morbidity not seen to the same extent in their lean peers. Extremely obese children have been found to have upper respiratory infections more frequently. Intertrigo may also be a problem. Obese children withstand heat stress less well. Slipped femoral capital epiphyses are more common in markedly overweight children. But none of these complications is of major importance in the mildly to moderately obese child.

The psychologic impact of being obese in childhood must not be overlooked. Many obese children, especially adolescents, have a great sense of isolation and rejection in a society in which obesity is increasingly unacceptable. For some, overeating may

> The psychologic impact of being obese in childhood must not be overlooked.

be a way of coping with stress and dealing with frustration. The degree to which certain personality traits are the cause rather than the result of obesity is uncertain.

THE RELATIONSHIP OF CHILDHOOD OBESITY TO ADULT OBESITY

The major current concern about obesity in childhood is that it will lead to obesity later in life.

Perhaps the major current concern about obesity in childhood is that it will lead to obesity in later life, thereby increasing the longterm risk to the individual of diabetes and cardiovascular disease and their complications. Because of the great difficulty in treating obesity once it is established, investigators began to look at its origin in an effort to try to prevent it. Asher (1966) found that 44% of a group of 269 children who were at least 25% overweight for their age and height had been obese since infancy. Other studies also linked obesity in childhood with that in adulthood.

Research in the mid–1960s provided a physiologic basis for the progression of obesity in later life from that in childhood. They estimated the number of fat cells and the amount of lipid per cell in a group of obese adults and compared these values with those obtained from a control group. The lipid content of fat cells in obese subjects was approximately 50% greater than that in control subjects. Fat-cell number, however, was estimated to be 300% above control. Similar determinations for nine infants and children suggested that fat-cell number tended to increase until adolescence but not beyond. Studies such as these led to the concept of hyperplastic and hypertrophic obesity. Obesity with its onset in childhood was characterized by an increased number of fat cells, whereas obesity beginning after adolescence resulted primarily in an increased amount of fat per cell. It was suggested that large numbers of fat cells acquired by the obese child could never be lost, making control of obesity in later life more difficult.

These studies have been validly criticized for a variety of methodologic reasons. Equally important, because no longitudinal studies of fat-cell size and cell number have been carried out, it is impossible to say whether the increased cell number encountered in obese adults was a response to overeating in childhood or was genetically predetermined. Finally, no theory has been proposed to explain why it should be more difficult to lose weight if the same amount of fat is packaged in more cells rather than in fewer.

One study frequently quoted to show that obesity in later childhood results from that in infancy is that of Eid (1970). It classified 474 infants according to their rates of weight gain during the first 6 months as rapid, moderate, or slow gainers. Children growing above the 90th percentile were placed in the rapid-weight-gain group. Follow-up was carried out 6 to 8 years later to determine the prevalence of obesity, defined as 20% overweight for age. The subsequent prevalence of obesity in the rapid-weight-gain group was 9.4%. This compared with prevalences of 3% and 1.9% in the other two groups. The rapid-gain group, however, was also taller and skinfold data suggested that children in this group were in fact probably no fatter than those in the other two groups. Finally, it should be noted that 90% of children classified as rapid weight gainers in infancy were not classified as overweight at 6 to 8 years.

Charney et al. (1976) related the weight of 366 adults to their weights at 6 months of age. Of the group that had been above the 90th percentile at 6 months of age, 36% were 10% or more above desirable weight as adults. Only 14% of infants below the 90th percentile were overweight to this degree as adults. Other studies suggest that the risk of remaining obese as an adult after being obese in childhood or adolescence is probably greater for the female than for the male. This increased propensity may be related to the normal differences in changes of fatness that take place during adolescence.

It is clear that some obesity beginning in childhood persists through adolescence and into adult life, and that the thin child does appear to be less likely to be overweight as an adult. It would be surprising if this were not the case. It is also clear that most children who are obese as infants will outgrow this during childhood and that the child who is obese is not inevitably destined to be obese in later life.

> The relationship of childhood obesity to obesity in the adult is not as well established as it once appeared to be.

MANAGEMENT OF OBESITY

The treatment of obesity has proven to be exceedingly difficult and more often than not unsuccessful. In theory treatment is amazingly simple. The energy balance equation must be altered so that energy utilization exceeds energy intake. Because of the complex cultural and social factors that influence how and what we eat, effecting a change in eating habits is exceedingly difficult, even under the best of circumstances. The parents of a younger child may not share the practitioner's concern about the child's obesity and consequently may lack motivation to follow any prescribed diet. Even well-motivated parents may find themselves in a situation in which the child's eating patterns and the significance of food within the family are so ingrained that any serious effort at curtailing food consumption is disruptive to the family, very quickly becoming unacceptable. These difficulties in management are compounded in the adolescent by the psychologic changes that normally take place during puberty.

Management begins with a careful dietary history or, preferably, a food diary for several days. This allows calorie intake to be estimated and, of equal importance, gives insight into the food preferences of the child and the family. Devising a diet that reduces energy intake without seriously disrupting the individual family's eating habits may require the help of a skilled nutritionist. Admonitions to "put the child on skim milk" or "cut out carbohydrates" rarely accomplish anything. A decrease of portion size and an emphasis on foods that are low in energy density but known to be liked and eaten is preferable. A diet that reduces energy intake to 80%–85% of that estimated by recall of food diary is a reasonable way to begin. This will have to be adjusted upward or downward depending on the response.

A marked reduction in calorie intake is ill-advised during infancy and early childhood. Rapid weight loss is unnecessary and undesirable at these developmental stages. A reasonable goal is the cessation of weight gain rather than weight reduction. If level weight can be maintained, the child will slowly outgrow the obesity. In extreme obesity, especially in older children, weight reduction is not an unreasonable goal. Gradual weight reduction, not to exceed about 0.5 lb per week, depending on the child's age, is desirable. Weight lost at this slow rate is more likely to be lost as fat than is weight lost exceedingly rapidly; rapid weight loss may require catabolism of protein stores as well as fat. Total fasting and the so-called protein-sparing modified fast have been used extensively in the treatment of adult obesity and occasionally in the treatment of children. It should be carried out only in specialized centers by investigators having a specific interest in and knowledge of the subject.

Appetite suppressants are not appropriate for the management of childhood obesity. Amphetamines, the drugs most frequently used, may cause the child to be insomniac. In addition, although the drugs may suppress appetite, they do not effect a change in eating habits. Studies of their use in childhood suggest that they offer no advantage over a placebo in effecting and maintaining weight reduction.

Admonitions to "put the child on skim milk" or "cut out carbohydrates" rarely accomplish anything.

A marked reduction in calorie intake is ill-advised during infancy and early childhood.

Suggested Reading

Asher, P. 1966. Fat babies and fat children. *Arch. Dis. Child.* 41: 672–673.

Charney, E. M.; Goodman, H. C.; McBride, M. et al. 1976. Childhood antecedents of adult obesity: do chubby infants become obese adults. *N. Engl. J. Med.* 295:6–9.

Edholm, O. G.; Fletcher, J. G.; Widdowson, E. M.; and McCance, R. A. 1955. The energy expenditure and food intake of individual men. *Brit. J. Nutrition* 9:286–300.

Eid, E. E. 1970. Follow-up study of physical growth of children who had excessive weight gain in first six months of life. *Br. Med. J.* 2:74–76.

Garn, S. M.; and Clark, D. C. 1976. Trends in fatness and the origins of obesity. *Pediatrics* 57:443–456.

Hegsted, D. M. 1974. Energy needs and energy utilization. *Nutr. Rev.* 32:33–38.

Hirsch, J.; and Knittle, J. L. 1970. Cellularity of obese and non-obese human adipose tissue. *Fed Proc* 29:1516–1521.

Hirsch, J., Knittle, J. L. and Salans, L. B. 1966. Cell lipid content and cell number of obese and nonobese human adipose tissue (abstract). *J. Clin. Invest.* 45:1023.

Miller, D. S.; and Mumford, P. 1967. Gluttony. An experimental study of overeating low- or high-protein diets. *Am. J. Clin. Nutr.* 20:1212–1222.

Pisacano, J. C.; Lichter, H.; Ritter, J.; and Siegal, A. P. 1978. An attempt at prevention of obesity in infancy. *Pediatrics* 61:360–364.

Waxman, M.; and Stunkard, A. J. 1980. Caloric intake and expenditure of obese boys. *J. Pediatr.* 96:187–193.

Weil, W. B., Jr. 1977. Current controversies in childhood obesity. *J. Pediatr.* 91:175–187.

Appendix A: Restricted Diets*

GLUTEN-FREE DIET

A gluten-free diet is indicated only in patients with a firm diagnosis of celiac disease. The use of therapeutic trials of gluten-free diets in children with chronic diarrhea may delay appropriate diagnosis of other conditions. Wheat, buckwheat, rye, oats, and barley all contain gluten. It is a subfraction of gluten, gliadin, that causes damage to the intestinal mucosa in sensitive individuals. A gluten-free diet leads to a prompt reversal of symptoms and signs of the disease. Although older children and young adults may not have a florid recrudescence of symptoms when gluten is reintroduced, biopsies of the small intestine show that this reintroduction does induce damage. Consequently, in celiac disease a gluten-free diet should be continued indefinitely. Many mothers with gluten-sensitive children prefer to cook "gluten-free" for the entire family rather than to prepare separate meals for the child with gluten enteropathy.

Gluten-Free Diet for Infants

All three baby food manufacturers will provide a pamphlet listing product ingredients and identifying those products containing

*This appendix was partially adapted from the *Manual of applied nutrition*, 6th ed., 1973, Nutrition Department, The Johns Hopkins Hospital, Janette Carlsen Martin, editor, The Johns Hopkins University Press.

wheat or other gluten-containing cereals. Because product formulations change from time to time it is suggested that copies obtained from the companies be updated periodically. The addresses are listed at the end of the Appendix. There follows a current list of gluten-free baby foods.

Foods permitted	*Foods omitted*
Standard infant formulas (some celiacs may be relatively lactose intolerant at the time of diagnosis)	Wheat cereal Oat cereal Barley cereal High-protein cereal Mixed cereal Oatmeal
Soy formulas	
Fruit juices	
Rice cereal (Beech-Nut or Heinz)†	
Single-ingredient fruits, vegetables, and meats	

Gluten-Free Diets for Older Children

The lists that follow give guidelines for products with and without gluten. With the number of convenience foods on the market it is impossible to be all-inclusive. Ultimately there is no substitute for careful label reading before food is purchased.

Foods permitted	*Foods omitted*
Meat: Beef, lamb, pork, veal, fish, or poultry prepared with allowed foods	Prepared meats such as scrapple, sausage, frankfurters, bologna, luncheon meat, and commercial hamburger, which may contain cereal fillers; meat loaf made with prohibited foods; croquettes; canned meat mixtures; gravy and cream sauces thickened with prohibited flours

---

†At the present time, Gerber adds barley malt flour to its rice cereal.

Foods permitted (continued)	*Foods omitted (continued)*
Cheese: As desired; cheese products made with permitted flours	Cheese products made with prohibited flours
Eggs: As desired	
Milk: Relative lactose intolerance at the time of diagnosis is not uncommon	Commercial chocolate milk, which may have cereal additives, malted milk
Fruits: As desired	
Vegetables: Prepared plain, or creamed with allowed flours	Any creamed or prepared with prohibited flours
Soups: Any clear broth or those made with allowed foods, thickened with cream, cornstarch, potato, soybean, or rice flour	Any prepared with prohibited flour
Bread and Cereal Products: Those made from arrowroot, cornmeal, wheat starch, soybean, rice, potato, or gluten-free wheat flour only; rice sticks; sago; tapioca, cereals made from corn or rice, such as corn flakes, Corn Kix, cornmeal, hominy grits, Rice Krispies, puffed rice, rice flakes unless malt flavoring is added; rice; gluten-free rice wafers, gluten-free bread, and low-protein pasta and porridge are available commercially; cornstarch	Whole wheat, graham, gluten, or white flours, bread, biscuits, rolls, muffins, crackers, pretzels, rusks, Zweiback, Rye Krisp, doughnuts, pancakes, waffles, or any product made with prohibited flours; bran or bran cereals, cream of wheat, farina, grapenuts, oatmeal, shredded or puffed wheat, Ralston, Wheatena, pablum, buckwheat, or other cereals derived from prohibited grains, wheat germ, macaroni, noodles, spaghetti, and other alimentary pastes; kasha, barley, sesame seeds, millet

Foods permitted (continued)	*Foods omitted (continued)*
Fats: Butter, margarine, cream, corn, peanut, safflower, or cottonseed oil; meat or poultry fat, mayonnaise and salad dressing made without prohibited flours; olives, nuts, peanut butter, olive oil	Boiled salad dressing, wheat germ oil
Desserts: Cornstarch, tapioca, or rice pudding, custard, junket, bavarian cream, blanc mange if thickened with cornstarch, gelatin, homemade ice cream, ice milk, ice, or sherbet made without prohibited flours; cookies and cakes made with allowed flours; meringues; fruit	Commercial ice cream with cereal additives; cake, pastry, cookies, pie crust, and pudding unless prepared with permitted flours, ice cream cones
Sweets: White, brown, or maple sugar; honey, molasses, sorghum, syrups; jelly, jam, preserves, marmalade; candy made without prohibited products; marshmallows	Candies containing prohibited products
Seasonings: Herbs, condiments, spices, salt, pepper, homemade catsup, chili sauce	Sauces and seasonings made with prohibited products
Beverages: See milk; pure cocoa, coffee, tea, fruit juices, carbonated beverages	Coffee substitutes, Postum, instant coffee; malted drinks, Ovaltine, ale, beer

LACTOSE-RESTRICTED DIET

As discussed in Chapter 9, very few people, especially children, are completely lactose intolerant. Because the age-dependent and race-dependent decline in lactase levels usually leaves the individual with about 15%–20% of maximal lactase activity, small amounts of lactose, especially as part of a meal are usually tolerated. The guidelines below list the obvious source of lactose. If symptoms do not abate on a lactose-restricted diet is is unlikely that the symptoms were due to lactose intolerance, although one cannot be certain of this fact until a lactose-free diet has been followed. We rarely find a lactose-free diet to be necessary for treatment of lactose intolerance.

We suggest removing almost all lactose initially so that a clear-cut symptomatic response can be observed, if it occurs. Small amounts of milk can than be added back to the diet—for example, on cereal, in creamed foods, in small amounts at mealtime, and in ice cream.

It must be emphasized that a lactose-restricted diet is not adequate therapy for children with galactosemia. This condition is rare, but any galactose, one of the component monosaccharides of lactose, is harmful to these children, and their diet must be lactose free. Most diet manuals provide an extensive list of lactose-containing products.

Lactose-Restricted Diets for Infants

Foods permitted	*Foods omitted*
Lactose-free formulas*	Lactose-containing formulas
Isomil	Enfamil
I-Soyalac	Enfamil Premature
Nursoy	Preemie SMA
ProSobee	Similac
Ensure	Similac Low Birthweight
Ensure Osmolite	Similac Special Care
Nutramigen	SMA
Portagen	
Pregestimil	

Solids — check manufacturers' handbooks. Addresses are listed at the end of the Appendix.

---

*Least expensive among these are the first four formulas, which are soy formulas. Formulas made with whole-milk protein, such as Portagen, may contain minute quantities of lactose. These amounts cause no problem for the lactose-intolerant infant but would be inappropriate for the infant with galactosemia.

Lactose-Restricted Diets for Older Children—Moderate Restriction

Foods permitted

Cheese
Yogurt

Foods omitted

Whole milk
Skim milk
Evaporated milk
Condensed milk } In large amounts
Dried milk
Ice cream
Goat milk

Older Children—More Strict Restriction

Listed below are typical foods that may contain lactose when prepared commercially. Like other restricted diets these are guidelines but do not substitute for careful label reading.

Ascorbic acid and citric acid mixtures

Buttermilk

Cakes and sweet rolls

Canned and frozen fruits and vegetables

Caramels, fudge, and coated candies

Cheese foods and spreads

Cookies and cookie sandwich fillings

Cordials and liquers

Cottage cheese and cottage-cheese dressings

Dietetic and diabetic preparations

Dried soups

French fries and corn curls

Health and geriatric foods

Ice cream

Infant formulas

Instant coffee

Instant potatoes

Meat products prepared with fillings, such as luncheon meats, frankfurters

Modified skim milk

Party dips

Pie crusts and fillings

Powdered coffee cream

Powdered soft drinks

Puddings

Salad dressings

Sherbets, frozen desserts, and ices

Sour cream

Spice blends

Starter cultures

Sweetened condensed milk

Sweetness-reducers in icings, candies, preserves, and fruit pie fillings

Tablets

Vitamin and mineral mixtures (lactose commonly used as a filler)

Note: Lactate, lactic acid, and lactalbumin do not contain lactose.

COW-MILK-FREE DIET

Rare infants and children will demonstrate hypersensitivity to milk protein when challenged in a double-blind fashion. For these children a milk-free diet is indicated.

Cow-Milk-Free Diet for Infants

Foods permitted (formulas)	*Foods omitted (formulas)*
Isomil	Enfamil
I-Soyalac	Enfamil Premature Formula
Nursoy	Ensure
ProSobee	Ensure Osmolite
Nutramigen	Portagen
Pregestimil	Preemie SMA
	Similac
	Similac Low Birthweight
	Similac Special Care
	SMA

Solids — whole-milk solids are added to a variety of baby foods, especially creamed products. Lists of product ingredients should be obtained from food manufacturers, whose addresses are listed at the end of this Appendix.

Cow-Milk-Free Diet for Older Children

Foods permitted	*Foods omitted*
Meat: beef, veal, lamb, pork, poultry	Creamed or breaded meat, fish, or poultry; some frankfurters and cold cuts; meats in gravies made with milk
Cheese: goat milk (may cross react)	All cow-milk cheeses
Eggs: any prepared with allowed foods	Eggs prepared with milk or milk products
Milk: goat milk (may cross react), soy formulas, meat-based formulas, protein-hydrolysate formulas	Cow milk (whole, skim, condensed, evaporated, buttermilk); yogurt; ice cream, sherbet; malted milk; whey; casein
Fruit: all fresh, canned, frozen	None unless prepared with milk or cream
Vegetables: all fresh, canned, or frozen, except as noted	Any creamed, breaded or buttered; instant potatoes
Soups: clear soups	Cream soups, chowders
Bread and cereal products: any that do not contain milk or milk products; macaroni, noodles, spaghetti, rice, popcorn made with allowed fats	Prepared mixes such as muffins, biscuits, waffles; instant or dry cereals to which milk solids have been added
Fats: margarines and dressings that do not contain milk or milk products; oils, shortenings, bacon, nuts, nut butters	Margarines and dressings containing milk or milk products; cream cheese, butter, peanut butter with milk-solid fillers
Desserts: water-and-fruit ices, gelatin, homemade cakes, pies, cookies made with milk-free (soy) formula in place of milk	Most commercial cakes, cookies, mixes, custard, ice cream, sherbet; any containing chocolate
Sweets: jelly, marmalade, jam, sugar, pure sugar candy	Any made with chocolate or cocoa, butterscotch, caramels

Beverages: fruit juices, coffee, tea, carbonated beverages, other soft drinks

Chocolate, cocoa, milk, malted milk

ADDRESSES FOR SPECIFIC INFORMATION

Baked gluten-free rice bread	Ener-G-Foods, Incorporated 1526 Utah Avenue, South Seattle, Washington 98134
Beech Nut strained and junior foods (consult company for product analysis)	BeechNut Food Corp. Fort Washington, Pa 19034
Cellu gluten-free bread mix	Chicago Dietetic Supply, Incorporated Department 25, P. O. Box 529 LaGrange, Illinois 60525
Cellu gluten-free flours, wafers, cakes, and cookies	Chicago Dietetic Supply, Incorporated Department 25, P. O. Box 529 LaGrange, Illinois 60525
Cellu gluten-free wheat starch	Chicago Dietetic Supply, Incorporated Department 25, P. O. Box 529 LaGrange, Illinois 60525
Gerber strained and junior foods (consult company for product analysis)	Gerber Products Company Fremont, Michigan 49412
Heinz strained and junior foods (consult company for product analysis)	H. J. Heinz Company Pittsburg, Pennsylvania 15230
Rice flour	Byrd Mill Company Richmond, Virginia 23220
Rice cakes	Chico San, Incorporated 1262 Humboldt Avenue Chico, California 95926
Rice wafers—Devonsheer	Devonsheer Melba Corporation Carlstadt, New Jersey 07072

Appendix B: Nutrition History for Infants

GENERAL INFORMATION

Name: _____

Date: _____ Date Admitted: _____

Parents' names: _____

Address: _____

Phone: _____

Birth Wt.: _____ L: _____ GA: _____

Age: _____ Sex: M   F

Diet order: _____

DX: _____

CURRENT STATUS

Presenting nutritional problem: _____

Wt.: _____ (%tile) L: _____ (%tile) HC: _____ (%tile)

Wt/L: (%tile) IBW/L: _____ Growth pattern: Slow_____ Steady_____ Other_____

Laboratory data: _____ Meds: _____

FEEDING SITUATION

Informant: _____

_____

Fed: Breast milk: _____ Cow milk: _____

Formula (kind): _____with Fe:___ Ready-to-feed:___ Powdered: ___ Liq. Conc.: ___

Method of formula prep: _____

Formulas tried	Age	Time span	Reason for discontinuing

Total formula taken each

day: _____

Supplements	Age	Amt.	Problem	Bottle	Spoon
Cereal					
Baby fruits					
Baby vegetables					
Baby meats					
Crackers					
Mashed food					
Chopped food					
Regular food					

Likes: _____

_____

_____

Dislikes: _____

_____

_____

Are baby foods bought? _____ Home prepared? _____ Who feeds child? _____

How long is the usual feeding period (in minutes)? _____

Has your child ever received vitamins? _____ Brand? _____ Amt? _____

Age vitamin supplements began: _____ Ended: _____ Home meds: _____

Has your baby ever been on a special diet? _____ Reason: _____

Have you ever had diet/nutrition education for your child? _____ By whom? _____

Does your child have any of the following?

Vomiting _____ Sucking problems _____

Diarrhea _____ Swallowing problems _____

Constipation _____ Physical handicaps _____

Allergies _____ Sleeping problems _____

Shortness of breath _____ Other _____

Appetite:

Good _____ Fair _____ Poor _____ Fluctuates _____

Summary of typical day's intake:

Total calories _____   kcal/kg _____

Total protein _____   Pro/kg _____

Total carbohydrate _____   Total fat _____

Typical intake	Time/place	Food pattern	Feeds every _____ hours

FAMILY SITUATION

Father's occupation: _____   Mother's occupation _____

Siblings and ages: _____

Others residing in household: _____

Available:

Food stamps _____   Crippled children's _____

WIC _____   Garden _____

Other _____

Other Pertinent Information: _____

ASSESSMENT: _____

PLAN: _____

Appendix C: Nutritional Status Assessment

NAME: _____

HISTORY NUMBER: _____

AGE: _____ SEX: _____

SUGGESTIVE PHYSICAL SIGNS

General appearance: _____

Thin _____ Well-nourished _____ Obese _____ Edematous _____

Other: _____

ANTHROPOMETRICS

Date _____ Date _____

Measurements	Actual	Centile	% Median*	Actual	Centile	% Median*
Height for age (cm)						
Weight for age (kg)						
Weight for height (kg)						
Head circumference (cm)						
Arm circumference (cm)						
Triceps skinfold (mm)						
Calculated values						
Arm-muscle area (sq cm)						
% body weight as fat						

LABORATORY DATA   Date _____   Date _____

	Actual	*Normal*	*% Norm*	*Actual*	*Normal*	*% Norm*
Serum total protein (g/dL)						
Serum albumin (g/dL)						
Hemoglobin (g/dL)						
Hematocrit (%)						
T.I.B.C. (μg/dL)						
Serum transferrin (mg/dL)						
24-hr urinary creatinine (mg)			†			†
Other: _____						
_____						

DIET HISTORY

	Actual	*Req'd*	*% Req'd*	*Actual*	*Req'd*	*% Req'd*
Energy intake (kcal/kg)						
Protein intake (g/kg)						
Other: _____						
_____						

PERTINENT MEDICAL INFORMATION: _____

_____

PERTINENT SOCIAL INFORMATION: _____

_____

ASSESSMENT(S): _____

_____

*Patient's value as a percentage of the 50th percentile value for age.

†Creatinine height index.

Appendix D: Calorie Count—Food Record

NAME: _____   DATE: _____

Please record all food and fluid consumed, including snacks. Record solid foods eaten in terms of fractions of amounts served, such as ½ or ¾. Record fluids in terms of mL consumed. The nutritionist will calculate the nutrient values in the foods.

Time	Food or fluid	Amount Consumed	Protein (g)	Carbo-hydrates (g)	Fat (g)	Energy (kcal)
	Nutrient totals					

Index

Abdominal pain, 185–186
Absorption
  protein, 219-*220*
  fat, 220-223, *221*
  carbohydrate, *223*
Additives, 109-111, 148
Adolescence
  nutrient requirements, *126*
Advertisements, T.V., 122-123
Albumin concentration, 14, 201,
  204, 208, 214
Alimentation, parenteral, 173,
  174
Allergy
  allergens in foods, 113
  milk, 86-87, 188-194
  peel oil, 96
  prevention, 62, 87
Amino acids
  absorption, 219-220
  essential, 24-27
  plasma, 14-15
  reference pattern, *26*-27
  score, 27
Amylase, 209, 223, 243
Amylopectin, 33-34
Amylose, 33-34
Anemia
  cow milk associated, 168-169

copper deficiency, 47
criteria, 164, *165*, 166
folic acid deficiency, 41, 171
hemolytic, 38, 171, 173
iron deficiency, 80-81, 95,
  163-165
marasmus, 201
vitamin B_6 deficiency, 40
vitamin B_{12} deficiency, 40,
  172-173
vitamin E deficiency, 38, 173
zen macrobiotics, 145
Anorexia, 128
  nervosa, 213-216
Anthropometrics, 4-13
Antibodies, to cow milk, 189
Appetite, toddler, 119-120
Arachidonic acid, 32
Ascorbic acid, *see* Vitamin C

Baby foods, *see* Solid foods
Beeturia, 165
Behavior, in iron deficiency,
  166
Beikost, *see* Solid foods
Bile acids, 209, 221-222, 242
Biliary atresia, 237
Bioavailability
  calcium-vegetarian diets, 141

iron, 59, 141-142, 152-*155*,
  157-158
Biotin, *37*, 42
Biologic value, 28
Blood loss, intestinal, 95, 168-169
Body composition, reference
  fetus, 244
Body image, 127-128
Bonding, 63
Botulism, 114
Bovine serum albumin, 168-169
Brain, growth after malnutrition,
  210-213
Breast Feeding, 55-78
  acute diarrhea, 231
  allergy, 61
  breast size, 64
  contraception, 72
  contraindications, 64
  demand, 65
  duration, 55, 72, 102
  fluoride supplementation, 70
  formula supplementation, 71
  growth rate of infant, 9
  hepatitis B, 65
  infant mortality, 56
  iron intake, 157
  jaundice, 70-71
  nutritional adequacy, 57-60

NOTE: Numbers in italics indicate tables and figures.

Breast Feeding (continued)
  prevalence, 55
  solid foods as supplement, 102
  trends, 55
  uterine involution, 63
  vegetarianism, 146
  vitamin supplementation, 69
  water, additional, 70
  weaning, 73
Breast milk
  calorie content, 57
  Ca:P ratio, 44
  carbohydrate content, 57
  compared to formula, 57-60
  composition, 58, 73
  cystic fibrosis, 236
  free fatty acids, 71
  iron content, 59, 157
  maternal medication, 73-78,
    75-77
  premature feeding, 247-249
  protein content, 29, 57
  renal solute load, 51, 59
  storage, 71
  vitamin B_{12}, 139
  vitamin D, 60
Breath hydrogen, see Hydrogen
Brewers yeast, 139
Bulimia, 214
Bulkiness of diet, 136, 141
B vitamins, 39-41

Calciferol, see Vitamin D
Calcium, 43-44, 248
  absorption, 36, 177, 243
  content in foods, 106, 130,
    142, 251
  intakes, vegetarians, 141
  phosphorous ratio, 43, 44
  requirement, 45, 247
Caries, dental, 93, 97
Calorie, 23-24
  balance, 257-259
  content in baby foods, 107, 108
  content in cereals, 106
  content in fast foods, 129, 130
  count, 18, 279
  effect on iron intake, 160, 162
  empty, 24
  intakes, 31, 136
  requirement, 25, 124-126, 235,
    245
  value, protein, fat, carbohy-
    drate, 24

Carbohydrate
  absorption, 223, 243
  components, 33
  osmolality, 49
  renal solute load, 49
  specialized formulas, 224-225
Carotenes, 35, 139, 214
Casein, 229
Celiac disease, 172, 203, 266
Cereal, 26, 136, 147
  calorie density, 103
  infant, 97, 105, 106, 107
  introduction, 104
  iron, 102, 159
  phosphorous, 44
  zen macrobiotics, 143
Ceruloplasmin, 14, 47, 174
Cholecalciferol, see Vitamin D
Cholestasis, dietary management,
    237
Cholesterol, 59, 83
Chromium, 47
Chronic nonspecific diarrhea,
    see Diarrhea
Clostridium difficile, 230
Cobalamin, see Vitamin B_{12}
Colic, 87, 97
Colitis
  milk, 190
  ulcerative, 239
Colostrum, 61
Commercial baby foods, see
    Solid foods
Complementarity, 136-137
Condensed milk, 81
Congestive heart failure, 237
Contraception, breastfeeding, 72
Copper
  absorption, premature, 243
  ceruloplasmin, 14, 47, 174
  deficiency, 47, 173-174
  requirement, 45, 47
Cow milk, 24, 189
  calcium:phosphorous, 44
  free diet, 109, 271
  intestinal blood loss, 80-81,
    95, 153, 168-169
  iron deficiency, 168-169
  nonfat, 109
  renal solute load, 51
  tetany of newborn, 44
Creatinine, 15
  height index, 15
Critical micellar concentration,

221, 233, 243
Crohn's Disease, 40, 172
Cup, introduction, 98
Cystic fibrosis, 202, 236
Cystine, 236

Dental caries, see Caries
Desserts, 108
Dextrins, 33, 34
Diarrhea
  acute infections, 231-233
  antibiotic, 230
  chronic, malnutrition, 233-235
  chronic nonspecific, 185
  folate deficiency, 171
  osmolality of diet, 49
Dietary recall, 16-17
Dieting, 127-128
Digestibility
  cereals, 107, 147
  processing, 148
  proteins, 26, 28, 137
  vegetarian diet, 136, 137
Digestion
  carbohydrate, 223
  fat, 220-223
  protein, 219-220
Dinners, infant, 108

Edema, 203, 204, 205, 208
  cystic fibrosis, 236
  vitamin E deficiency, 173
Eggs, 113
Energy, see Calorie
Enterohepatic circulation, 139
Enteropathy, cow milk associ-
    ated, 191
Essential fatty acids, see fatty
    acids
Evaporated milk, 81
Exercise, 259-260

Failure to thrive, see Marasmus
Fast food, 129-131
Fat, 30-32
  absorption, 220-223, 221, 222,
    242
  breast milk, 58
  calorie content, 24
  content, fast foods, 129, 130
  content, vegetarian diet, 136
  osmolality, 49
  renal solute load, 49
  specialized formulas, 224

Fatfold thickness, *see* Skinfold thickness
Fat soluble vitamins, *see* Vitamins A, D, E, K
Fatty acids
  essential, 32, 85, 136, 246
  polyunsaturated (PUFA), 32, 38, 247
Ferrioxidase, 47, 174
Fiber, 33, 34, 141
Flatulence, foods causing, 113
Fluoride, 70, 93, *94*
Folacin, *see* Folic acid
Folate, *see* Folic acid
Folic acid
  deficiency, 170-172
  goat milk, 86
  hemolysis, 171
  premature, 247
  requirement, *37*
  vitamin B_{12}, 40
Food allergy, *see* Allergy
Food diary, 16-17
Food habits, 123
Food intake, 103, 121-123, 257
  adolescence, 127
  assessment, 16-18
  unsalted baby foods, 110
Food processing, 147-148
Formula
  composition, 83, *84*, 85, *250*
  evaporated milk, 81-83
  iron fortified, 96
  modified cow milk, 83-85
  premature infant, 250
  renal solute load, 51
  skim milk, 85
  soy based, 87-*89*, 146, 193, 236
Formula feeding
  choice, 90
  cost, 82
  duration, 95
  growth rate, 92
  intakes, 91, *92*
  intolerance, 97, 235
  sterilization, 93-94
  vitamin supplementation, 93
  warming, 96
Fruits, infant, 107-*108*

Galactosemia, 269
Gastrointestinal blood loss, 153, 168-169
Globulins, 204

Glucose polymers, 229
Gluten, 109, 266-268
Goat milk, 41, 86, 168, 170
Goldman's Criteria, 189
Gomez Classification, 206-207
Growth
  adolescence, 124, *125*, 161-162
  breast-fed infant, 102
  catch-up, 209-210
  iron deficiency, 166
  preadolescence, 124
  premature infant, 244, 249
  standards, 7-9, 138, 206
  toddler, 118, 119
  vegetarian, 138
  zen macrobiotic, 145

Hair, zinc content, 46
Head circumference, 7
Height, 4-6, 8, 9, 15
Heiner's Syndrome, 191
Hematocrit, 15, 163-164
  anorexia nervosa, 214
  kwashiorkor, 204
  marasmus, 201
  normal, 163-*164*
Hemoglobin, 15
  iron, 153, 156
  marasmus, 201
  mass, 152
  normal, 163-*164*
Hepatitis
  B and breastfeeding, 65
  neonatal, 237
Honey, 114
Human milk, *see* Breast milk
Hypervitaminosis
  A, 35
  D, 36
Hypogeusia, 46
Hypoglycemia, marasmus, 201
Hypokalemia, 204, 205
Hyponatremia, 201, 204
Hypoproteinemia, 236
Hydrogen breath test, 183-184

Infantometer, 5
IgA, human milk, 60
Intestinal biopsy, 182
Intestinal blood loss, *see* Gastrointestinal blood loss
Intolerance
  lactose, 177-188
  milk protein, 188-192

Iodine, *45*, 47
I.Q., after malnutrition, 210-213
Iron
  absorption, 42, 150, 152-155, 157-158, 166, 174, 243
  balance, 152
  bioavailability, 59
  breastfed infant, 102, 157
  content, foods, 59, 102, *106, 130, 142*, 159, 251
  deficiency, 80-81, 95, 162-169
  density, 127, *160*
  fixed losses, 152
  formula feeding, 93, 102, 158-159
  heme, 127, 142
  nonheme, 142, 154
  requirement, 126-127, 152-153, 156-162, *161*, 247
  stores, 157
  vegetarians, 141-143, 147
  vitamin E, 173
Isoniazid, vitamin B_6, 40

Jaundice, 70-71
Joule, 23
Juices, 96, 113
Junior foods, 114-115
Junk food, 129-131

Kokoh, 145
Kwashiorkor, 14, 145, 170, 174, 201-205

Lactase, 177-179, 209, 243, 246
Lactation, 65-66, 73, 153
Lactobezoar, 252
Lacto-ovovegetarian, 134
Lactovegetarian, 134
Lactose, 33
  breast milk, 57
  digestion, 177
  intolerance, 88, 177-188
  malabsorption, 181, 186-188
  premature formulas, 249
  restricted diet, 269
Lean body mass, 152, 161-163, 170
Legumes, 26
Length, 4-8
Let-down reflex, 66, 97
Linoleic acid, 32, 246
Linolenic acid, 32
Lipase, 209, 220, 242

Lysine, 26, 136

Macrobiotics, *see* Zen Macro-
    biotics
Malabsorption
    acute diarrhea, 233
    cow milk associate, 190-191
    folic acid deficiency, 170-171
    formulas for treatment, 224-230,
        226-229
    protein-energy malnutrition,
        209
    vitamin B_{12} deficiency, 172
Malnutrition, *see* Protein-energy
    malnutrition
Maltose, 33
Marasmic-Kwashiorkor, 205
Marasmus, 14, 145, 170, 198-
    201, 233-235
Maternal deprivation, 211-212
McLaren Score, 207-*208*
Meats, *108*-109
Mediation, maternal re breast-
    feeding, 75-77
Medium chain triglycerides,
    221-222, 224, 229, 249
Megavitamins, 149-150
Menarche, 127
Menstruation, 127, 152, 214
Mental development, after PEM,
    210-213
Mental function, iron deficiency,
    166
Methemoglobinemia, 113
Methionine, 24, 26, 88, 136, 138
Micelle, 221
Microflora, colonic, 181, 188,
    230
Midarm circumference, 12
Milk
    allergy, *see* Allergy
    condensed, 81
    cow, *see* Cow milk
    evaporated, 81
    free diet, 109, 271
    human, *see* Breast milk
    let-down, 66, 97
    nonfat, in baby foods, 109
    secretion, 65
    skin, 85
Minerals
    intake, vegetarians, 141-143
    major, 43-46
    osmolality, *49*

renal solute load, *49*
requirement, premature, 246-247
supplementation, 93
trace, 46-47, 243
Modified starch, 107, 110-111
Monosodium glutamate, 111

Natural foods, 114, 143, 147
NCHS growth charts, 206
Necrotizing enterocolitis, 172, 252
Neutropenia, 174
Niacin, *37*, 41
Nightblindness, 35
Nitrates, 111, 113
Nitrites, 113
Nitrogen, 27-28
Nonheme iron, *see* Iron
Nutrient requirement, premature,
    244-247
Nutritional history, 4, 16-17,
    135, 274-276
Nutritional Status, 4-13, 123-124,
    277-278

Obesity, 9, 11, 85, 123
    childhood re adult, 262-263
    cultural attitudes, 260-261
    definition, 255
    exercise, 259-260
    genetic, 259
    management, 263-264
    morbidity, 261-262
Oral contraceptives, vitamin
    B_6, 40
Oral rehydration, 231-*232*
Organic foods, 148-149
Osmolality, 48-*49*, *84*, *89*
Overweight, 8
Oxalates, 141, 154
Oxygen consumption, 258
Oxytocin, milk let-down, 66

Pagophagia, 165
Pantothenic acid, *37*, 42
Parenteral alimentation, 173, 174,
    234, 236
Peanut butter, 119
Peel oil, 96, 113
Pellagra, 41
Peptidase, 219
Peroxide hemolysis test, 173
Phenylalanine, 24
Phosphorous, 44, *45*, 247, 248,
    251

Phytates, 43-44, 141, 154, 159
Polyunsaturated fatty acids
    (PUFA), 32, 38, 247
Ponderal index, 255
Potassium, *45*-46, 201, 204-205
Prealbumin, 14
Pregnancy, Fe requirement, 153
Premature infant
    folate deficiency, 170-171
    gastrointestinal function, 242-
        244
    nutrient requirements, 244-247
    vitamin E deficiency, 172
Preschool child, 118
Preschool nutrition survey, 167
Prolactin, 65
Protease, 219, 242
Protein, 24
    absorption, 219-220, 242
    amino acid score, 27
    animal, 25-28
    baby foods, 106, 108
    breast milk, 58
    calorie value, 24
    content, selected foods, *136*
    cow milk, 58
    effect on calcium excretion, 44
    efficiency ratio (PER), 27, 129
    fast foods, 129, *130*
    intakes, 30, *31*, 136
    kcal %, 138
    modifications, specialized
        formulas, 224
    osmolality, *49*
    quality, 25-28, 107, 136
    quantity, 136
    recommended dietary allow-
        ance, *25*
    renal solute load, *49*
    requirement, 28, 29, 124, *126*,
        137-138, 245-246
    serum, 14
    soy, 87, 97, 246
Protein-Energy malnutrition,
    197-217
    anemia, 170
    classification, 205-208
    gastrointestinal changes, 209
    growth, subsequent, 209-210
    mental development, subsequent,
        210-213
Protein-sparing modified fast, 264
Protrusion reflex, 104
Psychosocial dwarf, 199

Puberty, 124-125, 161-162
PUFA, *see* Fatty acids
Pyridoxine, *see* Vitamin B_6
Pyridoxal phosphate, 40

Radioallosorbent test (RAST), 189
Recommended Dietary Allowance, 19-20, 118, 124-125
  calories (energy), *25, 126*
  minerals, *45, 126*
  protein, *25, 126*
  vitamins, *37, 126*
Reference fetus, 244, 248
Regurgitation, 97
Renal solute load, 49-*53, 51*
  breast milk, 59
  cereals, infant, 106-108
  commercial formulas, *84, 89*
  evaporated milk formula, 81
Requirements, *see* Individual nutrients
RDA, *see* Recommended Dietary Allowance
Riboflavin, *see* Vitamin B_2
Rickets
  premature infant, 248-249
  vegetarianism, 140-141
  zen macrobiotics, 145
Rose hips, 148

Salt, table, 45, 110-*112*
Schilling test, 173
Scurvy, 42
Serum total protein, 14
Short-gut, 235-236
Skim milk, *see* Milk
Skin testing, 189
Skinfold thickness, 5, 10-12, *256-257*
Sodium, *45-46*
  breast milk, 59
  kwashiorkor, 204
  marasmus, 201
  premature infant, 246, 249
  recommended dietary allowance, *45*
Solid foods
  additives, 109-111
  calorie (energy) content, *108*
  developmental readiness, 103-104
  homemade, 111-112
  introduction, 100-105
  iron source, 102

junior foods, 114-115
  meats, 109
  modified starch, 110-111
  not fed to infants, 112-114
  protein content, *108*
  salt, added, 110
  storage, 111, 114
  strained foods, 109, 115
  sugar, added, 110
  tolerance, 101
  warming, 115
Soy-based formula, *see* Formula
Soy milk, zen macrobiotics, 145
Soy protein, *see* Protein
Specific dynamic action, 257
Starch, 33
Starvation stools, 232
Steatorrhea, 173, 222, 237
Sterilization, 93-94, 111
Stool pattern, 70
Stunting, 8, 207
Sucrose, 33, 110

Table foods, 115
Taste, 103
Taurine, 24-25, 57, 83, 246
Teenager, *see* Adolescence
Television, 121
Tension-Fatigue Syndrome, 191-192
Ten State Nutrition Survey, 31, 167
Tetany, 44
Thiamin, *see* Vitamin B_1
Thiamin pyrophosphate, 39
Threonine, 26
Tocopherol, *see* Vitamin E
Total body water, 255
Trace minerals, *see* minerals
Transferrin, 14, 204
Triceps skinfold, *see* Skinfold
Triglycerides, 31, 220-223, *221*
Tryptophan, 41
Tyrosine, 24

Ulcerative colitis, 239

Vegans, 134, 145
Vegetable oil, 32
Vegetables, infant, *108*
Vegetarianism, 132-150
  breastfeeding, 69
  calcium, 141
  iron, 141-143

management, 145-147
  types, 134
  vitamin B_{12}, 69, 172
  vitamin D, 140-141
Vitamins, 34-43, 93, 118, 139-141, 147, 247
Vitamin A (retinol), 34-36, *37*, 129-130, 139, 149, 214
Vitamin B_1 (thiamin), *37*, 39, 126
Vitamin B2 (riboflavin), *37*, 39-40
Vitamin B_3 (niacin), *37*, 41
Vitamin B_6 (pyridoxine), *37*, 40
Vitamin B_{12} (cobalamin), *37*, 40-41
  adolescence, 126
  anemia, 172-173
  breast milk, 139
  folate deficiency, 171
  premature infant, 243
  short gut syndrome, 236
  vegetarianism, 139-140
  vitamin C, 150
Vitamin C (ascorbic acid), *37*, 42-43, 148-149
  evaporated milk, 93
  fast foods, 129, *130*
  fruit juices, 96
  vegetarianism, 139
  toxicity, 149
Vitamin D (cholecalciferol), 36-*37*
  adolescence, 126
  breast milk, 60
  evaporated milk, 93
  premature infant, 247
  toxicity, 149
  vegetarianism, 140-141
Vitamin E (alpha tocopherol), 32, *37*, 38
  deficiency, 173
  premature infant, 173, 247
  toxicity, 149
Vitamin K, 38-39

Wasting, 8, 207
Waterlow classification, 207
Weaning, 73
Weight, 6-9, *128*
Whey:Casein ratio, 57, 83-84, 246, 249
Whole cow milk, *see* Milk
WIC, 82, 91

Yang, 143
Yin, 143

Zen macrobiotics, 143–145
Zinc, *45*–47, 243